OBESITY SYMPOSIUM
Proceedings of a Servier Research Institute Symposium held
in December 1973

OBESITY SYMPOSIUM

Proceedings of a Servier Research Institute Symposium held
in December 1973

Edited by

W. L. BURLAND
MB, ChB, DCH

*formerly Medical Director, Servier Laboratories
and Servier Research Institute, Greenford,
Middlesex, and Honorary Clinical Assistant,
Paediatric Unit, St. Mary's Hospital Medical
School, London.*

PAMELA D. SAMUEL
BSc (Nut.)

*Servier Laboratories and Servier Research Institute,
Greenford, Middlesex*

and

JOHN YUDKIN
MA, PhD, MD, MRCP

*Emeritus Professor of Nutrition,
University of London*

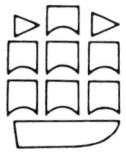

CHURCHILL LIVINGSTONE
Edinburgh London and New York 1974

CHURCHILL LIVINGSTONE

Medical Division of Longman Group Limited

Distributed in the United States of America by
Longman Inc., New York and by associated
companies, branches and representatives throughout
the world.

© **Longman Group Limited 1974**

All rights reserved. No part of this publication
may be reproduced, stored in a retrieval system, or
transmitted in any form or by any means, electronic,
mechanical, photocopying, recording or otherwise,
without the prior permission of the publishers
(Churchill Livingstone, 23 Ravelston Terrace, Edinburgh).

First published 1974

ISBN 0 443 01214 8
Library of Congress Catalog Card Number
Printed in Great Britain.
Computer Typesetting by Print Origination,
Bootle, Merseyside L20 6NS

Contents

Preface viii
List of Participants x

1. Introduction
   JOHN YUDKIN 1

2. The Varieties of Human Obesity: Some Lessons from Experimental Medicine
   G. A. BRAY 6

   Discussion

3. Obesity and Cardiovascular Disease. The Framingham Study.
   W. B. KANNEL and T. GORDON 24

4. Prevalence of Obesity in London: Obesity as a Risk Factor in Coronary Heart Disease.
   I. M. BAIRD 52

   Discussion

5. Obesity in the African
   B. K. ADADEVOH 60

6. The Problem of Obesity in Developing Countries: Its Prevalence and Morbidity
   R. RICHARDS and M. deCASSERES 74

   Discussion

7. Critical Periods in Childhood Obesity
   C. G. D. BROOK   85

   Discussion

8. Psychological and Social Factors in the Pathogenesis of Obesity.
   J. T. SILVERSTONE   105

   Discussion

9. Neurological Mechanisms Regulating Appetite
   B. K. ANAND   116

10. Insulin Requirements for Satiety Centre Activity
    A. F. DEBONS and I. KRIMSKY   146

    Discussion

11. Energy Balance and Obesity
    D. S. MILLER   160

12. The Effects of Exercise in Human Obesity
    P. BJÖRNTORP   171

    Discussion

13. The Human Adipocyte and Its Disorders
    D. J. GALTON   192

14. Hormones and the Adipocyte: Factors Influencing the Metabolic Effects of Insulin and Adrenaline
    L. B. SALANS and S. W. CUSHMAN   204

    Discussion

15. Peripheral Metabolism of Carbohydrate in Obesity and Diabetes
    MARGARET J. WHICHELOW   217

16. Endocrine and Metabolic Alterations Associated with Overfeeding and Obesity in Man
    E. S. HORTON, E. DANFORTH, Jr., E. A. H. SIMS

and L. B. SALANS 229

Discussion

17. A Preventive Programme for Obesity Control
    JOHANNA T. DWYER and J. MAYER 252

18. The Low-Carbohydrate Diet
    JOHN YUDKIN 271

19. Further Follow Up Experience After Prolonged Therapeutic Starvation
    CATHERINE J. CAMPBELL, I. W. CAMPBELL, J. A. INNES, J. F. MUNRO and ANNE L. NEEDLE 281

20. A Review of the Medicinal Treatment of Obesity
    PAMELA D. SAMUEL and W. L. BURLAND 293

21. Psychological Variables in the Control of Obesity
    P. LEY, P. W. BRADSHAW, J. A. KINCEY, J. COUPER-SMARTT and MARILYN WILSON 317

22. Untraditional Treatment of Obesity
    F. QUAADE 338

23. Treatment of Obesity: Round Table Discussion 353

    Summary
    W. J. H. BUTTERFIELD 366

24. Summary of Meeting
    C.C. BOOTH 369

    Index 373

List of Participants

Professor B.K. Adadevoh: *Metabolic Research Unit, Endocrine Metabolic Research Laboratory, Department of Chemical Pathology, University of Ibadan, Ibadan, Nigeria.*
Dr. B. Aggerbeck: *A/S Alfred Benzon, Copenhagen, Denmark.*
Dr. B.K. Anand: *Department of Physiology, All-India Institute of Medical Sciences, New Delhi, India.*
Dr. Margaret M. Ashwell: *Clinical Research Centre, Northwick Park Hospital, Harrow, Middlesex.*
Dr. I.M. Baird: *West Middlesex Hospital, Isleworth, Middlesex.*
Dr. Helle Bechgaard: *A/S Alfred Benzon, Copenhagen, Denmark.*
Mr. L. Beregi: *Departement Recherche Chimie, Science Union & Co., Suresnes, France.*
Dr. P. Björntorp: *First Medical Service, Sahlgren's Hospital, University of Gothenburg, Gothenburg, Sweden.*
Mr. B.P. Bliss: *Department of Surgery, Charing Cross Hospital (Fulham), London.*
Professor C.C. Booth: *Royal Postgraduate Medical School, Hammersmith Hospital, London.*
Dr. G.A. Bray: *Department of Medicine, Harbor General Hospital Campus, University College of Los Angeles, Torrance, California, U.S.A.*
Dr. C.G.D. Brook: *Department of Growth and Development, Institute of Child Health, London.*
Dr. W.L. Burland: *Servier Research Institute, Greenford, Middlesex.*
Professor W.J.H. Butterfield: *The University, Nottingham.*
Mr. D.B. Campbell: *Servier Laboratories Limited, Greenford, Middlesex.*
Dr. S. Carlstrom: *Medical Department, University Hospital, Lund, Sweden.*
Dr. J. Couper-Smartt: *Child and Family Psychiatry Clinic, Cam-*

bridge.

Dr. D. Craddock: *South Croydon, Surrey.*

Dr. A.F. Debons: *Department of Nuclear Medicine, Veterans Administration Hospital and State University of New York Downstate Medical Center, Brooklyn, New York, U.S.A.*

Dr. J. Duhault: *Departement Recherche Pharmacologie, Science Union & Co., Suresnes, France.*

Dr. J.V.G.A. Durnin: *Institute of Physiology, The University, Glasgow.*

Dr. Johanna T. Dwyer: *Department of Nutrition, Harvard School of Public Health, Boston, Massachusetts, U.S.A.*

Mr. J.A. Edwards: *Servier Laboratories Limited, Greenford, Middlesex.*

Dr. R.S. Elkeles: *Department of Medicine, University Hospital of Wales, Cardiff.*

Dr. Elizabeth Evans: *Department of Nutrition, Queen Elizabeth College, London.*

Dr. D.J. Galton: *Diabetes Research Laboratory, St. Bartholomew's Hospital, London.*

Dr. J.S. Garrow: *Clinical Research Centre, Northwick Park Hospital, Harrow, Middlesex.*

Professor B. Guy-Grand: *Clinique Medicale, Hotel Dieu, Paris.*

Mr. D. Harvey: *Department of Surgery, Charing Cross Hospital (Fulham), London.*

Dr. E.S. Horton: *Department of Medicine, University of Vermont College of Medicine, Burlington, Vermont, U.S.A.*

Dr. A.N. Howard: *Department of Investigative Medicine, University of Cambridge.*

Dr. W.B. Kannel: *National Heart and Lung Institute, National Institutes of Health, Framingham, Massachusetts, U.S.A.*

Professor H. Keen: *Department of Medicine, Guy's Hospital Medical School, London.*

Mr. J.A. Kincey: *Department of Clinical Psychology, Manchester Royal Infirmary, Manchester.*

Dr. D. Lemonnier: *Institut Scientifique et Technique de l'Alimentation, Conservatoire National des Arts et Metiers, Paris.*

Dr. B.A. Lewis: *Department of Chemical Pathology, Royal Postgraduate Medical School, Hammersmith Hospital, London.*

Dr. P. Ley: *Department of Clinical Psychology, The University of Liverpool, Liverpool.*

Dr. June K. Lloyd: *Department of Child Health, Institute of Child Health, London.*

Dr. J.D.F. Lockhart: *Servier Research Institute, Greenford, Middle-

sex.
Miss Sheila Macrae: *Servier Laboratories Limited, Greenford, Middlesex.*
Mr. D.S. Miller: *Department of Nutrition, Queen Elizabeth College, London.*
Dr. A. Mordo: *Les Laboratoires Servier, Neuilly-sur-Seine, France.*
Miss Pamela Mumford: *Department of Nutrition, Queen Elizabeth College, London.*
Dr. J.F. Munro: *Eastern General Hospital, Edinburgh.*
Dr. J.C. Petrie: *Department of Therapeutics and Clinical Pharmacology, University of Aberdeen, Aberdeen.*
Dr. F. Quaade: *Bispebjerg Hospital, Copenhagen, Denmark.*
Dr. P.H.W. Rayner: *Department of Paediatrics and Child Health, Children's Hospital, Birmingham.*
Mrs. Celia J. Reuter: *Servier Laboratories Limited, Greenford, Middlesex.*
Dr. R. Richards: *Department of Medicine, University of the West Indies, Mona, Kingston, Jamaica.*
Dr. Brigitte Riveline: *Les Laboratoires Servier, Neuilly-sur-Seine, Paris.*
Dr. L.B. Salans: *Department of Medicine, Endocrine-Metabolism Division, Dartmouth Medical School, Hanover, New Hampshire, U.S.A.*
Miss Pamela D. Samuel: *Servier Research Institute, Greenford, Middlesex.*
Dr. J.P. Sedgwick: *High Wycombe, Bucks.*
Dr. J.T. Silverstone: *St. Bartholomew's Hospital, London.*
Dr. M. Stock: *Department of Nutrition, Queen Elizabeth College, London.*
Dr. J.M. Stowers: *Diabetic Out-Patient Department, The Royal Infirmary, Aberdeen.*
Dr. J. Tremolieres: *Laboratory of Human Nutrition, Hospital Bichat, Paris.*
Dr. R. Vroom: *Servier Nederland bv, Den Haag, Holland.*
Mr. K.J. Walker: *Servier Laboratories Limited, Greenford, Middlesex.*
Dr. M.V. Wells: *The General Hospital, Nottingham.*
Dr. Margaret J. Whichelow: *Department of Medicine, Guy's Hospital Medical School, London.*
Miss Jean White: *Servier Laboratories Limited, Greenford, Middlesex.*
Dr. Elsie M. Widdowson: *Dunn Nutritional Laboratory, Cambridge.*
Professor V. Wynn: *Alexander Simpson Laboratory for Metabolic Research, St. Mary's Hospital Medical School, London.*

Dr. D. York: *Department of Physiology and Biochemistry, University of Southampton, Southampton.*
Professor John Yudkin: *Queen Elizabeth College, London.*

The Following authors of papers presented at the Symposium did not attend the meeting in person:

Mr. P.W. Bradshaw: *Department of Psychology, University of Otago, New Zealand.*
Dr. Catherine J. Campbell: *formerly from Edenhall Hospital, Edinburgh.*
Dr. I.W. Campbell: *formerly from Eastern General Hospital, Edinburgh.*
Dr. S.W. Cushman: *Department of Medicine, Endocrine-Metabolism Division, Dartmouth Medical School, Hanover, New Hampshire, U.S.A.*
Dr. M. DeCasseres: *Department of Medicine, University of the West Indies, Mona, Kingston, Jamaica.*
Dr. E. Danforth, Jr: *Department of Medicine, University of Vermont College of Medicine, Burlington, Vermont, U.S.A.*
Dr. T. Gordon: *National Heart and Lung Institute, National Institutes of Health, Bethesda, Maryland, U.S.A.*
Dr. J.A. Innes: *Eastern General Hospital, Edinburgh.*
Dr. I. Krimsky: *Department of Nuclear Medicine, Veterans Administration Hospital and State University of New York, Downstate Medical Center, Brooklyn, New York, U.S.A.*
Dr. J. Mayer: *Department of Maternal and Child Health, Harvard School of Public Health, Boston, Massachusetts, U.S.A.*
Dr. Anne L. Needle: *formerly from Edenhall Hospital, Edinburgh.*
Dr. E.A.H. Sims: *Department of Medicine, University of Vermont College of Medicine, Burlington, Vermont, U.S.A.*
Marilyn Wilson: *Senior Occupational Therapist, United Liverpool Hospitals.*

Preface

Daniel Lambert who appeared on the front cover of the Servier Research Institute's symposium programme* was Britain's most famous heavyweight. He weighed 739 lb (336 kg) and died in 1809 aged 39 years. William Campbell was fractionally heavier at 750 lb (341 kg) and only 22 when he died in Newcastle in 1878.

It is surprising that the early deaths of these and other record-making heavyweights did not encourage greater medical interest in obesity. Until comparatively recently man's only interest in obesity was for cosmetic reasons. The presence of 66 physicians, scientists and nutritionists at the first Servier Research Institute Symposium on Obesity indicates how much opinion has changed and that obesity now ranks alongside other serious conditions that similarly increase morbidity and mortality.

The symposium proceedings were edited and appear in the chapters that follow. Contributions were devoted to all aspects of the subject and indicate that experiment, research and inquiry are progressing on a wide front. In particular they include the cause and maintenance of obesity, its association with diabetes and cardiovascular disease in developed countries and its emergence in developing countries. Obesity in infancy and childhood is discussed and the influence this may have on the prevalence of the condition in adult life. Central nervous mechanisms, alterations in peripheral endocrine activity and metabolism, psychology and treatment are all reviewed and brought up to date.

Obesity is a complex subject and there is still much to identify. Some may look to the adipocyte for new answers, others to the gut. It is to be hoped that the symposium and this book will have served to bring together current knowledge and act as a stimulus for further study.

We are grateful to all the participants, chairmen and contributors, and to Mrs. Pamela Kyffin for her invaluable assistance in the administration of the symposium and with the preparation of the manuscript.

W.L.B.
P.D.S.
J.Y.

*by kind permission of the Leicester Museum and Art Gallery

1. Introduction

JOHN YUDKIN

Obesity differs in several important respects from all other diseases. Firstly, in the affluent countries it is far more prevalent than is any other disease, except perhaps diagnosed and undiagnosed atherosclerosis. Secondly, it is a condition in which almost every individual, whether affected or not, has strong and often unshakeable views as to its cause and its likely cure. Thirdly, most views held by lay people are very different from those held by research workers, whilst practising physicians are at least as likely to share the views of the layman as they are to share those of the research worker. Part of the failure to prevent and cure obesity stems I believe from a failure to try and understand the nature of these two cultures; unless we do, we shall not be able to bridge the gap between them.

I deliberately speak of bridging the gap, since we shall find that lay opinion, often assumed to be entirely irrational, is not always so; we shall also find that the conventional wisdom is not always infallible. Let us then compare the answers we might obtain to three common questions relating to obesity, from the man in the street and from the man in the research laboratory or clinic. These are:-
 1. Is a change of diet necessary for the treatment of obesity?
 2. Does dietary restriction inevitably lead to diminished obesity?
 3. What controls food intake?

We shall find, as I have intimated, that the practising physician may have views that sometimes lean to those of the layman and sometimes to those of the specialist.

1. Is a change of diet necessary for the treatment of obesity? Many of the varieties of slimming cures offered to the public, usually through advertisements in newspapers, magazines, television and radio, come within the law since they do not claim explicitly that obesity can be cured solely by the use of special garments, baths and massage, or by electrical or vibratory treatment. But it is certain that the majority of the public who are induced to buy these preparations or treatments believe that they need not bother a great deal if at all about dietary restriction.

Orthodox teaching on the other hand insists that dietary restriction is virtually essential for the reduction of adiposity. The only exception that might be agreed is an increase in physical activity without an increase in dietary intake. However, this is usually considered to be unrealistic in view of the relatively small utilization of energy in relation to the degree of activity that the obese individual can be expected to add to his ordinary activities. As Derek Miller points out in Chapter 11, this conventional view must be challenged though it is still true that most non-dietary treatments are of little value.

The practising physician can be expected to accept the orthodox view, but in one area he often agrees with the patient in believing in the efficacy of what in fact is ineffective treatment. I refer here to the use of diuretics and of hormones. The elimination of water, even assuming that this is water excessively retained by the body, has nothing to do with the removal of the excess fat that constitutes obesity. As for hormones, it is well known that real deficiency of thyroid is characterized by very evident features; obesity is by no means the most evident, nor indeed is it always present. Chorionic gonadotrophin, whenever it has been properly examined, has been shown to be without value in the treatment of obesity. Nevertheless, many physicians agree with their patients in believing that diuretics and hormones have a place in the treatment of obesity.

2. Does dietary restriction invariably lead to decreased obesity?
Leaving aside new work regarding the role of physical activity, it is agreed that a necessary condition for reducing body fat is dietary restriction. But this immediately raises the question of whether or not dietary restriction is also a sufficient condition.

The conventional view is certainly that with physical activity constant a reduction of energy intake must inevitably lead to loss of weight. This view is held so strongly that failure of a patient to lose weight is accepted as proof that he has not reduced his food intake. It is held that one kilogram of adipose tissue will be lost when food intake is reduced by some 7000 Kcal; thus, a reduction of food intake by as little as 500 Kcal a day should reduce body weight by 2 kg in a month. If this does not occur then it is held that it must be because the individual is not in fact reducing his food intake as he claims.

The layman is quite convinced however that many people can reduce their intake by much more than 500 Kcal a day, and yet lose little or no body weight. Certainly it is true that many of the examples cited by the layman are due to non-adherence to the prescribed diet, though it usually requires very close observation to illustrate this. Yet it is becoming clear that, within unexpectedly wide limits of food intake, body weight can in fact remain very constant, and that examples do exist both of increased food intake not leading to increased body weight, and of reduced food intake not leading to reduced body weight.

This is less implausible than at first appears. There is no doubt that some people do have the facility of disposing of increased energy intake by an increase in heat production: the phenomenon of thermogenesis. Some of these people then have a body weight that is no greater than it would be with a lower energy intake. Reduction of their energy intake to their true requirements, from that where excess is being used in thermogenesis, will therefore not lead to any significant weight reduction.

Thermogenesis may be considered as an adaptation to energy intake above requirement. In addition, there is evidence that the body can adapt to intakes below normal requirements, partly by unconscious restriction of activity, and partly by a reduction in basal metabolism. Here then is another mechanism that would allow body weight to be maintained though energy intake is reduced.

The description I have given exaggerates the situation, in that there is a limit to the amount of excess energy intake that can be accounted for by thermogenesis and clearly a limit to the degree of adaptation that can occur to a low intake. Moreover, the adaptations are not complete or immediate, so that there is always some increase or decrease in body weight before a plateau is reached. However, apart from this, we must accept that some people can maintain a fairly constant body weight with an energy intake that is not constant. Thus, in this instance, the lay view is correct and the accepted texts are wrong. Individuals need not necessarily gain weight to any degree if they overeat, or necessarily lose weight to any degree if they reduce their food consumption.

3. *What controls food intake?* Here too there is a difference in viewpoint between the scientist and the layman. Most workers who are investigating mechanisms of regulation of food intake are concerned with the energy content of the food. It is assumed that these mechanisms set a level of hunger and appetite that determine the number of calories that are to be consumed.

The non-scientist on the other hand is well aware that the amount that one eats depends upon many factors other than the satisfaction of a pre-set energy demand. He knows, for example, that there is a distinction, often ignored in the text book, between hunger and appetite—the one an unpleasant sensation largely satisfied by any food that is at least not abhorrent, the other a pleasant sensation that can only be satisfied by particular and palatable foods. If the foods that are available are unpalatable, he is likely to stop eating them before his energy needs are completely met; if the foods are very highly palatable, he is likely to eat them long after his energy needs are satisfied, and so risk the development of obesity.

There are other factors determining energy intake that are more likely to be recognized by the lay person than by the specialist. One is the social occasion; many fat businessmen know that at least part of their problem is due to the frequent and excessive lunches that they consume. Another source of excessive energy intake is habituation to alcohol.

On the other hand, there are some beliefs about determinants of food intake that are quite unfounded and yet are by no means confined to the non-scientist. Perhaps the commonest is that which recommends that the most obvious food component to be reduced in order to reduce caloric intake is fat, since it yields more than twice the amount of energy for a given weight than does protein or carbohydrate. This implies that an important factor regulating food intake is the weight of food. It implies that a person will be just as likely to consume 10 g of fat as to consume 10 g of sugar or 10 g of bread (or 20 g of bread if we ignore the moisture content). I know of no evidence that this is so. On the contrary, there is evidence that satiety requires far larger quantities of carbohydrate than of fat or protein. Yet the advice to reduce fat intake because of its high energy concentration is given as frequently by the specialist as it is by the physician and by the lay writer.

More recently, the dangers of obesity in infancy arising from the too early introduction of solid foods have been emphasized and the emphasis seems to have been entirely on the physical state of the food, ignoring its chemical composition. I find it difficult to believe that for example egg or meat are as likely to cause obesity as is a cereal food. More particularly, there has been little comment on the much more serious practice of giving babies frequent sweetened drinks, or of adding sugar to the cereal.

I have attempted here to make two points. Firstly there is often a considerable gap between what the layman believes about the cause and cure of obesity, and what the specialist believes; what the practising physician believes is sometimes closer to the one and sometimes to the other. Secondly, there are several examples where the layman's belief is nearer to reality than is that of the professional nutritionist.

But what matters more than people's beliefs is people's behaviour. How do we account, for example, for the behaviour of the fat woman who spends two weeks in a health farm, where at great expense she partakes of a ridiculously small diet, but in the evening takes off to a local restaurant for a four-course dinner? This psychological area of the problem of obesity has seen even less research than has the physiological area; let us hope that a major result of this symposium will be to encourage more research in both areas.

2. The Varieties of Human Obesity: Some Lessons from Experimental Medicine

G. A. BRAY

Investigators interested in the field of obesity have a number of models from which to choose. For ease of classification, these models can be divided into five major groups (Table 2.1):
    Obesity following ventromedial hypothalamic injury
    Endocrine imbalance
    Physical inactivity
    Nutritional obesity
    Genetic obesity
Detailed studies on many of these experimental forms of obesity have provided insight into some of the mechanisms by which human obesity develops (Bray, 1973, 1974). In this chapter I shall discuss hypothalamic obesity and genetic obesity in some detail.

EXPERIMENTAL HYPOTHALAMIC OBESITY

Bilateral injury to the ventromedial hypothalamus is followed by obesity in mice (Montemurro, 1971), rats (Hetherington & Ranson, 1942), cats (Ingram, 1952), monkeys (Hamilton, 1973), birds (Lepkovsky, 1973) and man (Babinski, 1900; Bray, 1974; Frohlich, 1901). Such injury can be caused in many ways (Table 2.1). The most widely studied model is the rat in which electrolytic lesions are used to damage the ventromedial hypothalamus (Brobeck, 1964; Stevenson, 1969), but microsurgery (Jansen & Hutchison, 1969) and chemical injury with gold thioglucose (Brecher & Waxler, 1949), 4-nitroquinoline-1-oxide (Yamamoto *et al*, 1970) and bipiperidyl mustard (Rutman *et al*, 1967) have also been used. In man, the principal lesions leading to hypothalamic obesity are trauma, inflammatory disease and tumours (Bray, 1973, 1974).

    Several features of the syndrome which follow effective ventromedial hypothalamic lesions are summarized in Table 2.2. Hyper-

Table 2.1.

Classification of Obesities

Human	Experimental Animals
I. *Hypothalamic*	
1. Tumours	
a. solid (Fröhlich-Babinski syndrome)	1. Electrolytic
b. leukaemia	
2. Inflammatory	2. Microsurgical
3. Trauma	
4. Increased intracranial pressure	3. Chemical
(Empty sella, pseudotumour cerebri)	
II. *Endocrine*	
1. Cushing syndrome	
2. Insulinoma	1. Excess corticosteroids
3. Castration	2. Hyperinsulinaemia
4. Stein-Levinthal syndrome	3. Castration
5. Pregnancy	
III. *Inactivity*	
IV. *Genetic*	
1. Laurence-Moon-Biedl syndrome	1. Dominant inheritance
2. Hyperostosis frontalis interna	(A^{iy}, A^{vy}, A^y)
3. Alström's syndrome	2. Recessive inheritance
4. Prader-Willi syndrome	(ob, db, db/ad, fa)
5. Juvenile onset (?)	3. Polygenic
V. *Dietary*	
	1. Gorging
	2. High fat diet
VI. *Drugs*	
1. Phenothiazines	
2. Oestrogens	
3. Cyproheptadine	
VII. *Essential*	

phagia is characteristic of this syndrome in mature animals (Brooks & Lambert, 1946; Tepperman *et al*, 1943), but does not occur in weanling rats (Goldman *et al*, 1970). In the adult rat, food intake rises by as much as 50 to 100 per cent after hypothalamic injury and this appears to be the major aetiological factor in the obesity (Tepperman *et al*, 1943). Prevention of hyperphagia by appropriate paired feeding of lesioned rats to lean controls reduces most or all of

8   OBESITY SYMPOSIUM

the obesity (Brooks & Lambert, 1946). In weanling rats hyperphagia is not observed nor is there an acceleration in the rate of weight gain (Bernardis & Frohman, 1971). However, there is an increase in total body fat in both weanling and adult animals indicating that the metabolic alterations produced by hypothalamic injury and which lead to obesity do not require hyperphagia for their manifestation (Goldman *et al*, 1970). The animal with hypothalamic obesity

Table 2.2

Abnormalities following bilateral ventromedial injury in the experimental animal

1. Hyperphagia
2. Finicky appetite
3. Diminished spontaneous activity
4. Hypometabolism (variable)
5. Abnormal oestrus behaviour and gonadal atrophy
6. Enlarged pancreatic islets
7. Hyperinsulinaemia
8. Enlarged fat cells
9. Enhanced lipogenesis
10. Stunted growth

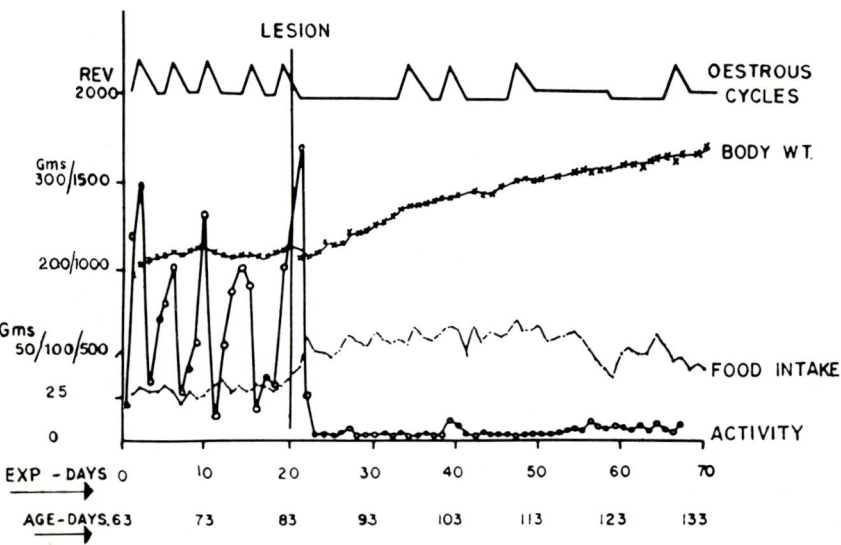

Figure 2.1

The effects of hypothalamic injury in the rat. Following the introduction of hypothalamic lesions, the food intake increases and there is a gradual rise in body weight. Oestrus cycles which were regular before surgical intervention become irregular and spontaneous activity is decreased. (Adapted from Brooks & Lambert, 1946).

displays several other features including laziness or decreased physical activity, a finicky appetite and frequent aggressiveness. The rage reaction and aggressiveness seem to go hand-in-hand with the injury to the ventromedial hypothalamus. Several of these features are depicted in Figure 2.1 taken from Brooks & Lambert (1946). After injury, food intake rises, physical activity falls, body weight rises and the animals show a decreased metabolic rate and alterations in the oestrus cycle. More recent studies have shown an increase in the size of the pancreatic islets (Kennedy & Parker, 1963) and hyperinsulinaemia (Frohman et al, 1969; Hales & Kennedy, 1964; Han, 1968). Increased fat stores comprise almost all of the weight gained after hypothalamic injury (Stevenson, 1969). This increased storage of fat occurs almost, if not entirely, as a result of enlargement of already existing fat cells (Hirsch & Han, 1969). That is, hypothalamic obesity represents hypertrophy rather than hyperplasia of fat cells.

The hyperinsulinaemia is of particular interest and may play an important role in the pathogenesis of this syndrome. The initial suggestion of altered insulin metabolism was provided by the observations of Kennedy & Parker (1963) who showed enlargement of the islets of Langerhans in rats with hypothalamic injury and obesity. Such a finding suggested elevated secretion of insulin. Subsequently, Hales & Kennedy (1964) showed increased insulin levels and this has been confirmed by many other groups of workers (Frohman et al, 1969; Han, 1968). Of particular interest is the fact that the rise of insulin occurs within the first two to three days following ventromedial injury at a time before the animals become obese (Han, 1968). Moreover, paired feeding of animals with ventromedial lesions to the same level as those who have been sham-operated does not prevent the hyperinsulinaemia (Slaunwhite et al, 1972). Thus, the increase in insulin does not depend on increased food intake. These findings suggest the possibility that injury to the ventromedial hypothalamus has altered insulin metabolism and that it is the hyperinsulinaemia which leads to many of the metabolic features of this syndrome.

Further support for the role of insulin in the pathogenesis of hypothalamic obesity comes from studies with insulin injections. MacKay and his collaborators (1940) demonstrated that injections of long-acting protamine zinc insulin could produce weight gain and obesity in experimental animals. When animals are made obese with injections of insulin, body weight will return to normal when the insulin injections are stopped (Hoebel & Teitelbaum, 1966). If bilateral ventromedial lesions are produced and injections of insulin stopped body weight remains elevated (Boebel & Teitelbaum, 1966).

The mechanism by which insulin produces its effect on food intake appears to involve an interaction with the lateral hypothalamus. If glucose is injected into the lateral hypothalamus, food intake does not occur when insulin is injected peripherally (Booth, 1968). Moreover, if lateral hypothalamic lesions are induced, rats become hypoglycaemic and die after receiving insulin but do not display hyperphagia. This experimental evidence strongly suggests that the effects of insulin on hyperphagia are mediated through glucose utilization and/or glucose concentration as sensed by localized regions of the lateral hypothalamus.

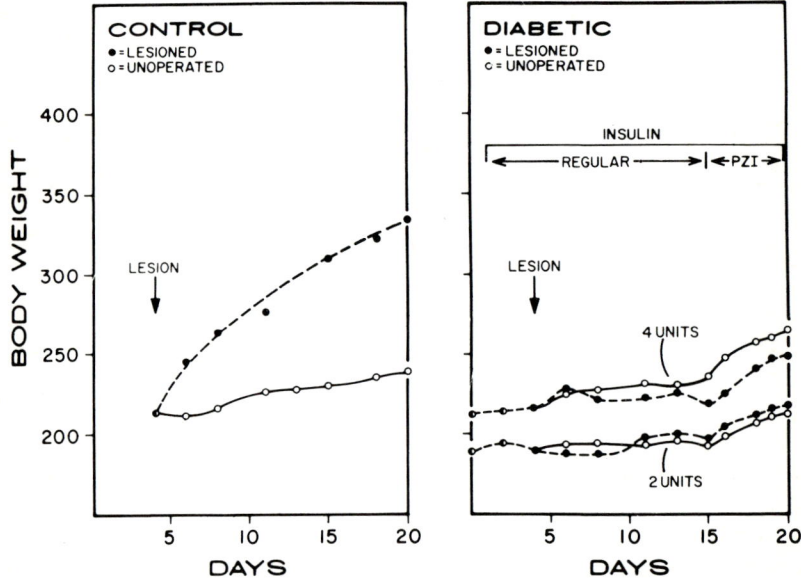

Figure 2.2
Hypothalamic obesity in the diabetic rat. The increase in body weight following such injury compared to an unlesioned rat is shown on the left-hand panel. The effects of hypothalamic injury in diabetic rats treated with two or four units of insulin per day are shown on the right-hand panel. Hypothalamic injury did not lead to either hyperphagia or an acute weight gain in the diabetic rats. (Adapted from York & Bray, 1972).

A second line of evidence to indicate the importance of hyperinsulinaemia in the development of hypothalamic obesity has been provided by experiments which destroy the pancreatic islets and thus abolish hyperinsulinism. Such studies have been conducted using several experimental approaches including injections of alloxan (Friedman, 1972), injections of streptozotocin (Goldman *et al*, 1972; York & Bray, 1972), and surgical pancreatectomy (Young & Liu, 1965). In all cases the results have been similar. There is little or no increase in food intake when the ventromedial nuclei of diabetic rats are damaged. Thus, ventromedial hypothalamic lesions do not produce the same degree of hyperphagia nor do they produce obesity in animals that cannot increase insulin secretion. This is illustrated in Figure 2.2. In this study, rats received streptozotocin several days before their bilateral ventromedial lesion. Following hypothalamic injury in the control animals, hyperphagia occurred and body weight increased. In the diabetic group, similar lesions did not produce hyperphagia and the increase in body weight was similar to the animals without lesions.

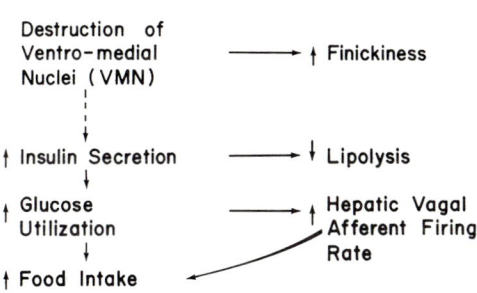

Figure 2.3
Pathogenic sequence for hypothalamic obesity. Following destruction of the ventromedial nucleus, hyperinsulinaemia is produced which stimulates glucose utilization and/or hypoglycaemia thus leading to enhanced food intake and the eventual appearance of obesity.

From the published evidence the following pathogenetic sequence for hypothalamic obesity can be constructed (Fig. 2.3). Destruction of the ventromedial nucleus leads to increased insulin secretion in response to ingested food. The hyperinsulinaemia leads to increased glucose utilization and possibly hypoglycaemia. The increased utilization of glucose and/or hypoglycaemia are sensed by the lateral hypothalamus and lead to increased food intake and obesity.

HUMAN HYPOTHALAMIC OBESITY

The reports by Babinski (1900) and Fröhlich (1901) at the turn of the century focused attention on the obesity which occurs with hypothalamic injury. Since then more than 100 cases have been described in which the onset of obesity was associated with a hypothalamic lesion (Bray, 1973, 1974) and I have been able to study eight such patients. One young patient developed obesity in association with a dermoid cyst of the third ventricle. She initially presented with obesity at six months of age. Her weight rose sharply and has remained consistently above the 97th percentile. At age 14, the time of her last visit, her weight was in excess of 250 lb. The second patient probably had tuberculosis with hypothalamic involvement and showed a rapid weight gain of 100 lb in her final year of life.

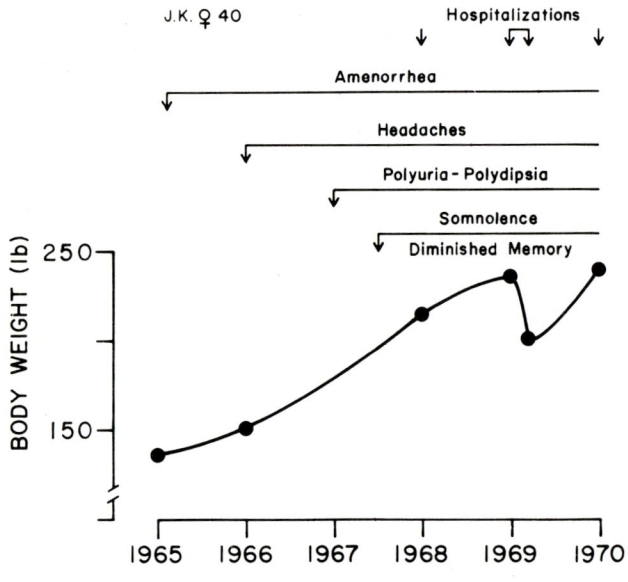

Figure 2.4
Human hypothalamic obesity. J.K. was a 40 year old female who developed a craniopharyngioma at age 36. Following the onset of her initial symptoms, there was a gradual increase in weight, which only decreased during a period of hospitalization lasting three months. Among her other symptoms were diabetes insipidus, hypopituitarism, diminished memory and somnolence.

The third patient was found to have a chordoma at the base of the clivus. These tumours arise from the embryological notochord and in the adult the residuum of this tissue is found in the nucleus pulposus of the intervertebral disc. Occasionally, they become malignant. Although most of these tumours are observed in the region of the coccyx, about a third of them are intracranial. This patient showed onset of obesity following neurosurgical exploration. The fourth patient had a lipoma of the interpenduncular fossa. The fifth had a craniopharyngioma, and gained weight steadily (Fig 2.4). This tumour which develops from embryological remnants along the stalk of the hypophyseal duct is the most common cause of hypothalamic obesity in man (Bray, 1973). In this series, however, there was only one patient with such a tumour, and the only man in the series had an aneurysm of the internal carotid artery. Following the insertion of a clip, he gained 100 lb in six months. Before this his weight had been constant at less than 160 lb. The final patient had a meningoma of the right optic nerve.

Patients with hypothalamic obesity are rare. A review of the literature has elicited 336 other causes of obesity due to tumours, only 68 of which provided enough data for analysis of weight gain. Fifty-nine of these patients developed hypothalamic obesity before 40 years of age. Craniopharyngioma was the most common pathological lesion. The obesity appears to be due to hypertrophy of the fat cells, although hyperplasia of fat cells may have occurred in one patient. In addition to obesity, all patients had one or more additional symptoms. Headache, visual impairment and abnormalities of the reproductive system (amenorrhoea in women, loss of libido in men and failure of sexual development in children) were the most commonly associated symptoms. Polyuria, diabetes insipidus, somnolence and behaviour disorders were also reported but with considerably lower frequency. Thus, hypothalamic obesity in man, when it occurs, is almost invariably associated with other manifestations of intracranial disease. There were no patients who weighed over 300 pounds in whom a hypothalamic lesion was clearly the cause of their obesity. Indeed, there were only two who weighed between 275 and 300 pounds. One can thus conclude that patients weighing over 250 pounds rarely have obesity due to hypothalamic injury. Moreover, none of the patients with hypothalamic obesity gained more than 125 pounds. Thus, hypothalamic obesity in man is a hypertrophic form of the obesity associated with increased food intake and weight gain and is almost always associated with other signs or symptoms of intracranial hypothalamic disease.

In summary studies on the pathogenesis of hypothalamic obesity in experimental animals have suggested that insulin is the key factor in this process. A similar pathogenetic mechanism may also apply to the development of hypothalamic obesity in man.

GENETIC OBESITY

As can be seen in Table 2.1, several varieties of genetic obesity have been described. These are inherited by many different modes (Bray & York, 1971). The yellow obese mouse inherits obesity as an autosomal dominant with three varieties. Among the animals which inherit obesity as an autosomal Mendelian recessive trait are four different varieties, the obese mouse (ob/ob) adipose mouse (ad/ad) and diabetic mouse (db/db) and the 'fatty' rat (fa/fa). The adipose mouse originally described by Falconer & Isaacson (1959) appears now to be an allelomorph of the diabetic mouse and has a new gene

Table 2.3

Comparison of metabolic and regulatory obesity in the fatty and the Zucker rat

Parameter	Control Rat	Fatty Rat	Hypothalamic Obesity
Body weight g	252	583	479
Food Intake g/d	13.1	18.2	18.1
Liver Weight g	9.4	19.6	17.5
g/100 g body wt	3.7	3.4	3.6
Cardiac Weight mg	810	1270	1230
Plasma Glucose mg/100 ml	156	139	145
Free Fatty Acids μEq/l	1268	1486	1251
Insulin μU/ml	45	124	—
Triglyceride mg/100 ml	76	616	598
Cholesterol mg/100 ml	114	85	92
Osmolality mOsm/ml	293	313	—
Oxygen Consumption ml/O_2/g 0.7/h	7.35	6.22	—
Urine Volume ml/d ml/O_2/g 0.7/h	9.6	13.7	10.4
with Pitressin ml/d	6.7	10.8	7.9
Adipose Tissue			
Cell Size (nl)	0.78	0.98	—
No. of Fat Cells x 10^6	16.4	41.0	—
Thyroid Function			
Weight mg	19.9	20	21
RAI uptake %	29.8	17.1	19.8
PBI μg/100 ml	1.9	1.6	1.9
Serum TSH μU/ml	32.4	37.3	42.8
Reproductive Function			
Vaginal Opening, d	38.6	54.0	—
Oestrus Cycle d	4.1	6.0	—
Plasma FSH ng/ml	61	60	—
Plasma LH ng/ml	225	174	—
Uterine Weight mg	418	291	—
Pituitary			
Weight mg	12.8	6.96	10.9
Thyrotropin mU/mg	104.1	149.8	85.6
LH μg/mg	16.5	24.5	—
FSH μg/mg	1.85	3.24	—

symbol db^{AD}/db^{AD}. A third group of rodents with polygenic inheritance are illustrated by the New Zealand obese mouse and the Japanese KK mouse. These animals were bred for obesity through many generations. A fourth variety of inherited obesity is that seen in hybrid mice such as the Wellesley mouse or the C3F1 hybrid. The parents of both strains are lean as are the pure bred offspring. When the two lines are crossed, however, the f_1 offspring become obese at the time of sexual maturation. The desert rodent presents the final group of obesities in which environmental factors are acting on a genetically susceptible background to produce obesity. These animals will develop hyperphagia and obesity when exposed to foods of high caloric density but not when fed their usual diet of greens.

Some of the genetic forms of obesity may provide a good model for obesity in man, particularly the juvenile onset form. Humans whose obesity begins in childhood have an increased total number of adipocytes (Hirsch & Knittle, 1970; Salans *et al*, 1973) and so do the

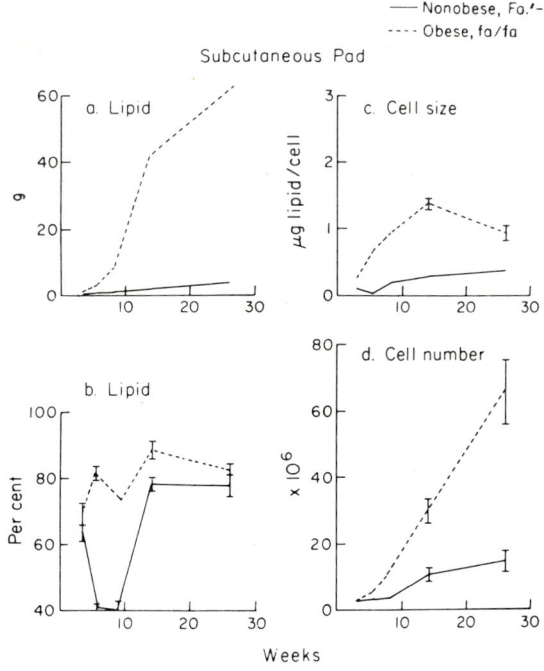

Figure 2.5
Body weight, fat content and body fat in the fatty rat. At four to six weeks of age there is little difference in the number of adipocytes in the lean and fatty rats. After that age there is a sharp and steady increase. (Reproduced by permission, Johnson *et al*, 1971).

fatty rat and the obese (ob/ob) mouse. Several features of the fatty rat are illustrated in Table 2.3. The abnormalities observed in these animals suggest three possible mechanisms for their obesity. These are

  Derangement of adipose tissue
  Abnormalities of hypothalamic function
  Derangements of insulin

The adipocytes in the fatty rat are enlarged as they are in essentially all forms of obesity (Bray, 1969; Johnson, 1971). In addition, these rats have an increased total number of adipocytes (Johnson et al, 1971). Figure 2.5 shows body weight, total body fat and the size and number of adipocytes in the fatty rat (Johnson et al, 1971). Before six weeks of age, the number of adipocytes appears to be similar in lean and 'fatty' rats, but after that age there is a steady increase in the total number of adipocytes with little further increase in the size of individual cells. Thus, the fatty rat is an example of hypercellular obesity which is transmitted as a Mendelian recessive trait.

The functional characteristics of these adipocytes have been compared with adipocytes from lean rats. The release of glycerol as a marker for breakdown of triglycerides from adipose tissue incubated *in vitro* is clearly related to the size of fat cells regardless of the animal from which they come (York & Bray, 1973a). In Figure 2.6 glycerol release is shown for a group of lean animals and for four groups of 'fatty' rats of comparable age. These 'fatty' rats were maintained on either *ad libitum* diets or on diets which were

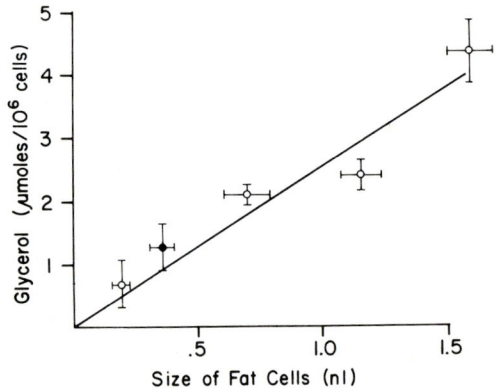

Figure 2.6
Glycerol release by adipocytes from the fatty rat. Size of and glycerol release from adipocytes from normal rats (solid circles) and fatty rats (open circles). Differences in the size of adipocytes for fatty rats were produced by various periods of food restriction. (Reproduced by permission, Bray et al, 1974).

partially, slightly or severely restricted in order to produce adipocytes of different size. Prior to study each group had been on an *ad libitum* diet for 10 days. Glycerol release increased as the size of the adipocyte increased. The increased total number of adipocytes in the fatty rats did not appear to alter the function of individual cells (Bray *et al*, 1974; York & Bray, 1973a).

Differences in the lipogenesis of these adipocytes have also been demonstrated and are related to the age of the animals (Bray *et al*, 1974; York & Bray, 1973b). At six weeks of age the fatty rats had a greater release when fat was incubated with adrenaline (Fig. 2.7). The basal and stimulated release of glycerol were both increased in rats at 18 weeks of age. Examination of these data show that when the numbers were expressed in terms of the total number of adipocytes, the differences between the two groups of animals were relatively small.

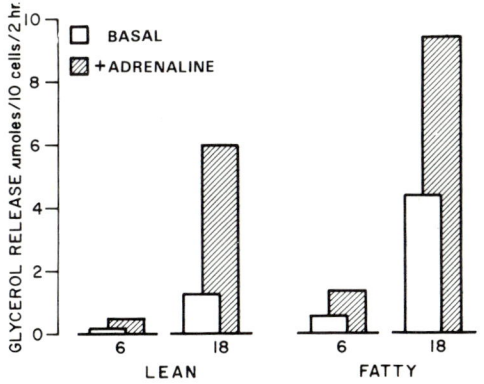

Figure 2.7
Effects of adrenaline on glycerol release from adipocytes at 6-18 weeks of age in lean and fatty rats. Adrenaline 1 μ g (cross-hatched bar) enhanced the release of glycerol at both ages, but the absolute effect was greater in the older rats. Although fatty rats showed slightly greater basal release at both ages, the effect of age was greater than the difference between the fatty and lean animals.

When one examines lipogenesis, however, the effects of age become very prominent (Fig. 2.8). In six-week old animals, incorporation of radioactivity from glucose into fatty acids was 300 times greater in adipocytes from fatty rats than in those from lean animals (Bray, 1974; York & Bray, 1973b). A clear-cut effect of insulin was present in both groups but particularly in the enlarged fat cells of the young fatty rats. By 18 weeks of age these differences had largely disappeared suggesting that aberrations in the metabolism of adipose tissue are present at a very early age in the genetically obese rat. The observations raise the possibility that deranged metabolism of multiplying adipocytes may play an important role in the development of the hypercellularity of the adipose tissue in these animals which becomes manifest after six to eight weeks of age.

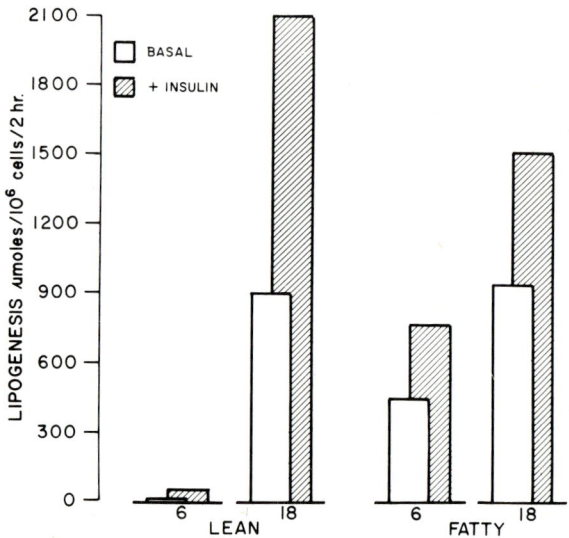

Figure 2.8

Lipogenesis by the adipocytes from fatty and lean rats. The effects of insulin (1 milliunit) is shown by the cross-hatched bars in lean rats (left-hand bars) and fatty rats (right-hand bars). At 6 weeks of age, little radioactivity was incorporated into fatty acids by adipocytes from the lean rat while clearly measurable quantities were incorporated into the adipocytes of fatty rats. Insulin had a significant effect in the fatty rat but a very small effect in the lean animals at this age. By 18 weeks of age, there was little difference between the basal lipogenesis in either fatty or lean animals and the stimulation by insulin appeared greater in the lean animals.

A second group of abnormalities in the fatty rat are associated with hypothalamic function. These are summarized in Table 2.3. The uterus of the fatty rat is significantly smaller than that of the lean animal (Saiduddin et al, 1973). The uptake of radioactive iodine and turnover of thyroid hormone are reduced in the fatty rat as compared to its lean counterpart (York et al, 1972a) whereas urine volume is significantly greater in the fatty rat even when animals are pair fed (York & Bray, 1971). Finally, fatty rats are hyperphagic (Bray & York, 1972). These four observations suggest the possibility of a hypothalamic abnormality underlying the obesity. This could manifest itself in one of two ways: either as primary hyperphagia with most of the other abnormalities resulting from the obesity, or as a diffuse defect in hypothalamic function of which hyperphagia is only one manifestation. We have examined the possibility that hyperphagia is the primary cause for the obesity and all other defects. Pair feeding or restricted food intake does not restore to normal either thyroid or reproductive function in any animals (Bray et al, 1973). It thus appears that primary hyperphagia will not account for these abnormalities in the fatty rat. The possibility of a more diffuse hypothalamic aberration is currently under investigation.

The third mechanism which might account for obesity is hyperinsulinaemia. The fatty rat has increased insulin (York et al, 1972b; Zucker & Antoniades, 1972). This has been examined in rats on different dietary intakes. The fatty rat, whether pair fed or fed *ad libitum*, has significantly higher levels of insulin than the lean rat. One explanation for the abnormality in the fatty rat would be similar to that presented for hypothalamic obesity. This hypothesis has been tested by comparing rats with hypothalamic injury to fatty rats. The evidence would suggest that lesions in the ventromedial nucleus *per se* are not the pathogenetic mechanism in the fatty rat (Bray & York, 1972).

Insulin resistance or alterations in the structure of insulin remain possible explanations of the pathogenesis of obesity in the fatty rat. The elevated insulin levels which are measured by radioimmunoassay may not be biologically active. There are no bioassays of insulin-like activity. The possibility of a defect in insulin action still remains a realistic possibility, particularly with the abnormalities observed in the early phases of development of the syndrome. In summary, the fatty rat presents a model of obesity similar in a number of ways to the juvenile form of human obesity. Adipocytes appear to function in relation to the size of the fat cells and are not influenced by their increased number.

REFERENCES

BABINSKI, M.D. (1900) Tumeur du corps pituitaire sana acremegalie et avec de developpement des organes genitaux. *Rev. Neurol.*, **8**, 531.
BERNARDIS, L.L. & FROHMAN, L.A. (1971) Effects of hypothalamic lesions at different loci on development of hyperinsulinemia and obesity in the weanling rat. *J. Comp. Neurol.*, **141**, 107.
BOOTH, D.A. (1968) Effects of intrahypothalamic glucose injection on eating and drinking elicited by insulin. *J. Comp. Physiol. Psychol.*, **65**, 13.
BRAY, G.A. (1969) Studies on the composition of adipose tissue from the genetically obese rats. *Proc. Soc. Exptl. Biol. Med.*, **131**, 111.
BRAY, G.A. (1973) Types of human obesity—a system of classification. *Obesity Bariat.*, **2**, 146.

BRAY, G.A. (1974) Some clinical aspects of obesity. The varieties of obesity. In *Treatment and Management of Obesity*, Ed. Bray, G.A. & Bethune, J.E. Ch. 5, Section II. Maryland: Harper & Rowe (in press).
BRAY, G.A. LUONG, D. & YORK, D.A. (1974) Regulation of adipose tissue mass in the genetically obese rodents. *Exerpta Medica* (in press).
BRAY, G.A. & YORK, D.A. (1971) Genetically transmitted obesity in rodents. *Physiol. Rev.*, 51, 598.
BRAY, G.A. & YORK, D.A. (1972) Studies on food intake of genetically obese rats. *Am. J. Physiol.*, 223, 176.
BRAY, G.A. YORK, D.A. & SWERDLOFF, R.S. (1973) Genetic obesity in rats. I. The effects of food restriction on body composition and hypothalamic function. *Metabolism*, 22, 435.
BRECHER, G. & WAXLER, S.H. (1949) Obesity in albino mice due to single injection of gold thioglucose. *Proc. Soc. Exptl. Biol. Med.*, 70, 498.
BROBECK, J.R. (1964) Mechanism of the development of obesity in animals with hypothalamic obesity. *Physiol. Rev.*, 26, 541.
BROOKS, C.M. & LAMBERT, E.F. (1946) A study of the effect of limitations of food intake and the method of feeding on the rate of weight gain during hypothalamic obesity in the albino rat. *Am. J. Physiol.*, 147, 695.
FALCONER, D.S. & ISAACSON, J.H. (1959) Adipose, a new inherited obesity of the mouse. *J. Heridity*, 50, 290
FRIEDMAN, M.I. (1972) Effects of alloxan diabetes on hypothalamic hyperphagia and obesity. *Am. J. Physiol.*, 222, 174.
FRÖHLICH, A. (1901) Ein fall von tumor der hypophysis cerebri ohne akromegalie. *Wie. Klin. Rund.*, 15, 883.
FROHMAN, L.A., BERNARDIS, L.L., SCHNATZ, J.D. & BURCK, L. (1969) Plasma insulin and triglyceride levels after hypothalamic lesions in weanling rats. *Am. J. Physiol.*, 216, 1496.
GOLDMAN, J.K., SCHNATZ, J.D., BERNARDIS, L.A. & FROHMAN, L.A. (1970) Adipose tissue metabolism of weanling rats after destruction of ventromedial hypothalamic nuclei: Effect of hypophysectomy and growth hormone. *Metabolism*, 19, 995.
GOLDMAN, J.L., SCHNATZ, J.D., BERNARDIS, L.L. & FROHMAN, L.A. (1972) Effects of ventromedial hypothalamic destruction in rats with pre-existing streptozotocin-induced diabetes. *Metabolism*, 21, 132.
HALES, C.N. & KENNEDY, G.C. (1964) Plasma glucose, non-esterified fatty acids and insulin concentrations in hypothalamic-hyperphagic rats. *Biochem. J.*, 90, 620.
HAMILTON, C.I. (1973) Physiologic control of food intake. *J. Am. Diabetic Assoc.*, 62, 35.
HAN, P.W. (1968) Obesity in force-fed hypophysectomized rats bearing hypothalamic lesions. *Proc. Soc. Exptl. Biol. Med.*, 127, 1057.
HETHERINGTON, A.W. & RANSON, S.W. (1942) The spontaneous activity and food intake of rats with hypothalamic lesions. *Am. J. Physiol.*, 136, 609.
HIRSCH, J. & HAN, P. (1969) Cellularity of rat adipose tissue: effects of growth, starvation and obesity. *J. Lipid Res.*, 10, 77.
HIRSCH, J. & KNITTLE, J.L. (1970) Cellularity of obese and nonobese human adipose tissue. *Fed. Proc.*, 29, 1516.
HOEBEL, B.G. & TEITELBAUM, P. (1966) Weight reduction in normal and hypothalamic hyperphagic rats. *J. Comp. Physiol. Psychol.* 61, 189.
INGRAM, W.R. (1952) Brain stem mechanisms in behaviour. *Electro-*

encepholagr. Clin. Neurophysiol., **4**, 397.

JANSEN, G.R. & HUTCHISON, C.F. (1969) Production of hypothalamic obesity by microsurgery. *Am. J. Physiol.*, **217**, 487.

JOHNSON, P.R., ZUCKER, L.M. CRUCE, J.A.F. & HIRSCH, J. (1971) Cellularity of adipose depots in the genetically obese Zucker rat. *J. Lipid Res.*, **12**, 706.

KENNEDY, G.C. & PARKER, R.A. (1963) The islets of Langerhans in rats with hypothalamic obesity. *Lancet*, **2**, 981.

LEPKOVSKY, S. (1973) Newer concepts in the regulation of food intake. *Am. J. Clin. Nutr.*, **26**, 271.

MACKAY, E.M., CALLOWAY, J.W. & BARNES, R.H. (1940) Hyperalimentation in normal animals produced by protamine insulin. *J.Nutr.*, **20**, 59.

MONTEMURRO, D.G. (1971) Inhibition of hypothalamic obesity in the mouse with diethyl stilbestrol. *Can. J. Physiol. Pharmacol.*, **49**, 554.

RUTMAN, M.N., LEWIS, F.S. & BLOOMER, W. (1967) Metabolic investigations during the development of obesity in bipoperidyl mustard treated mice. *Trans. N.Y. Acad. Sci.*, **30**, 224.

SAIDUDDIN, S., BRAY, G.A., YORK, D.A. & SWERDLOFF, R.S. (1973) Reproductive function in the genetically obese fatty rat. *Endocrinology*, **93**, 1251.

SALANS, L.B., CUSHMAN, S.W. & WEISSMAN, R.E. (1973) Studies of human adipose tissue: Adipose cell size and number in nonobese and obese patients. *J. Clin. Invest.*, **52**, 929.

SLAUNWHITE, W.R., GOLDMAN, J.K. & BERNARDIS, L.L. (1972) Sequential changes in glucose metabolism by adipose tissue and liver of rats after destruction of the ventromedial hypothalamic nuclei: Effect of three dietary regimens. *Metabolism*, **21**, 619.

STEVENSON, J.A.F. (1969) Neural control of food and water intake. In *The Hypothalamus*, Ed. Haymaker, W., Anderson, E. & Nauter, W.J.H. p. 524. Springfield, Ill.

TEPPERMAN, J., BROBECK, J.R. & LONG, C.N.H. (1943) The effects of hypothalamic hyperphagia and of alterations in feeding habits on the metabolism of the albino rat. *Yale J. Biol. Med.*, **15**, 855.

YAMAMOTO, S., MIZUTANI, T. & KANEUCHI, G. (1970) Obesity induced in mice injected intracerebrally with 4-nitroquinoline 1-oxide or 4-hydroxyaminoquinoline 1-oxide. *Proc. Soc. Exptl. Biol. Med.*, **133**, 303.

YORK, D.A. & BRAY, G.A. (1971) Regulation of water balance in genetically obese rats. *Proc. Soc. Exptl. Biol. Med.*, **136**, 798.

YORK, D.A. & BRAY, G.A. (1972) Dependence of hypothalamic obesity on insulin, the pituitary and the adrenal gland. *Endocrinology*, **90**, 885.

YORK, D.A. & BRAY, G.A. (1973a) Genetic obesity in rats. II. The effect of food restriction on the metabolism of adipose tissue. *Metabolism*, **22**, 443.

YORK, D.A. & BRAY, G.A. (1973b) Adipose tissue metabolism in six week old fatty rats. *Horm. Metab. Res.*, **5**, 355.

YORK, D.A., HERSHMAN, J.M., UTIGER, R.D. & BRAY, G.A. (1972) Thyrotropin secretion in genetically obese rats. *Endocrinology*, **90**, 67.

YORK, D.A., STEINKE, J. & BRAY, G.A. (1972) Hyperinsulinemia and insulin resistance in genetically obese rats. *Metabolism*, **21**, 277.

YOUNG, T.K. & LIU, A.C. (1965) Hyperphagia, insulin and obesity. *Chinese J. Physiol.*, **19**, 247.

ZUCKER, L.M. & ANTONIADES, H.N. (1972) Insulin and obesity in the Zucker genetically obese rat 'fatty' *Endocrinology*, **90**, 1320.

DISCUSSION

Dr. Anand. When lesions are made in the region of the ventromedial nucleus hyperphagia occurs, but endocrine changes are also produced. This is the area which acts as a funnel through which all these factors may affect the hypophysis. Remarkable variations of insulin, thyroid and corticosteroid activity occur. Dr. Bray suggests that in some animals hyperinsulinaemia results. Studies in monkeys showed the opposite effect; when ventromedial lesions were made, diabetes mellitus with low insulin and high blood sugar concentrations developed. It has, however, been shown that such effects are independent of the glucose levels. If the connections to the hypothalamus are blocked no changes in the endocrine concentrations occur, but hyperphagia still results. It is thus possible to produce hyperphagia in obesity by blocking the connections to the hypothalamus without changes in insulin. Such an effect cannot then be insulin-dependent. On the other hand, insulin will produce variable effects dependent on the amount of glucose available. If there is insulin and excess glucose, then inhibition of hypothalamic activity will be produced. However, if there is insulin and a small amount of glucose available, glucose utilization is decreased and the hypothalamus will be active. Increased glucose utilization as a result of increased activity will produce exactly the opposite effect, inhibiting the hypothalamus rather than stimulating it. All this makes an extremely good hypothesis, but we may be dealing with drives and motivations which may not be completely independent of these endocrine effects.

Dr. Bray. The most difficult and inadequately understood aspect of the ventromedial nucleus is where output goes. Dr. Anand is absolutely right in saying the hyperphagic syndrome can be produced by microsurgical lesions between the ventral and lateral nucleus. However, this is no assurance that the tracts go in that direction. It has been suggested that microsurgical lesions below the ventromedial nucleus, not involving it, will produce the same syndrome. Other studies showed that injection of 6-hydroxydopamine into noradrenergic pathways passing down the brain stem from the ventromedial nucleus can also do this. It is not clear whether the ventromedial nucleus and the fibre tracts which are lateral to it really run laterally. My guess is that they only partly do so, and the ventromedial hypothalamic syndrome involves two components, hyperphagia and finickiness. These, I think, will be shown to be completely dissociable experimentally. It is only the hyperphagic component which I contend is an insulin-dependent component.

Dr. Debons. In connection with Dr. Bray's hypothesis, once ventromedial lesions are made hyperphagia is induced; this in itself could account for the hyperglycaemia and increased insulin output by the β-cells. If lesioned animals are pair-fed they still develop hyperinsulinaemia.

Dr. Bray. Yes, that has been confirmed in published data. If the animals are starved it does not happen but if they are pair-fed or tube-fed it does.

Mr. Miller. Can I challenge this concept that the hypothalamic lesion produces obesity by means of hyperphagia? Certainly the bigger, fatter animals have eaten more food, but I would expect bigger animals to eat more food than small animals. However if food intake is divided by body weight, or by weight to the three-quarters, these animals will be shown to be eating less than normal. Your last comment about pair-feeding and insulin would support my reasoning. Have you tried to measure the metabolic rate of these animals because it may well be that hypothalamic lesions are affecting metabolism in general, rather than simply producing hyperphagia. A good model for this hypothesis is the animal with hypothalamic damage due to monosodium glutamate—in this case the animals are the same weight as the controls, eat the same amount of food, but finish up with twice as much fat in their carcasses. There can be no argument about the body weights because they are the same.

Dr. Bray. In answer, there are several pertinent points. Firstly, the ventromedial hypothalamic lesioned animals have been examined *in extenso* for many years. The conclusion from work conducted more than 20 years ago by Dr. Anand and others suggested that hyperphagia was a major factor for the adult animal. More recent studies in the weanling animal suggest a second metabolic component—this is part of my thesis. If the weanling rat is lesioned, there is obesity without hyperphagia and without a change in body weight. The animal does not eat any more and gains no more weight than its unlesioned control, but it becomes significantly fatter. Thus, I think there are two components: there is a hyperphagic component which precedes the increase in weight in the adult animal, but it is also possible to have an increase in fat in pair-fed animals or weanling animals without hyperphagia.

3. Obesity and Cardiovascular Disease. The Framingham Study.

W. B. KANNEL and T. GORDON

Obesity is the most prevalent metabolic disorder in affluent societies. Despite wide recognition of the adverse health consequences of obesity, including cardiovascular dysfunction, digestive disturbances, diabetes mellitus, skin ailments and degenerative arthritis, its prevalence remains high.

In this chapter, we intend to examine the prevalence of obesity, time trends in weight, the biologic concomitants of weight gain and the cardiovascular consequences of obesity. The Framingham cohort, which provides most of the substance of this report, consists of 5209 men and women originally aged 30–62 years at entry in 1948. This cohort has been followed biennially for the development of cardiovascular disease in relation to a variety of personal attributes, including relative weight, measured at each examination. The methods, sampling procedures, response rates and criteria for disease used have been detailed elsewhere (Kannel & Gordon, 1968). Follow-up has been reasonably complete with about 85 per cent taking every possible examination within the 18 years of follow-up. Only two per cent have been completely lost to follow-up.

METHODS

Weights were assessed on each examination with a clinical beam scale, with subjects clothed only in an examination gown without shoes or street dress, except that men wore trousers. Weights were measured in pounds and ideal weight for height was derived from tables published by the Metropolitan Life Insurance Company. Relative Metropolitan weight used as a measure of obesity in this report represents actual weight divided by the appropriate 'desirable' weight for height and expressed as a percentage. Skinfold thickness was also measured but not on every occasion.

Analytical Procedures

The relation of relative weight at each biennial examination to cardiovascular morbidity and mortality was ascertained for the age group 45–74 years for each sex, adjusting for the variable age composition of each relative weight subgroup. Age adjustment was accomplished by the indirect method Shurtleff (1974).

The strength of the association is evaluated by computing regression coefficients—bivariate, taking only age into account, and multivariate, also taking into account other major contributors to cardiovascular disease such as systolic blood pressure, serum cholesterol, electrocardiographic left ventricular hypertrophy (ECG-LVH), blood glucose and smoking. Where relative weight is considered without taking associated risk factors into consideration, the regression of the cardiovascular events on relative weight is estimated by the method of Walker & Duncan (1967), to which the reader should refer for further explanation (also see footnote).

Clinical Criteria

The clinical endpoints considered include:

Coronary heart disease (including angina pectoris, myocardial infarction, the coronary insufficiency syndrome and sudden death).

Atherothrombotic brain infarction (ABI) (focal neurological deficits of abrupt onset without evidence of haemorrhage or other processes which might cause such deficits).

Intermittent claudication based on a history of cramping calf discomfort provoked by walking and relieved promptly by rest.

Congestive heart failure requiring a combination of major and minor criteria.

Further diagnostic details for all cardiovascular events including congestive failure are available elsewhere (Shurtleff, 1970).

Criteria for obesity

There is no clear demarcation of obesity from leanness. The ideal

---

$P(X) = \dfrac{1}{1+e^{-(a+Bx)}}$ where P is the probability of the cardiovascular event in two years and X is the relative weight. This procedure provides an estimate of B (the regression coefficient) and a (the intercept) in the equation for the logistic function. Where other variables are taken into account, the exponent becomes:
$-(a + B_k + Z_i X_i Z_i)$. The analytical methods used for measuring the strength of the association of relative weight and cardiovascular disease taking into account associated variables are multivariate discriminant analysis (Fisher, 1936) and logistic regression (Walker & Duncan, 1967).

degree of fatness is not established and probably varies in different socioeconomic groups if survival is used as a yardstick. In areas where the food supply is intermittent and the climate frigid, obesity is probably beneficial. In affluent societies with a constant surfeit of rich food and drink, obtained at small energy cost and protected against extremes of weather, survival is more likely in those as lean as possible.

Table 3.1
Correlations of various measures of obesity with relative weight* (Examination 5)

Age (years)	No. of persons	Subscapular Skinfold	Arm Girth	Ponderal Index
MEN				
40–49	627	0.68	0.82	0.96
50–59	489	0.68	0.79	0.95
60–69	282	0.60	0.75	0.95
WOMEN				
40–49	813	0.74	0.85	0.97
50–59	676	0.67	0.80	0.97
60–69	417	0.69	0.78	0.97

*according to Metropolitan Life Insurance Company table of ideal weights.

Assessment of the influence of obesity on cardiovascular incidence is clouded by the assertion that relative weight is an imprecise measure of adiposity (Seltzer, 1969). However, relative weight and skinfolds are highly correlated (Table 3.1) and whether relative weight, skinfold thickness or weight gain after completion of musculo-skeletal growth are used to assess obesity, the results as regards incidence of cardiovascular disease are virtually identical (Table 3.2). Since no critical value of fatness can be identified at which cardiovascular morbidity or atherogenic traits occur, it is best to consider the problem in terms of degree of overweight rather than as a categorical entity of obesity. Of course, there are rare individuals in whom gross excess of body fat leads to a definable clinical entity but such persons are not the subject of this report.

PREVALENCE OF OBESITY

Fatness is characteristic of affluent populations and tends to increase with age. Estimates of obesity in the United States of America come largely from three sources: life insurance data, the national health survey and epidemiologic surveys (Gordon & Kannel, 1973; Lew,

Table 3.2
Standardized univariate regression coefficients[1] for the prevalence of coronary heart disease on various measures of adiposity Framingham Study, 10 year follow-up

Age (years)	Relative Weight	Subscapular Skinfold	Arm Girth	Ponderal Index
MEN				
40–49	0.3667*	0.3618*	0.2459	0.2778
50–59	0.2406*	0.2296	0.1636	0.2554*
60–69	0.1966	0.2807	0.3684*	0.1346
Average	0.2655+	0.2816+	0.2420+	0.2298+
WOMEN				
40–49	0.4489*	0.2374	0.4808	0.3571
50–59	0.3511*	0.2969*	0.0746	0.3384*
60–69	0.1393	0.4078+	−0.0079	0.1303
Average	0.2871+	0.3291+	0.1039	0.2623+

[1] Regression coefficients estimated by method of Cornfield et al (1961)
Average $\beta = \dfrac{\Sigma \beta_1 / V_1}{\Sigma \frac{1}{V_1}}$ where β_1 is the age-specific standardized regression coefficient and V_1 is its variance
* Significant. $P < 0.05$
+ Significant. $P = 0.01$

1948; Lew, 1969; National Health Surveys, 1964, 1965, 1967, 1970; Shurtleff, 1974). These indicate that obesity is very prevalent, but it is difficult to obtain precise or uniform estimates because definitions of the condition vary. Life insurance companies define optimal or desirable weight as that associated with the best chance of survival. Currently, by this criterion they find that of insured adult men aged 30 to 39 years, half are at least 10 per cent overweight and a quarter at least 20 per cent overweight. At 50 to 59 years of age the corresponding figures are 60 per cent and 33 per cent (Lew, 1969). The percentages in women are somewhat lower under the age of 40, the same between the ages of 40 and 49 years, and greater after 49 years.

Using the criterion of 20 per cent above *average* weight, 12 per cent of adult men and 16 per cent of women are obese (Fig 3.1). If the insurance criteria of optimal weight are applied to the National Health Examination Survey data for 1960-1962 almost 30 per cent of men and women are 20 per cent above *optimal* weight. The average Framingham subject was about 20 per cent above optimal weight and more than 15 per cent of the men and 20 per cent of the women had relative weights at least 35 per cent above optimum. As many as 3 per cent of men and 9 per cent of women were massively obese, i.e. 50 per cent above optimal weight (Gordon & Kannel, 1973).

Considered categorically, with common definitions, obesity is second to none of the other major risk factors in atherosclerotic cardiovascular disease in frequency (Figure 3.2). While obesity is not as powerful an independent contributor to cardiovascular disease as the other factors, it assumes special importance because it is to some extent a determinant of the major risk factors of hypertension, hyperlipidaemia and diabetes mellitus. About 40 per cent of persons aged 40 to 49 have one or more atherogenic traits which promote cardiovascular disease. The proportion tends to increase with relative weight (Figure 3.3).

Trends in Weight

An examination of cross sectional Framingham data (Table 3.3) indicates that young men tend to weigh more than older men. In women the situation is different. Young women weigh less than middle-aged women. Between the ages of 60 and 75 years, weight in women decreases slightly; after age 75 it drops sharply, as it does in men.

Longitudinal cohort curves (Table 3.4) reveal that the age differences noted in cross-sectional data are largely due to secular, or

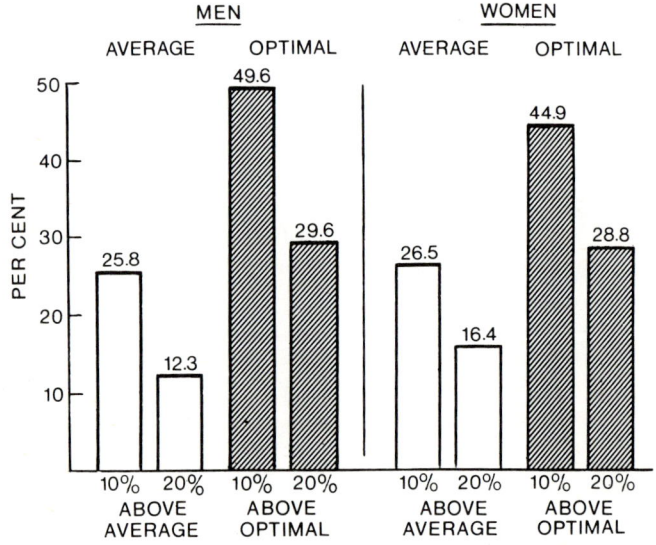

Figure 3.1
Prevalence of obesity in the population of the United States. Men and women aged 18-79 years (Source: National Health Survey, 1960-1962).

Table 3.3

Secular trends in relative weight
Men and women 29-79 years: Framingham study

Mean Metropolitan Ideal Relative Weight

AGE AT EXAM 1 (yr)	Exam Number:	1948-52 1	2	3	4	5	6	7	8	9	1966-70 10
MEN	29-34	117.3	119.6	123.9	—	—	—	—	—	—	—
	35-39	118.5	119.0	119.9	122.3	122.0	128.2	—	128.0	133.0	—
	40-44	118.8	119.6	120.4	120.9	121.6	122.1	123.6	123.1	123.6	125.0
	45-49	119.4	119.3	119.8	120.6	120.6	121.5	121.9	122.3	122.6	123.9
	50-54	120.8	121.1	121.2	120.7	120.9	120.7	121.0	121.0	120.9	122.6
	55-59	118.3	119.4	121.7	123.0	121.0	120.7	120.1	121.1	119.2	119.4
	60-64	122.3	119.6	118.3	118.3	118.9	119.9	121.1	119.8	118.6	119.6
	65-69	—	98.0	116.7	119.1	119.0	118.5	118.6	118.0	118.4	118.2
	70-74	—	—	—	—	117.5	123.2	119.7	119.0	117.8	118.0
	75-79	—	—	—	—	—	—	—	—	—	—
WOMEN	29-34	110.8	109.2	106.9	—	—	—	—	—	—	—
	35-39	116.1	114.3	114.7	113.8	110.9	117.7	—	114.3	116.5	—
	40-44	118.2	117.4	117.5	117.4	116.0	115.4	115.6	119.4	118.8	115.9
	45-49	123.9	122.0	119.7	118.9	118.2	119.4	118.9	121.2	121.4	120.8
	50-54	127.8	126.1	124.6	124.5	121.1	119.4	119.6	120.5	120.4	121.4
	55-59	129.9	128.1	126.6	125.7	125.8	123.0	122.5	124.0	124.2	122.0
	60-64	134.5	130.0	128.0	127.4	126.5	125.4	125.2	125.9	122.5	124.3
	65-69	—	—	129.6	131.0	126.3	125.6	125.1	124.9	124.4	123.3
	70-74	—	—	—	—	128.8	132.5	125.4	122.2	122.5	120.5
	75-79	—	—	—	—	—	—	—	—	—	—

Table 3.4

Trend in relative weight with age over 18 years
Men and women 29-62 years at Exam 1: Framingham study

Years of follow up: AGE AT EXAM 1 (yr)		2	4	6	8	10	12	14	16	18
					Mean Metropolitan Ideal Relative Weight					
MEN	29-34	117.3	119.0	120.0	121.1	121.5	122.0	122.4	122.9	122.9	124.5
	35-39	118.5	119.4	120.2	121.4	121.1	121.7	122.2	123.2	122.8	123.2
	40-44	118.8	119.8	120.3	121.1	121.0	120.7	120.6	121.3	120.5	120.8
	45-49	119.4	119.6	120.5	120.8	120.1	120.6	120.2	120.6	119.1	118.9
	50-54	120.8	121.2	121.7	122.0	120.7	119.9	120.1	119.4	118.0	118.4
	55-59	118.3	118.2	117.9	117.8	117.7	118.4	118.3	118.9	118.4	118.2
	60-62	122.3	121.0	123.8	121.5	122.6	124.7	123.2	124.1	120.7	124.6
WOMEN	29-34	110.8	111.1	113.0	113.7	113.7	115.4	116.6	118.1	118.7	119.3
	35-39	116.1	116.7	117.6	118.6	118.4	119.4	120.7	121.3	121.8	121.9
	40-44	118.2	119.0	119.3	119.6	119.7	119.7	119.7	120.7	121.1	121.3
	45-49	123.9	123.9	123.2	124.6	123.6	122.9	123.0	122.8	123.3	122.7
	50-54	127.8	126.5	126.5	126.6	125.3	125.3	125.6	125.3	123.5	123.2
	55-59	129.9	128.5	127.3	128.3	127.2	125.9	124.6	125.1	124.1	122.3
	60-62	134.5	134.4	134.3	130.7	129.5	131.8	130.6	128.4	123.5	126.4

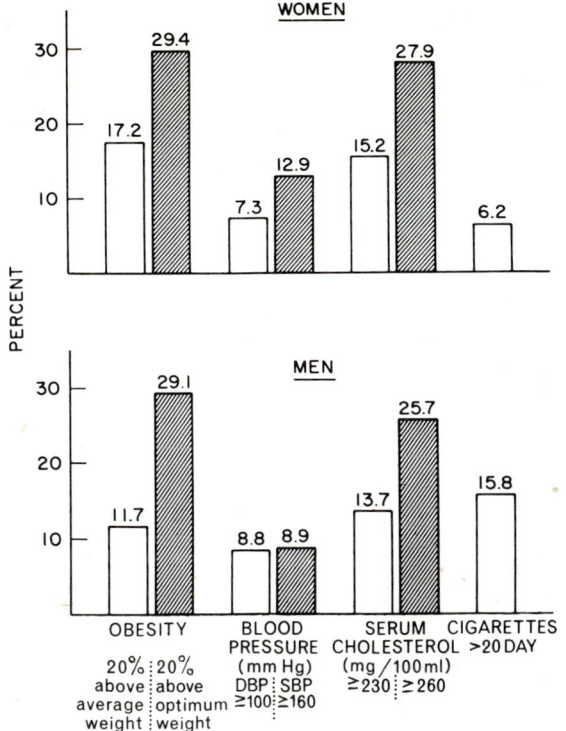

Figure 3.2
Comparative prevalence of major cardiovascular risk factors in general United States population. Men and women aged 45-54 years
(Source: National Health Survey, 1960-62).
DBP = diastolic blood pressure
SBP = systolic blood pressure

cohort, differences. Men born later in this century are consistently heavier at any age than those born earlier. With women the converse is true (Table 3.4, Figure 3.4). On the other hand, both men and women become heavier as they grow older, up to the age of 55. Beyond middle age they tend to lose weight.

Examination of weight fluctuation in the Framingham cohort reveals that weight in adults at one age is closely related to weight later in life. Weights at the beginning of the study had a correlation of 0.75 with weight 18 years later. While there was a relatively large average difference of more than 21 lb between the highest and lowest weights in 18 years, this reflects chiefly short-term fluctuation, and persistent changes occur rather slowly.

DETERMINANTS OF OBESITY

The secular trends noted in relative weight suggest that life style plays an important role in determining obesity. Despite even greater affluence, women are lighter than formerly suggesting a response to change in fashions. However, despite powerful psycho-social forces, including fashion, youth cultism and health consciousness, weights tend inexorably to creep up with age in both sexes. Social forces and group influences are powerful not only in the development of obesity, but also in its control. Obese families tend to generate obese children, and group therapy seems to be more successful in controlling obesity than individual therapy.

In the Framingham cohort spouses share a tendency to obesity. Among 1242 spouse pairs of single continuous marriages, 15 per cent of the husbands of obese women were overweight, a proportion double that of the spouses of non-obese women (Figure 3.5). A probable explanation is the tendency for spouses to share nutrient

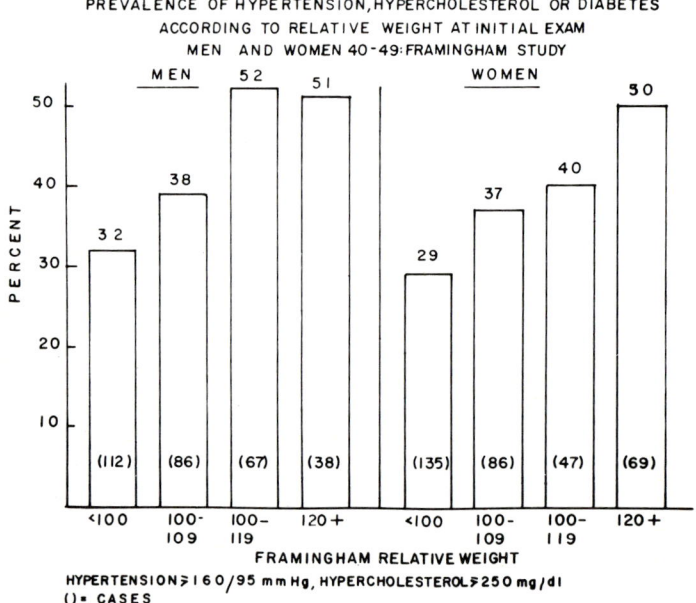

Figure 3.3

intakes in quantity and quality (Table 3.5). However, since there was little tendency for spouse aggregation of obesity to increase with the duration of the marriage, assortive mating must be considered.

For one reason or another, obesity is very much a family affair. Conditioning as well as genetic factors acting early in life seem to play an important role. Equating leanness with ill-health is a parental attitude which provokes overfeeding of children. They are prompted

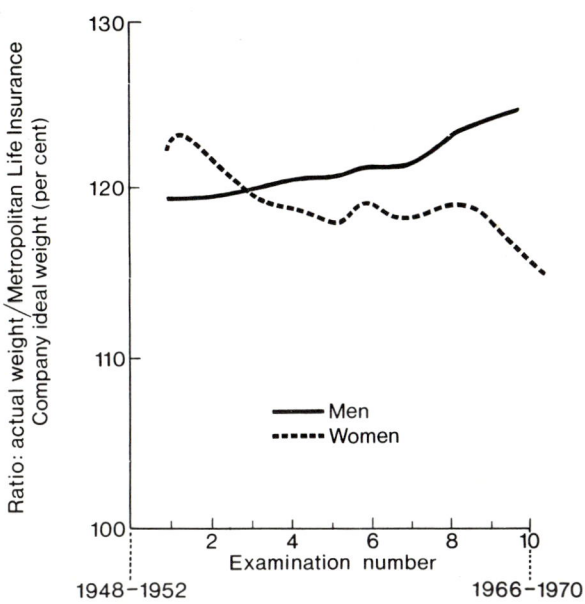

Figure 3.4
Changes in average weight in 10 years, Framingham study: persons aged 45-48 years

to empty their plates rather than to eat until they are satieted. Feeding has changed from a necessity to a form of pleasurable entertainment for the family.

Once established in childhood, there is some evidence to suggest that obesity tends to perpetuate itself. Research suggests that permanent hyperplasia of fat cells occurs and these cells become insensitive to insulin (Heald et al, 1965), and that the obese also experience a blunting of their ability to regulate intake precisely to their need for calories (Campbell et al, 1971). Such metabolic derangements accompanying obesity may be an adaptive response to overfeeding as well as the factor which tends to perpetuate it. In any event, the more pronounced the obesity and the earlier in life it becomes established, the more it resists management.

Table 3.5

Correspondence of nutrient intake and obesity status of spouses*

Husband's nutrient intake**	Kcalories /day	Mean Fat (g)	Intake of Wives Carbohydrate (g)	Plasma Cholesterol (mg/100ml)	Husband's Obesity Status (% ideal body weight)	Percent of Wives Obese
Low	1938	85	202	421	<100	9
Medium	2182	93	231	518	100-119	17
High	2369	111	254	546	≥20	22

* 278 couples—Framingham diet study
** these subgroups are tertiles of the distribution of nutrients

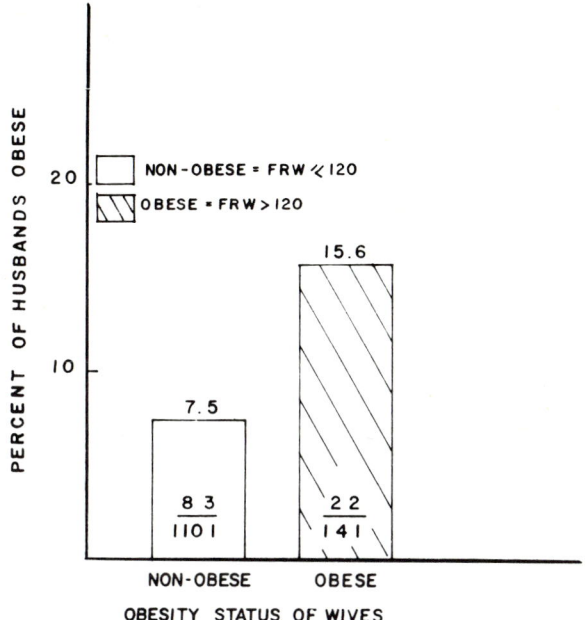

Figure 3.5
FRW = Framingham relative weight

BIOLOGICAL ACCOMPANIMENTS

Metabolic aberrations occur in most persons as they become obese. These include impaired glucose tolerance, inadequate mobilization of fatty acids, a sluggish free fatty acid response to exogenous insulin, resistance to ketosis and a diminished growth hormone response to hypoglycaemia, exercise and starvation (Heald *et al*, 1965).

Longitudinal data on the biological accompaniments of fattening in the general population are scarce. Such data from Framingham reveal that obesity is associated with a number of biological changes which operate to the detriment of the cardiovascular system. Weight gain is associated with a rise in serum lipids, an increase in blood pressure, impairment of glucose tolerance and a slight rise in plasma uric acid concentrations (Figure 3.6). This combination of atherogenic traits has a powerful influence on cardiovascular incidents

(Figure 3.7). On this account it is not surprising that obesity is associated with an excess of cardiovascular morbidity and mortality.

The effect of weight change on the level of atherogenic traits as determined longitudinally, therefore, merits a detailed examination. In men, for each 10 per cent decrease in weight there is, on the average, an 11 mg/100 ml reduction in serum cholesterol, a 5 mm reduction in systolic blood pressure, a 2 mg/100 ml reduction in blood glucose and a 0.4 mg/100 ml fall in serum uric acid. In women the changes are half this order of magnitude (Ashley & Kannel, 1974). While these relationships are not universal or dramatic from an individual point of view, they hold at all ages and are independent of the general level of adiposity. It is encouraging to note that weight loss is associated with a corresponding reduction in major atherogenic traits, and it is reasonable to hope that this has prophylactic significance.

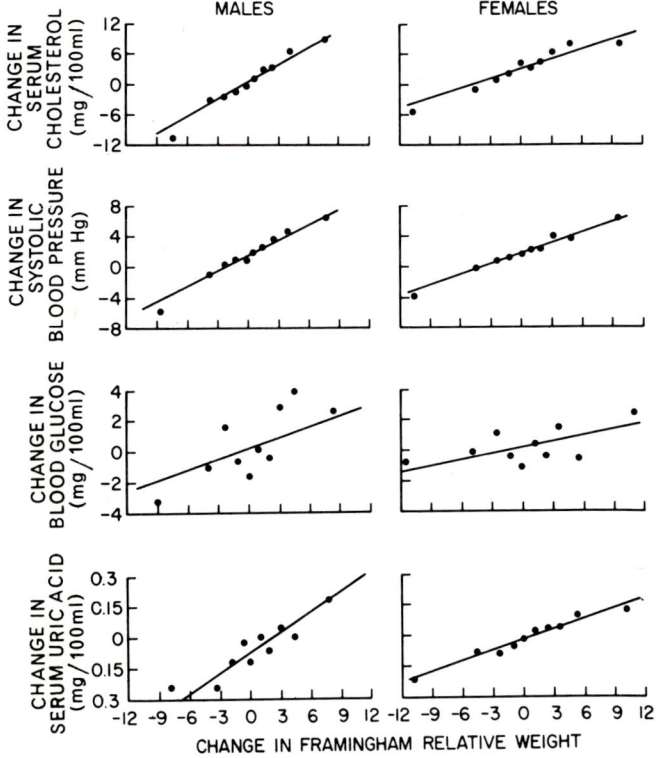

Figure 3.6
Changes in characteristic values with change in Framingham relative weight

OBESITY AND CARDIOVASCULAR DISEASE

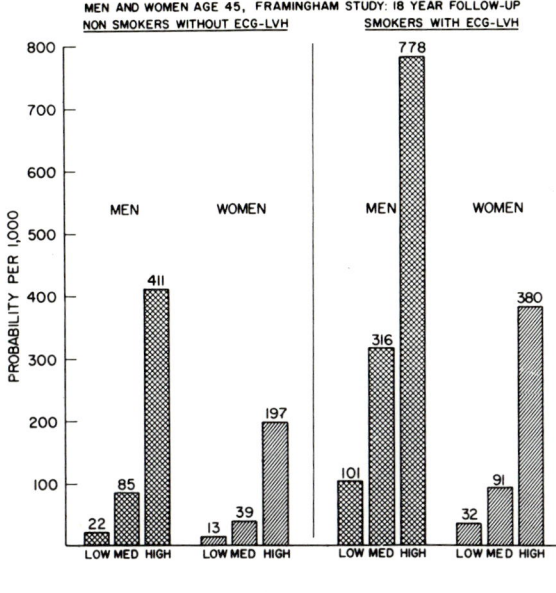

Figure 3.7
(serum cholesterol (CHOL), systolic blood pressure (SBP) and glucose intolerance)

AUTOPSY FINDINGS

In the Framingham autopsy series body weight is more strikingly related to left ventricular weight and thickness than to coronary atherosclerotic involvement, suggesting a greater impact on cardiac workload (Table 3.6). The effect of overweight on the heart seems greater in women than men. The effect on heart weight and thickness is statistically significant and independent of associated blood pressure, glucose and cholesterol. On the other hand, from the number of observations available the effect on coronary atherosclerosis is not statistically significant. These data suggest that obesity may impose more of a haemodynamic than an atherogenic threat to the circulatory apparatus. Other autopsy series also suggest only a modest atherogenic impact of obesity *per se* (Spain *et al*, 1963; Wilkins *et al*, 1959).

Table 3.6

Correlation of cardiac findings at autopsy with relative weight during life: Framingham study

	1 year before death (n = 55)			9 years before death (n = 66)		
	Age at Death	Weight	Relative Weight	Age at Death	Weight	Relative Weight
MEN						
Heart Weight	−0.059	0.145	0.203	−0.073	0.277*	0.343**
Left Ventricular Muscle Thickness	−0.082	0.275*	0.217	−0.068	0.375**	0.277*
Percent Intimal Involvement	−0.028	0.083	0.146	−0.026	0.126	0.180
Percent Luminal Insufficiency	0.060	−0.076	−0.012	0.052	0.035	0.093
WOMEN						
Heart Weight	0.267	0.207	0.223	0.249	0.435**	0.423**
Left Ventricular Muscle Thickness	0.253	0.200	0.244	0.315*	0.238	0.291
Percent Intimal Involvement	0.529***	0.108	0.150	0.609***	0.171	0.222
Percent Luminal Insufficiency	0.424**	−0.024	0.034	0.545***	0.134	0.195

*   Significant $P < 0.05$
**   Significant $P < 0.01$
*** Significant $P < 0.001$

MORTALITY

An examination of overall mortality in relation to relative weight or weight loss reveals the surprising finding—in the light of the foregoing—that leanness may be a risk (Figure 3.8). Closer scrutiny reveals the cause. An appraisal of the group sustaining large weight losses (10 per cent or more) which were not immediately preceded or followed by a large weight gain reveals a subgroup with a large excess mortality. This subgroup is comprised of persons whose weight loss was preceded by a medical illness which explains the loss. Mortality in this group was at least four times that of those whose weight loss was due to deliberate dieting (either prescribed or self-determined), or weight loss unexplained by medical history. Interestingly the latter weight losses were associated with no excess mortality.

Although taken at face value overall mortality in both sexes and cardiovascular mortality in men are both lower in the obese than in lean persons, coronary mortality in general and sudden death rates in particular are substantially higher in the obese (Figure 3.9). If selective factors are considered, these data are not inconsistent with the observations of life insurance companies that overweight con-

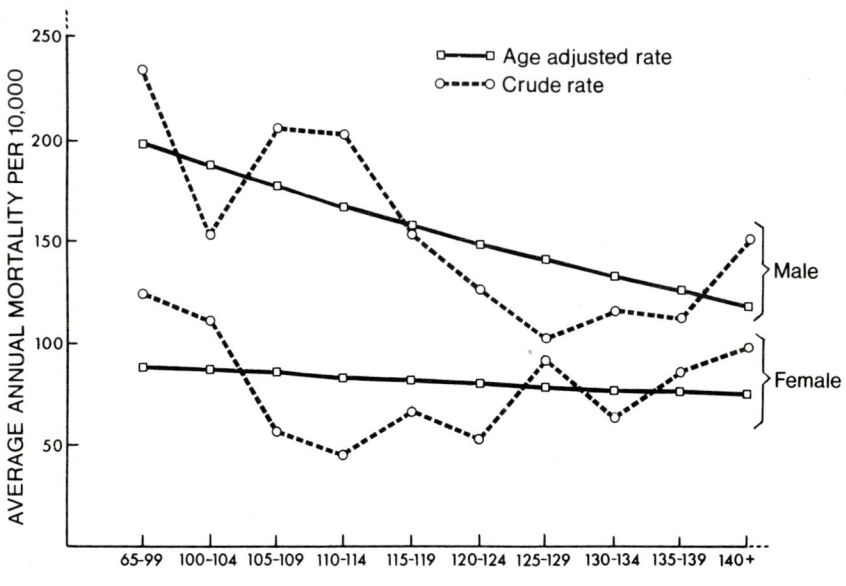

Figure 3.8
Risk of death according to relative weight. Men and women aged 45-74 years at examination, Framingham study: 18 year follow-up.

40 OBESITY SYMPOSIUM

tributes to earlier mortality, particularly from cardiovascular disease (Lew, 1948, 1969).

CARDIOVASCULAR MORBIDITY

Except for occlusive peripheral arterial disease in both men and women in the Framingham cohort, a higher incidence of all the major clinical manifestations of atherosclerotic cardiovascular disease was observed among the obese (Figure 3.10). The strength of the association can be judged from the size of the coefficients for the regression of the specified cardiovascular events on relative weight. As seen in Table 3.7 the association is about equal in strength in men for the various cardiovascular events, other than intermittent claudication. In women, the effect is definitely stronger for brain infarction and congestive heart failure (CHF) than for coronary heart

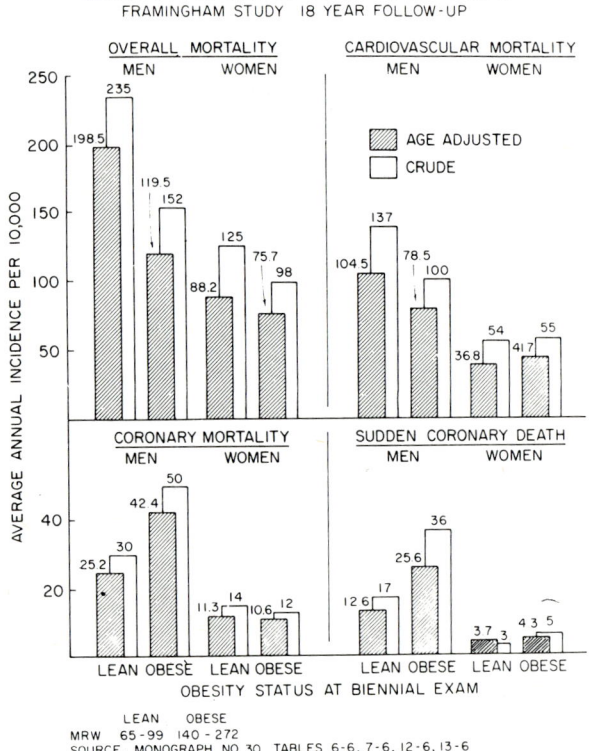

Figure 3.9
Obesity status. Men and women aged 45-74 years at examination. Framingham study: 18 year follow-up.

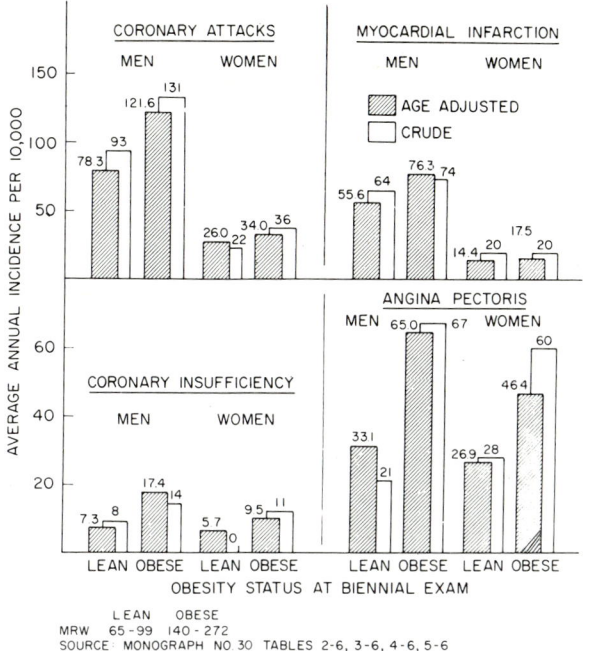

Figure 3.10
Framingham study: 18 year follow up.

disease (CHD) (Table 3.7, Figure 3.10). It is of interest that there is in men a strong, statistically significant negative relationship between relative weight and intermittent claudication (Table 3.7, Figure 3.10). This is not seen for angina pectoris, a symptom also provoked by physical exertion.

The net, or independent, effect of obesity can be ascertained from a comparison of the bivariate regression coefficient (accounting only for age) and multivariate regression coefficient (accounting as well for systolic blood pressure, cholesterol, glucose, cigarettes, ECG-LVH). Such comparison (Table 3.7) reveals in men a substantial reduction in the impact of obesity when its atherogenic accompaniments are taken into account for brain infarction and CHF but not CHD or intermittent claudication. In women, the net effect of obesity is small for ABI and cardiovascular events except CHF. In men, a significant and sizeable regression coefficient persists in the multivariate case for CHD (and a negative one for claudication); in women, for CHF only.

Table 3.7
Regression of cardiovascular morbidity on relative weight: Framingham study 18 year follow-up: men and women, 45–74 years

Cardiovascular Disease Entity	MEN Regression coefficients		WOMEN Regression coefficients	
	Bivariate$_{(1)}$	Multivariate$_{(2)}$	Bivariate$_{(1)}$	Multivariate$_{(2)}$
Atherothrombotic brain infarction	0.010	0.003	0.018**	0.009.
Intermittent claudication	−0.016*	−0.019*	0.005	−0.002
Congestive heart failure	0.012	0.006	0.018**	0.011*
Coronary Heart disease	0.012**	0.010**	0.009**	0.002

(1) Bivariate: Metropolitan relative weight and age
(2) Multivariate: Above plus systolic blood pressure, cholesterol, ECG-LVH, cigarettes and glucose

* Significant $P < 0.05$ level
** Significant $P < 0.01$ level

A more detailed examination of the relation of obesity to individual clinical manifestations of CHD reveals that, in men, all coronary manifestations are related to obesity (Figure 3.11). However, only angina and coronary attacks are significantly related with the numbers available (Table 3.8). Judging from the size of the regression coefficients, overweight is less strikingly related to myocardial infarction than to other coronary manifestations. In women, only angina and the coronary insufficiency syndrome are strikingly or significantly related to relative weight. In men, multivariate coefficients are only modestly reduced compared to bivariate, indicating that very little of the effect of obesity in promoting CHD can be attributed to coexisting atherogenic traits (Table 3.8). In women, on the other hand, a good deal of the effect in angina appears to be mediated through the associated atherogenic traits.

Risk of the major cardiovascular events rises in proportion to the degree of overweight so there does not appear to be any critical degree of obesity involved (Figure 3.12).

NET AND JOINT EFFECTS

While there is no secure basis for precisely estimating the net and

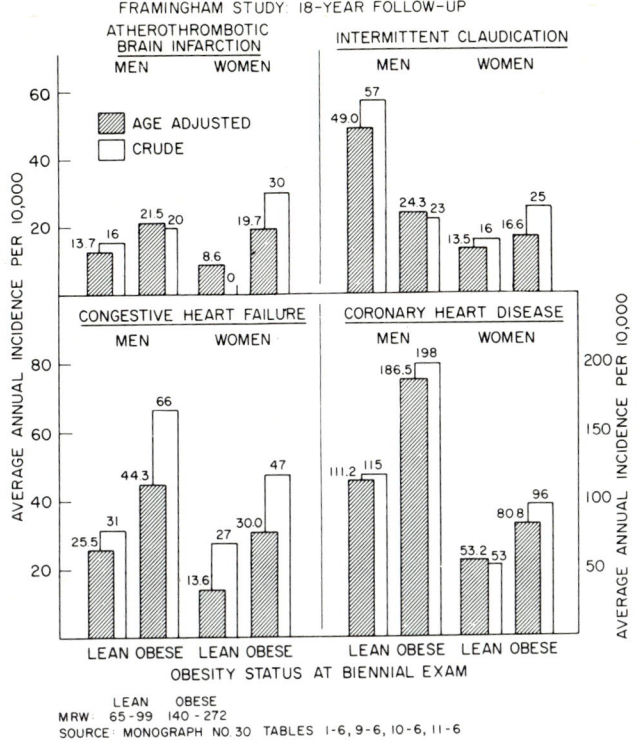

Figure 3.11
Risk of manifestations of coronary heart disease according to obesity status. Men and women aged 45-74 years at examination. Framingham study: 18 year follow-up.

joint effect of obesity in promoting cardiovascular disease or the potential benefit of correcting obesity it is clear that obesity is an important contributor to cardiovascular morbidity. Although there is some unique effect, obesity is clearly not a major independent predictor of cardiovascular incidence given knowledge of the major risk factors. This is not to say that overweight is an unimportant consideration in prophylaxis against cardiovascular disease, but rather that it is not particularly helpful in estimating risk.

Cardiovascular disease risk is best conceptualized as the joint result of multiple contributors, i.e. risk factors. 'Stroke' and congestive heart failure are largely a consequence of hypertension, yet at any level of blood pressure, risk of either varies widely depending on concomitant risk factors. Choice of the ingredients of a cardiovascular profile for estimating risk should take into consideration not

Table 3.8
Regression of incidence of manifestations of coronary heart disease (CHD) on relative weight: Framingham study 18 year follow-up. Men and women 45–74 years.

Clinical Manifestations of CHD	MEN Regression Coefficients Bivariate(1)	Multivariate(2)	WOMEN Regression Coefficients Bivariate(1)	Multivariate(2)
Coronary attacks	0.010*	0.008	0.006*	0.002
Myocardial infarction	0.007	0.006	0.004	−0.004
Coronary insufficiency	0.020	0.017	0.011	0.012
Angina pectoris	0.015*	0.014*	0.012*	0.003
Sudden death	0.016	0.014	0.003	0.005

* Significant $P < 0.05$ level
(1) Bivariate = metropolitan relative weight and age
(2) Multivariate = above plus systolic blood pressure, serum cholesterol, blood glucose, ECG-LVH and cigarette smoking.

only the strength of the association of a particular factor with disease, but also its independent contribution to risk. Also, it should ideally contribute to a variety of cardiovascular outcomes. For some cardiovascular outcomes, but not all, measures of overweight qualify as a useful ingredient of such a profile (Table 3.9).

BENEFIT OF WEIGHT REDUCTION

While not all concur (Keys *et al*, 1972), insurance companies have long been persuaded that overweight not only leads to increased mortality but that weight reduction in the obese leads to a decrease in this excess mortality. The evidence seems to warrant this conclusion despite questions about reinsurance of previously obese persons.

There is at present no secure basis for precisely estimating the benefit to be derived from correcting obesity. This requires a long-term controlled clinical trial. However, a few paper and pencil estimates may provide some perspective. Judging by the effect of weight loss on atherogenic traits, we might expect a 20 per cent reduction in weight in the obese to result in a 40 per cent reduction in the chances of coronary heart disease (Table 3.10). The effect

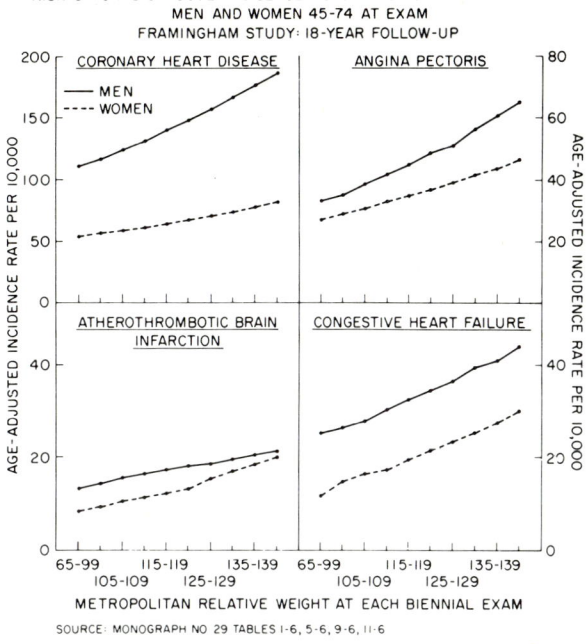

Figure 3.12
Risk of cardiovascular disease according to relative weight. Men and women aged 45-74 years at examination. Framingham study: 18 year follow-up.

should be slightly less pronounced in women and for older, rather than younger, persons. Another way to look at it is directly from an assessment of disease incidence. It is estimated that if everyone at Framingham above optimum weight were at ideal weight instead, the incidence of coronary heart disease would be about 25 per cent less and brain infarction and CHF 35 per cent lower. However it is not likely that the actual benefit realized will be this great since sustained weight reductions are hard to achieve and the methods employed are sometimes hazardous. Avoiding overweight would seem preferable to correcting it.

However, the relationship may well be a good deal more complex than such computations suggest, since the effect of the major identified risk factors on cardiovascular disease may be different in lean as compared to obese persons. To explore this, a six-variable discriminant function analysis of cardiovascular disease (age, systolic blood pressure, serum cholesterol, blood sugar, ECG-LVH, smoking) was carried out contrasting persons with relative weights under 90 and over 130 lb (Table 3.11). In lean men, systolic blood pressure

Table 3.9
T values of additional contribution of relative weight to discrimination of heart conditions by sex and age Framingham study: 16 year follow-up

	CHD*	ABI*	IC*	CHF*
MEN				
45–54	1.03	−0.34	−2.96**	1.11
55–64	2.37**	0.44	−0.52	0.74
65–74	0.46	0.46	−0.61	0.28
Average	2.46**	0.33	−2.15**	1.24
WOMEN				
45–54	0.40	2.52**	1.08	0.04
55–64	0.67	0.87	−1.01	3.80**
65–74	−0.45	0.80	−0.23	−0.64
Average	0.44	2.10**	−0.51	2.46**

* CHD = Coronary heart disease
ABI = Atherothrombotic brain infarction
IC = Intermittent claudication
CHF = Congestive heart failure

** Significant P = 0.05. In addition to relative weight the following variables are included in the linear discriminant function: systolic blood pressure, diastolic blood pressure, serum cholesterol, LVH-ECG, glucose intolerance and cigarette smoking

Table 3.10
Relative odds of coronary heart disease corresponding to a given change in relative weight
Framingham study

Change in relative weight	MEN (age in years)		WOMEN (age in years)	
	35–44	45–54	35–44	45–54
−20	0.57	0.62	0.62	0.83
−10	0.76	0.80	0.80	0.94
+10	1.38	1.31	1.31	1.20
+20	1.86	1.68	1.69	1.35

and blood sugar are significant contributors to the risk of cardiovascular disease. This is not true in obese men, suggesting that in men the type of hypertension and impaired glucose tolerance which accompanies obesity is different and unassociated with an excess cardiovascular morbidity and mortality.

In women, the effect of impaired glucose tolerance is reduced almost to half in the obese, but not to a statistically significant

Table 3.11
Discriminant coefficients for risk factors for cardiovascular disease in lean versus obese
Framingham study: 18 year follow-up

Risk Factor	Lean FRW<90	Obese FRW>130	T-value for contrast
MEN			
Age	0.0546*	0.0815*	−0.91
Systolic blood pressure	0.0340*	0.0079	2.10
Serum cholesterol	0.0025	0.0051	−0.43
Blood glucose	0.0193*	−0.0103	2.49
ECG-LVH	1.8233	2.1801	−0.15
Cigarette smoking	0.1199	0.1851	−0.30
No. of cases	70	20	
X^2 for generalized distance:	78.9	14.6	
WOMEN			
Age	0.1083*	0.0413*	2.78
Systolic blood pressure	0.0099	0.0139*	−0.46
Serum cholesterol	−0.0001	0.0092*	−2.11
Blood sugar	0.0199*	0.0122*	0.83
ECG-LVH	9.3066	2.8457*	3.28
Cigarette smoking	0.1142*	0.1185	−0.02
No. of cases	59	49	
X^2 for generalized distance:	134.5	58.0	

* $P < 0.05$
FRW = Framingham Relative Weight

degree with the numbers available. Blood pressure, however, is not innocuous in obese women. This contrast in the two sexes is puzzling.

In both sexes coefficients for serum cholesterol, ECG-LVH and smoking are as large in the obese as the lean and/or statistically significant in the obese suggesting they predispose both obese and lean persons to cardiovascular disease. In general the set of risk factors discriminates better in lean than obese persons in both sexes.

MECHANISMS

It seems clear that much of the increased risk associated with obesity is mediated through the accompanying atherogenic traits. However, in angina in men, but not in women, in brain infarction in women and in CHD there seems to be some **additional unique** effect. This may be an increased cardiac work load imposed by the obesity *per se* so that in persons with an already compromised arterial circulation to the heart and to the brain, ischaemic symptoms are more readily provoked in the obese.

The curious inverse relationship to intermittent claudication in men is paradoxical and may derive from a disinclination of obese men to exercise their lower limbs enough to elicit the symptom. However, it is curious that this does not apply to women or to angina pectoris in men. The inverse relationship of weight to overall and cardiovascular mortality may be a product of the tendency of seriously ill persons to lose weight in the terminal stages of illness.

The fact that there is a smaller net effect of obesity when its atherogenic accompaniments are taken into account does not mean that obesity is an unimportant innocent accompaniment of these more powerful contributors to cardiovascular disease. Because weight gain is associated with a worsening of atherogenic traits obesity may be one of the common causes of these promoters of cardiovascular disease. Weight reduction because it improves cardiovascular risk factors offers a potentially important means for improving cardiovascular health.

Still to be determined is the exact mechanism by which adiposity elevates blood pressure, serum lipids and uric acid and impairs glucose tolerance. The degree to which specific nutrients consumed in excess and positive energy balance *per se* is at fault remains to be established.

Also in need of further study are the determinants of obesity in the general population and the reason for the tendency for families to share the overweight problem. The role of genetics, psychosocial factors, exercise and nutrient composition of the diet need to be better elucidated.

PREVENTIVE IMPLICATIONS

Overweight is a major public health problem, contributing not only to cardiovascular disease but to other diseases such as diabetes mellitus, gout, gallbladder disease and arthritis (Kannel et al, 1969). Although this is well known, some investigators continue to doubt that obesity poses a serious threat to health and life (Keys, et al, 1972).

Conflicting reports concerning the role of obesity in cardiovascular disease contribute to the scepticism. Many investigators have been unable to support the belief that obesity is related to CHD because of inability to demonstrate that persons with recent myocardial infarction differ in weight from matched controls (Epstein, 1965; Sanders, 1959). Autopsy studies, including those in Framingham, have failed to show a striking quantitative relationship between adiposity and coronary atherosclerosis, particularly in non-hypertensives and women (Spain *et al*, 1963; Wilkins *et al*, 1959). Coronary angiographic findings also have not correlated particularly well with the degree of adiposity of patients undergoing the examination (Cramer *et al*, 1966). Life insurance data are often suspected of selective bias (Lew, 1969). A number of factors may contribute to these conflicting results. The coronary angiographic findings are usually obtained in persons with advanced disease or subjects with hyperlipidaemia (Cramer *et al*, 1966). In the Framingham data obesity is more strikingly related to sudden death and angina than to myocardial infarction. Furthermore, patients with recent myocardial infarctions tend to lose weight so that retrospective studies, including autopsies, underestimate the usual weight status. Conflicting results have also been attributed to differences in measures of obesity used. Some have found relative weight unrelated to CHD but could show an association with skinfold thickness (Paul *et al*, 1963; Sanders, 1959; Stamler *et al*, 1966). In Framingham relative weight correlated quite well with skinfold thickness, as well as skinfold thickness in one area of the body correlating with that in another area (Table 3.1). Skinfold thickness, as well as relative weight, is clearly related to the incidence of CHD (Table 3.2). It appears that however assessed, adiposity is related to coronary incidents in the general population.

There should be no lingering doubt that obesity contributes to cardiovascular morbidity and mortality. Public health measures designed to modify the life style that promotes sloth and gluttony would seem to be required to combat the general tendency for affluent populations to fatten. The chief determinants of adiposity in affluent populations require further study but it seems already clear that inactivity and overeating must play a prominent role. The use of dining as a form of entertainment and overfeeding in childhood seem to condition the adult for obesity (Salans *et al*, 1968). Effective means for preventing and treating obesity have yet to be developed.

Control of obesity in the individual prone to cardiovascular disease and in the general population would seem a legitimate enterprise for those interested in controlling the annual toll of cardiovascular mortality. Medical science would be well served by greater attention to overweight, its atherogenic metabolic effects and its haemodynamic effects on the cardiovascular apparatus. Weight control would appear to be the first method that should be employed in the correction of hypertension, hyperlipidaemia and impaired glucose tolerance of persons susceptible to cardiovascular disease. Control of overweight should improve the exercise tolerance of patients with established CHD or CHF.

REFERENCES

ASHLEY, F.W. & KANNEL, W.B. (1974) Relation of weight change to changes in atherogenic traits: The Framingham study. *J. Chron. Dis.* 27, 103.

CAMPBELL, R.G., HASHIM, S.A. & VAN ITALLIE, T.B. (1971) Studies of food intake regulation in man: responses to variations in nutritive density in lean and obese subjects. *New Eng. J. Med.*, 285, 1402.

CORNFIELD, J., GORDON, T. & SMITH, W.W. (1961) Quantal response curves for experimentally uncontrolled variables. *Bull. Int. Stat. Instit.*, 38, 97.

CRAMER, K., PAWLIN, S. & WERKO, L. (1966) Coronary angiographic findings in correlation with age, body weight, blood pressure, serum lipids and smoking habits. *Circulation*, 33, 888.

EPSTEIN, F.H. (1965) The epidemiology of coronary heart disease. A review. *J. Chron. Dis.*, 18, 735.

FISHER, R.A. (1936) The use of multiple measurements in taxonomic problems. *Ann. Eug. London*, 7, 179.

GORDON, T. & KANNEL, W.B. (1973) The effects of overweight on cardiovascular disease. *Geriatrics*, 28, 80.

HEALD, F., MULLER, P. & DANGELA, M. (1965) Glucose and free fatty acid metabolism in obese adolescents. *Am. J. Clin. Nutr.*, 16, 256.

KANNEL, W.B. & GORDON, T. (1968) The Framingham study, sections 1 and 2, Washington, D.C.

KANNEL, W.B., PEARSON, G. & McNAMARA, P.M. (1969) Obesity as a force of morbidity and mortality. In *Adolescent Nutritional Growth* p.57, Ed. Heald, F.P. New York: Appleton-Century-Crofts.

KEYS, A., ARAVANIS, C., BLACKBURN, H., VAN BUCKEM, F.S.P., BUSINA, R., DJORDEVIC, B.S., FINDANZA, F.F., KARVONEN, M.J., MENOTTI, A., PUDDU, V. & TAYLOR, H.L. (1972) Coronary heart disease: overweight and obesity as risk factors. *Ann. Int. Med.*, 77, 15.

LEW, E.A. (1948) Mortality statistics for life insurance underwriting. *JASA.*, 43, 274.

LEW, E.A. (1969) Importance of overweight in life insurance. *11th International Congress of COINTRA*, 277.

National Health Survey (Nation Center for Health Statistics) (1964) Blood pressure of adults by age and sex, United States, 1960-1962. PHS No. 1000, Series 11, No. 4, June.

National Health Survey (National Center for Health Statistics) (1964) Blood height and selected body dimensions, United States, 1960-1962. PHS No. 1000, Series 11, No. 8, June.

National Health Survey (National Center for Health Statistics) (1967) Serum cholesterol levels of adults, United States, 1960-1962. PHS No. 100, Series 11, No. 22, March.

National Health Survey (National Center for Health Statistics) (1970) Changes in cigarette smoking habits between 1955 and 1966. PHS No. 1000, Series 10, No. 59, April.

PAUL, O., LEPPER, M.H., PHELAN, W.H., DUPERTIUS, G.W., McMILLAN, A., McKEAN, H. & PARK, H. (1963) Longitudinal study of coronary heart disease. *Circulation*, **28**, 20.

SALANS, L.B., KNITTLE, J.L. & HIRSCH, J. (1968) The role of adipose size and adipose tissue insulin sensitivity in the carbohydrate intolerance of human obesity. *J. Clin. Invest.*, **47**, 153.

SANDERS, K. (1959) Coronary artery disease and obesity. *Lancet*, **2**, 432.

SELTZER, C.C. (1969) Overweight and obesity. The associated cardiovascular risk. *Minn. Med.*, **52**, 1265.

SHURTLEFF, D. (1970) Some characteristics related to incidence of cardiovascular disease and death. In *The Framingham Study*, Ed. Kannel, W.B. & Gordon, T. Section 26, Washington, D.C.

SHURTLEFF, D. (1974) Some characteristics related to incidence of cardiovascular disease and death. Framingham Study 18 year follow up. In *Framingham Study of Cardiovascular Disease* Section 30. DHEW Public. (NIH). 74.

SPAIN, D.M., NATHAN, D.J. & GELLIS, M. (1963) Weight, body type and the prevalence of coronary atherosclerotic heart disease in males. *Amer. J. Med. Sci.*, **245**, 63.

STAMLER, J., BERKSON, D.M. & LINDBERG, H.A. (1966) Coronary risk factors. *Med. Clin. N. Amer.*, **50**, 229.

WALKER, S.H. & DUNCAN, D.B. (1967) Estimation of the probability of an event as a function of several independent variables. *Biometrika*, **54**, 167.

WILKINS, R.H., ROBERTS, J.C.Jr., & MOSES, C. (1959) Autopsy studies in atherosclerosis III. distribution and severity of atherosclerosis in the presence of obesity, hypertension, nephrosclerosis, rheumatic heart disease. *Circulation*, **20**, 527.

4. Prevalence of Obesity in London: Obesity as a Risk Factor in Coronary Heart Disease

I. M. BAIRD

There is increasing evidence that obesity is common in infancy due to overnutrition in the first three months of life (Shukla *et al*, 1972). Knittle (1971) suggested that excess numbers of fat cells were one main cause of adult obesity. Brook *et al* (1972) found all obese individuals had an increase in the size of their fat cells, but only those who had gained weight excessively in the first year of life had an increased number of fat cells. It is possible that the post-war child, maturing earlier and being taller and heavier than the pre-war equivalent (Tanner *et al*, 1966), may show an increased trend towards early adult obesity due to an increased number of fat cells.

It is of importance to find out the prevalence of adult obesity within the United Kingdom at the present time, to correlate the incidence of obesity with age and social categories and to examine traditional views that coronary heart disease is related to obesity.

Scanty data are available about the heights and weights of the adult population in the United Kingdom. The tables commonly used in Britain are those constructed by the Society of Actuaries referring to 160,000 men and 30,000 women insured at standard risks by 11 American Life Assurance Companies from 1935 to 1954. Although helpful because of the large sample involved, the tables are heavily biased in favour of the higher socio-economic groups and refer predominantly to males.

Kemsley made a war-time study of the civil British population in 1943 (Kemsley, 1952), but since then only occasional surveys have been made available. Khosla & Lowe (1968) found heights and weights in an industrial population had increased since 1943. Montegriffo (1968) and Silverstone (1968) also found a high prevalence of adult obesity, although such samples may not be representative of other populations or areas. The Richmond study reported here was made in order to examine a random sample of height and weight data in a geographically defined population, and as a comparison made with previous United Kingdom studies. The prevalence of obesity can be determined within this population with special reference to age, sex and social status. The details of the methods used in the survey are given elsewhere (Baird *et al*, 1974). Richmond is in the South West of Greater London and has a population of about 174,000 of which 47 per cent are male and 53 per cent are female, a sex ratio close to the national figure.

Persons covered by the study were aged 16 to 64 years. Richmond contained a higher proportion of professional workers, employers and managers (26 per cent) than the national average of 15 per cent at the 1966 census. A random selection of three in 10 general medical practitioners and one in 10 of their patients provided the sample. All the subjects were written to and individually weighed at their doctors' surgery, with a Weylux model 400 weighing machine

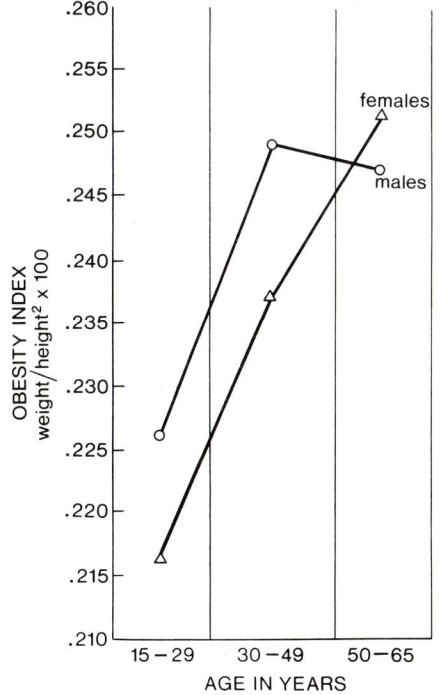

Figure 4.1
The rise in obesity index with age in males and females (Baird, I. McLean *et al.*, 1974).

accurate to the nearest 50 g. Height was also measured at the surgery to the nearest centimetre with a Weylux aluminium measure. Those who did not attend were visited in their homes.

There were 1334 persons in the sample, comprising a 1 per cent random sample of the Richmond population, 794 women and 540 men. There was a normal distribution of weights in both males and females. The prevalence of obesity as measured by the obesity index I_2 (weight in kg divided by the square of the height in cm multiplied by 100) showed a progressive rise with age in females (Figure 4.1) and a rise in males between the 15—29 year group and 30—49 year group, although the obesity index fell slightly in the older age group.

These results are very similar to those of the survey by Khosla & Lowe (1968) and indicate that young and middle aged men are both heavier and taller than men of the same age 30 years ago. Females in the lower social classes D and E have much higher average weights and higher obesity indices than females in social classes A and B (Table 4.1). There is no such trend in males and the I_2 is relatively constant (Table 4.2). The fall of I_2 is due to the fact that social class is positively correlated with height.

Table 4.1
The number (and percentage) in each weight group according to social class
(females)

	SOCIAL CLASS		
	A & B	C_1 & C_2	D & E
Underweight	12 (9.7)	81 (17.2)	16 (10.3)
Normal or <20% overweight	92 (74.3)	306 (65.0)	84 (54.2)
Obese, >20% overweight	19 (15.5)	84 (17.8)	55 (35.5)
Obesity Index (I_2)	0.233	0.235	0.253

Table 4.2

The number (and percentage) in each weight group according to social class.
(males)

	SOCIAL CLASS		
	A & B	C_1 & C_2	D & E
Underweight	7 (7.6)	40 (12.0)	16 (18.3)
Normal or <20% overweight	75 (80.5)	239 (71.8)	55 (63.2)
Obese, > 20% overweight	11 (11.9)	54 (16.2)	16 (18.4)
Obesity Index (I_2)	0.245	0.244	0.241

The Richmond study confirms the post-war phenomenon that with more generous dietary standards children are maturing into taller and heavier adults. The high incidence of 35.5 per cent of obesity in the females in social classes D and E gives rise to concern. This is much higher than the 15.5 per cent in classes A and B. Social pressure to stay lean may be stronger in the higher socio-economic groups and faulty eating habits the cause in the lower social classes. It may also reflect faulty early infant feeding patterns. Whatever the cause, the results indicate that these social groups predisposed to obesity need dietary education. Further surveys are now required to determine whether the trend towards obesity is uniform in most areas in Britain or whether some areas have a different pattern of obesity.

RELATIONSHIPS TO CORONARY HEART DISEASE (CHD)

Obesity is one well recognized risk factor for CHD. The Framingham study has shown an association between sudden death (probably a fatal cardiac arrhythmia), angina and obesity. However, the evidence of obesity being related to diagnosed myocardial infarction is less clear. Most physicians looking after coronary care units are not impressed by any high incidence of obesity in their patients admitted with myocardial infarction. Sanders (1959) explained this anomaly by finding a significant increase in body fat, although body weights were similar, when compared with control patients matched for age and sex admitted for other causes.

Keys (1972) using multivariate analysis of data from several countries found that no measure of relative weight or obesity made any significant contribution to future CHD when the factors of age, blood pressure, serum cholesterol and smoking were comparable. The prevalence of obesity rises steeply with age, as does the incidence of CHD, and it is possible that a classification of obesity using 'desirable weight' falsely attributes to obesity an arteriosclerotic process which is due to age alone. Other risk factors may also operate, such as vigorous exercise in leisure time (Morris et al, 1973) which is likely to be less in the obese group.

Females aged 45 to 60 years show a greater rise of CHD compared with females aged 15 to 45, correlating well with a rise in obesity index from 0.216 to 0.251 between the ages of 50 and 65 years, but changing hormonal factors are also a variable here.

Whether the incidence of CHD can be reduced by weight loss in obese subjects is difficult to determine. Christakis (1966) put subjects on a low fat diet, but a reduced serum cholesterol, increased exercise and reduced smoking may well have contributed to the reduced incidence of the new coronary episodes recorded in his group. The role of primary prevention of CHD in obese subjects by weight reduction and increased exercise needs clarifying by a longitudinal 'Framingham type' study in middle aged sedentary males and post-menopausal females. The difficulties in this type of epidemiological study are considerable.

After a myocardial infarction has occurred there are often compelling clinical reasons to lose weight quite apart from any theoretical secondary prevention of a further infarct. Increased exercise leads to improved peripheral blood distribution and return (Fisher *et al*, 1971; Helfant *et al*, 1971), and enzymatic adaptations may permit better work performance (Fisher *et al*, 1971). Angina pectoris is notably improved after weight reduction and therefore it is essential that obese patients be encouraged to lose weight after convalescing from myocardial infarction, as the quality of their life is certainly improved.

REFERENCES

BAIRD, I.M., SILVERSTONE, J.T., GRIMSHAW, J.J. & ASHWELL, M. (1974) Prevalence of Obesity in a London Borough. *Practitioner* 212, 706.

BROOK, C.G.D., LLOYD, J.K. & WOLF, O.H. (1972) Relation Between Age of Onset of Obesity and Size and Number of Adipose Cells. *Brit. Med. J.* 1, 25.

CHRISTAKIS, G., RINZLER, S.H., ARCHER, M., WINSLOW, G., JAMPEL, S. STEPHENSON, J., FRIEDMAN, G., FEIN, H., KRAUS, A. & JAMES, G. (1966) A Dietary Approach to the Prevention of Coronary Heart Disease—a Seven Year Report. *American J. Publ. Hlth*, 56, 299.

FISHER, M., NUTTER, D. SCHLANT, R. (1971) Hemodynamic Evaluation of Isometric Exercise Testing in Cardiac Patients. *Abstract, Circulation*, 44, (Supp. 11), 50.

HELFANT, R.H., DE VILLA, M.A. & MEISTER, S.G. (1971). Effect of Sustained Isometric Handgrip Exercise on Left Ventricular Performance. *Circulation*, 44, 982-993.

KEMSLEY, W.F.F. (1952) Body Weight at Different Ages and Heights. *Ann Eug.* 16, 316.

KEYS, A., ARAVANIS, C., BLACKBURN, H., VAN BUCKEM, F.S.P., BUSINA, R., DJORDEVIC, B.S., FINDANZA, F.F., KARVONEN, M.J., MENOTTI, A., PUDDU, V. & TAYLOR, H.L. (1972) Coronary Heart Disease; Overweight and Obesity as Risk Factors. *Ann. Int. Med.*, 77, 15.

KHOSLA, T. & LOWE, C.R. (1968) Height and Weight of British Men. *Lancet*, 1, 742.

KNITTLE, J.L. (1971) Childhood Obesity. *Bull. N.Y. Acad. Med.*, 47, 579.

MONTEGRIFFO, V.M.E. (1968) Height and Weight of a United Kingdom Adult Population with a Review of the Anthropometric Literature. *Ann. Hum. Gen., London*, 31, 389.

MORRIS, J.N., CHAVE, S.P.W., ADAM, C., SIREY, C., EPSTEIN, L. &

SHEEHAN, D.J. (1973) Vigorous Exercise in Leisure-Time and the Incidence of Coronary Heart Disease. *Lancet*, 1, *333.*

SANDERS, K. (1959) Coronary-Artery Disease and Obesity. *Lancet*, 2, 432.

SHUKLA, A., FORSYTH, H.A., ANDERSON, C.M. & Marwah, S.M. (1972) Infantile Over-nutrition in the First Year of Life: A Field Study in Dudley, Worcestershire. *Brit. Med. J.,* 4, 507.

SILVERSTONE, J.T. (1968). Psychosocial aspects of obesity. *Proc. Roy. Soc. Med.*, 61, 371.

TANNER, J.M., WHITEHOUSE, R.H. & TAKAISHI, M. (1966) Standards from birth to maturity for height, weight, height velocity and weight velocity: British children 1965. *Arch. Dis. Childh.*, 41, 454 & 613.

DISCUSSION

Dr. Bray. May I challenge Dr. Kannel to put into perspective the data about the importance of obesity as a risk factor? Dr. Keys and others have discussed the relationship and importance of obesity as a risk factor in coronary artery disease and from their data I am not sure that it is a risk factor at all. This is an area in which there is considerable difference of opinion.

Dr. Kannel. This is a logical, semantic issue rather than a substantive scientific one. I think what Dr. Keys is saying is that if a population is examined and its weight characteristics determined in general it will be found that the incidence of cardiovascular disease rises in proportion to the weight: that fat people do indeed develop more disease than lean people. He further states that if other risk factors contributing to the cardiovascular disease are taken into consideration, the effect of overweight is lost. Until this step everything is correct, but the next step which he takes is a logical fallacy I think. He says, therefore, that obesity is unimportant. If it can be shown, as it has been in the general population and in the metabolic ward, that as people gain weight so their blood lipids rise and their glucose tolerance becomes impaired, their blood pressure increases and their uric acid concentration rises these factors in turn promoting cardiovascular disease, then what Keys has shown is that he has identified precisely how obesity works to promote cardiovascular disease by promoting atherogenic traits. So to conclude that obesity is unimportant is incorrect. But it is true to say that if the blood pressure, the cholesterol and the glucose tolerance are known, then it does not help to also know that the patient is fat.

Professor Wynn. With regard to Dr. Kannel's remarks concerning obesity and atherogenesis, we want to know whether obesity *per se* causes an increased tendency to atherogenesis and heart disease. There are obese individuals who do not have metabolic abnormalities. Evidence would suggest that there is no definite increase in atherogenic heart disease in these people. In obese individuals the lipid patterns, insulin secretion and often glucose tolerance can be normalized without removing the obesity altogether. If an individual who is substantially overweight has a relatively small decrease in weight—achieved in particular by carbohydrate restriction—there are substantial changes in lipids, glucose and insulin levels. In my experience it is probably better to consider certain obese individuals who do not have hypertension or hyperlipidaemia or even abnormal glucose tolerance, and ask them whether they really want to slim. In metabolic terms weight loss may be irrelevant for some patients.

Professor Yudkin. All this is equally true for other single factors. Just as there are some people who are obese who do not develop coronary disease, there are some with high circulating cholesterol who do not develop coronary disease. My inclination is to agree with Dr. Kannel that here we have a semantic argument; if a man is fat he is more likely to have a coronary event. Whether it is through disturbances which accompany—not necessarily caused by—the overweight, is less important in the prevention of coronary disease.

Professor Keen. I should like to challenge Professor Wynn. He proposes that an obese individual without hypertension, hyperlipidaemia, hyperglycaemia or hyperinsulinaemia—I suppose there are a few such individuals—should be asked whether he is absolutely certain he wants to lose weight. Would he go further and say that, if he found an obese person with hypertension he would only treat the hypertension and not concern himself with the obesity? Would he try to lower the blood cholesterol, or to improve glucose tolerance also without bothering about the obesity if these were raised? After all, these are the true risk factors; why worry about the obesity which is not one, at least in this sense? I do suggest that treating the obesity is an easy way of treating several of these other problems.

Dr. Lewis. Could Professor Keen comment on the suggestion that diabetes mellitus is a risk factor for sudden death, as opposed to ischaemic heart disease in general?

Professor Keen. Dr. Lewis refers to Dr. Epstein's data and to those published by Ostrander which indeed suggest that sudden death is more common amongst diabetics, as a proportion of total cardiovascular mortality and morbidity. There are many good clinical studies which suggest that if a diabetic has a coronary occlusion he is more likely to die from it than the non-diabetic is. In others, however, including the Bedford study, all manifestations of coronary disease have been shown to be increased in the diabetic, including electrocardiographic changes in the absence of any clinical manifestations. There are various provocative tests, such as exercise, which have been applied to diabetic and non-diabetic populations, which also suggest that coronary occlusive disease, short of a clinical episode, is more commonly found in diabetics than in non-diabetics. Ostrander showed also that cerebrovascular disease was more common in the most hyperglycaemic quintile of the population, which lends confirmation to the view that it is not merely an electrical phenomenon which is involving the most hyperglycaemic group, but also either an actual change in the myocardium, or a change in the coagulability of the blood.

5. Obesity in the African
Socio-Medical and Therapeutic Considerations

B. K. ADADEVOH

Obesity in the African seems to have received very little attention although it is common knowledge that market women in West Africa are fat (Figure 5.1). Medical literature on the subject is scanty and in discussing nutrition and its problems in Africa, textbooks concentrate on undernutrition particularly in children. Documented medical history for all areas in Africa make no reference to obesity. Conferences on nutritional problems have also dealt exclusively with malnutrition, undernutrition and child feeding. This bias reflects the overall nutritional problems of developing countries where the majority of the population is under 15 years of age and *per capita* income is low. However, urbanization and socio-economic awareness are currently causing a change in the food availability and food habits of many inhabitants. In most the result is improved nutrition with the attendant risk of overnutrition and its associated diseases (Adadevoh, 1972). In this changing society, decreased utilization of energy also occurs particularly in the higher income group and since corpulence is accepted as a symbol of prosperity and abundance the incidence of obesity increases (Olupitan & Adadevoh, 1967).

Haddock (1969) concluded that obesity is not a negligible medical problem and that serious obesity is an appreciable problem in women in Accra Ghana. Owusu (1971) reviewing diabetes mellitus in Accra observed that over a five-year period a significant increase in the number of obese diabetic patients had occurred, both male and female. This may be a reflection of a raised standard of living. Mngola & Alouch (1973) have similarly observed that obesity is becoming a problem in East Africa where the majority, as in other areas of Africa, live on a high carbohydrate diet. Also the popular news media in Africa have recently published articles in their columns on obesity and disease, and the need to lose extra fat (Figure 5.2). The importance of obesity in association with, or in the

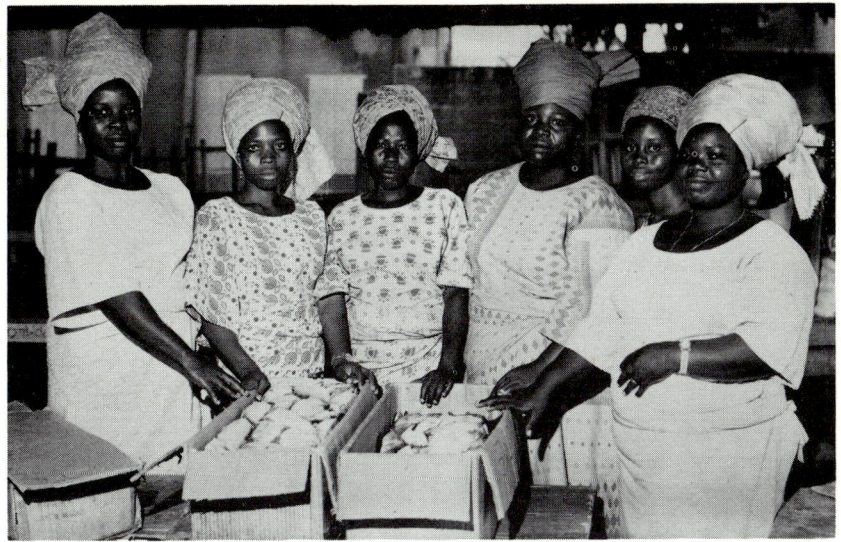

Figure 5.1
Women traders in a fish market in Dugbe Ibadan

genesis of, a number of diseases has likewise been recently emphasized in medical writings. These include diabetes mellitus, hypertension, osteoarthritis and gout (Bolodeoku *et al,* 1972; Fleishmann & Adadevoh, 1973; Haddock *et al,* 1972; Johnson, 1969; Osuntokun *et al,* 1971; Owusu, 1971; Seftel, 1961).

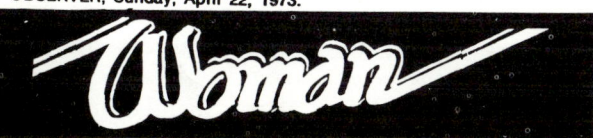

Figure 5.2
Abstract from Nigerian newspaper—woman's column

DIETARY HABITS

Although dietary habits vary widely amongst the African countries, tribes and villages, it is generally established that the African diet is rich in carbohydrates. Calorie intake for the most is low and protein falls short of the recommended allowance. In addition, the deficiency of calories and protein is more for the rural areas than for the urban areas (East African Conference on Nutrition and Child Feeding, 1969; West African Conference on Nutrition and Child Feeding, 1968). While nutrition surveys have revealed similar low calorie and protein intakes in Nigeria (Republic of Nigeria Nutrition Survey, 1967), they have also shown a wide variation in dietary habit and food intake because of agricultural resources and cultural differences (Adadevoh, 1972) (Tables 5.1 and 5.2).

Table 5.1
Average daily intake of calorie and protein
in different areas of Nigeria

Areas	Calories	Protein (g)
NORTH	1,778	43.7
WESTERN STATE	1,613	41.7
MID-WEST	1,545	49.2
EAST CENTRAL	2,470	66.8
SOUTH-EAST	2,111	58.0

(from Olusanya & Omololu, 1972)

The complex of traditional beliefs, attitudes and prejudices seen amongst Africans in the selection and use of foods, contributes to the imbalance in their diet. This affects mainly children and women, particularly during pregnancy and lactation, and contributes to the retardation in development seen amongst Africans (Adadevoh, 1972; Dovlo, 1972). The pregnant woman is discouraged from consuming oil or fatty foods for fear this might result in large babies and therefore difficult birth. These foods are however liberally allowed during lactation. Indeed, for most lactating mothers restrictions imposed during pregnancy are replaced by a relative over indulgence to promote adequate breast milk (Dovlo, 1972). In contrast, the adult African male is normally served with the best meals in terms of both quality and quantity.

In women, obesity seems to appear most frequently after the first child. Little alteration in weight occurs after the age of 25 years in

Table 5.2

The average daily percentage of calorie (and protein) contributed by the specific food groups in different areas of Nigeria

Food Groups	North	Western State	Mid-West	East-Central	South-East
CEREALS	54.4 (64.1)	20.6 (19.7)	11.0 (8.1)	5.3 (4.8)	5.2 (4.0)
STARCHY ROOTS	7.8 (5.0)	42.9 (9.1)	38.4 (17.7)	41.6 (15.3)	48.1 (11.0)
LEGUMES, NUTS AND SEEDS	1.9 (4.4)	11.4 (25.9)	11.5 (16.3)	28.9 (41.5)	21.3 (24.4)
VEGETABLES AND FRUITS	3.6 (4.4)	3.3 (4.6)	2.1 (1.8)	2.5 (5.7)	3.3 (4.1)
MEAT PRODUCTS	3.3 (10.5)	4.1 (14.6)	2.7 (7.1)	3.0 (13.6)	4.0 (20.7)
FISH PRODUCTS	— (—)	4.3 (24.5)	12.7 (49.0)	3.9 (18.2)	7.4 (35.8)
OILS AND FATS	10.9 (—)	11.4 (—)	21.6 (—)	12.0 (—)	10.0 (—)
BEVERAGES AND DRINKS	6.2 (0.2)	0.6 (0.2)	— (—)	2.7 (0.9)	0.7 (—)
COW'S MILK (NONO)	5.6 (11.4)	0.7 (1.4)	— (—)	— (—)	— (—)
SUGAR-CUBE	6.3 (—)	0.7 (—)	— (—)	0.1 (—)	— (—)

(Adapted from Olusanya & Omololu, 1972)

either men or women (Republic of Nigeria Nutrition Survey, 1967). Thus obesity may be expected to occur less frequently with age than in non-Africans

PHYSIQUE—HEIGHTS AND WEIGHTS

There are no generally accepted standards with which the physique of the African can be judged. Thus, the definition of obesity presents the usual problems of determining acceptable minimum anthropometric standards which distinguish between the normal and the obese (Butterfield, 1969; Editorial South African Medical Journal, 1969; U.S. Department of Health, 1966).

The African child has a relatively low birth weight but by six months most have attained body weights found in non-Africans. By the age of two years, however, a deficit in weight occurs which may be two kg or more (West African Conference on Nutrition and Child Feeding, 1968). The return to normal heights and weights found elsewhere at about four years of age is not generally observed. In the urban areas the degree of retardation in physique is less than in the rural areas (Figures 5.3 and 5.4). Between the ages of 15 and 22 years an increase in body weight occurs in the Nigerian averaging about 12.5 kg in males and 6.0 kg in females. Between the ages of 22 and 25 little change in weight occurs except that in a number of females post-partum obesity is seen. These changes are reflected in

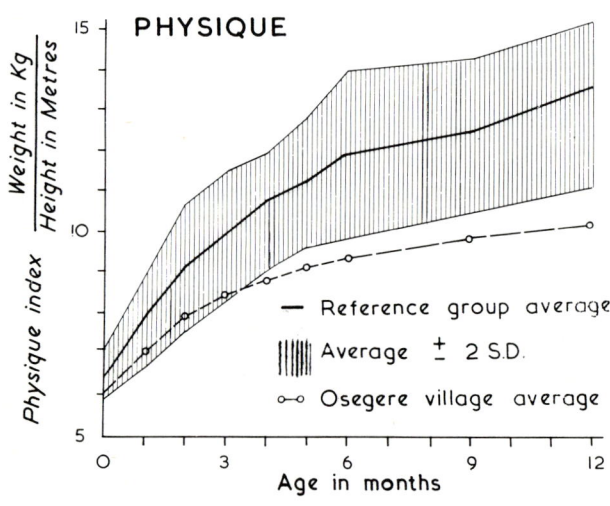

Figure 5.3
Physique—Nigerian children under one year. Reference group (urban), Osegere village (rural).

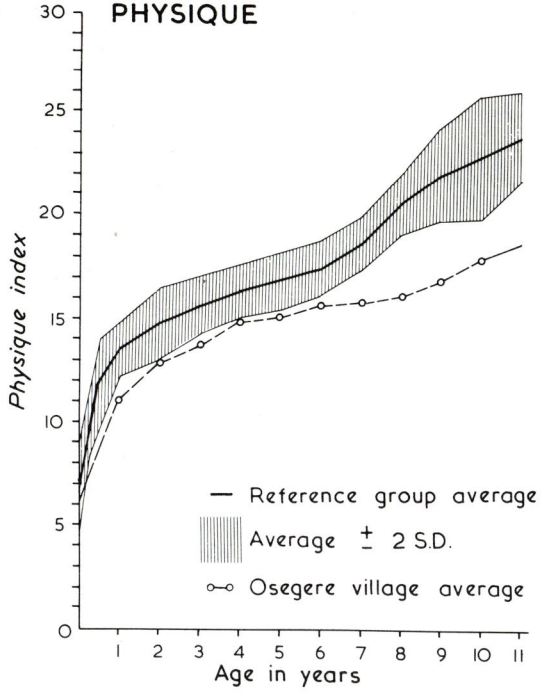

Figure 5.4
Physique—Nigerian children under 11 years. Reference group (urban), Osegere village (rural).

the skinfold measurements. Whilst in males a gradual increase occurs up the age of 45, in females a sharp increase occurs with a peak between 25 and 34 years and a decline after the age of 35—45 years. Skinfold measurements in females are on the average 1.3 to 2.0 times greater than those in males between the ages of five and 45 years (Adadevoh, personal observation; Republic of Nigeria Nutrition Survey, 1967). The relative obesity seen in the African female constitutes an acceptable symbol of beauty in most areas except perhaps the Masai tribe of East Africa. Indeed, amongst a number of tribes, premarital fattening in special 'fattening homes' is common practice since the bride must be presented showing not only evidence of a good level of nutritional care by her family but also fatness as a symbol of beauty. In some Central African tribes and possibly elsewhere, the accumulation of fat around the buttocks (steatopygia) at particular periods of life in the female is practised, coinciding with pubescent rites and the preparations for marriage. The method employed is not however stated (de Rachewiltz, 1964).

Heights and weights of some adult African groups have been

recorded for ages ranging from 20 to 40 years. Table 5.3 summarizes the findings which are difficult to compare in view of the wide differences in the methodology, and the dates of each study which do not allow for possible significant socio-economic changes in the interval. However, the data suggest that Africans have a lesser physique than non-Africans and point to the need for standard anthropometric indices for defining normal physique. Amongst the Zulus for example the relative overweight observed is due to excessive fat (Slome *et al*, 1960). Triceps skinfold thickness ranging from 9.4–11.5 mm in Zulu males aged 20–50 years and 21.6–22.1 mm in Zulu females compare with 6–8 and 9–14 mm in Nigerian males and females (Adadevoh, unpublished observation; Republic of Nigeria Nutrition Survey, 1967). In a group of 240 African labourers in Natal, Abramson & Gampel (1960) found 30.9 per cent with triceps skinfold thickness of under 5.0 mm. These figures indicate the extreme leaness of the average African when judged against the minimum triceps skinfold thickness of 16–23 mm in males and 28–30 mm in females, and the figure of 25 mm for subscapular skinfold in European males (Butterfield, 1969).

Table 5.3
Mean heights and weights of African adults

Study			Height (cm) M	F	Weight (kg) M	F
Orr & Gilks	(1931)	Kikuyu	164	152	51	44
		Masai	172	158	60	54
McGregor & Smith	(1952)	Gambians	167	158	55	52
Coles	(1957)	Ugandians	167	155	57	56
Moore & Roberts	(1957)	Tanzanians	163	152	54	47
Slome *et al*	(1960)	Zulus	166	156	70	71
Johnson	(1970)	Nigerians	168	158	60	58

PHYSIQUE–BIOCHEMICAL CORRELATES

While there have been conflicting reports on the association of physique with certain biochemical values, for example serum lipids and urinary steroids, information amongst Africans is generally lacking. Cholesterol concentrations have been widely reported to be low in the African. In respect to carbohydrate metabolism, diabetes mellitus and insulin concentrations, the picture is not entirely clear. Whilst the African female is invariably more obese than the male, diabetes mellitus appears to occur more frequently in males

Table 5.4
Matrix of simple correlation coefficients

	Age	Ponderax Index	Serum Cholesterol	Plasma Uric Acid
Age				
Ponderal Index	−0.0741			−0.1710**
Serum Cholesterol	0.0714	−0.1636*		
Diastolic Blood Pressure	0.0678	−0.0747	0.8944***	
Systolic Blood Pressure			0.0731	

Height 169.3 ± 0.33 cm;   Weight 60.8 ± 0.34 kg (Mean ± SEM)

* $p < 0.05$
** $p < 0.01$
*** $p < 0.001$

(Adadevoh, 1970; Adadevoh & Lukanmbi, 1972; Taylor, 1971).

Taylor (1971) studied three groups of 743 subjects from amongst low income and high income Nigerians and male Europeans resident in Nigeria. Amongst the Nigerians, mean cholesterol and phospholipid concentrations in males and females appeared to increase significantly after the age of 15 years. Thereafter, values for females were significantly higher than those for males. Triglyceride concentrations were however higher in the males, while no difference was observed in the mean cholesterol esters. In the high income Nigerians, total cholesterol, cholesterol esters and phospholipids were similar to those for the European group but significantly higher than in the low income Nigerians. Triglyceride was similar in both Nigerian groups and significantly higher for the European group. Fatty acid patterns also showed certain differences. It appears that socio-economic factors, leading to diets high in energy, protein and fat and to decreased energy requirements, may account for the differences in lipid pattern amongst the Nigerians.

Fleischmann & Adadevoh (1973) found no consistent correlation between uric acid concentrations, ponderal index, weight and height in 114 Nigerian villagers. However in males of 41 years and above, the mean blood uric acid significantly correlated with weight and height. Similarly in a study of biochemical parameters in 242 Nigerian soldiers aged 18—49 years (mean 24.6), significant correlations were found between ponderal index, cholesterol and uric acid (Table 5.4).

The importance of these observations in terms of the prevalence of disease, particularly those diseases associated with obesity, cannot at this stage be properly assessed in the absence of reports from most other African areas. However, it is noteworthy that several of these diseases, e.g. gout, atherosclerosis and cardiovascular dysfunctions and diabetes mellitus, still show a low prevalence according to clinical records.

PATTERN OF OBESITY

The increasing prevalence of obesity in adults has been reported (Haddock, 1969; Haddock et al, 1972; Mngola and Alouch, 1973; Olupitan & Adadevoh, 1967; Owusu, 1971) (Table 5.5). In these reports, the diagnosis of obesity was based essentially on general observation, height and weight, suggesting that these were obvious cases of simple obesity. Marginal obesity and particularly obesity in childhood seem to have received no attention even though it is recognized in Europe and America that childhood obesity forms an important reservoir for obesity in adults (Anderson, 1972; U.S. Department of Health, Education and Welfare, 1966). The assessment of the amount of fat in the African as an index of obesity has however been made difficult by the absence of acceptable anthropo-

Table 5.5
Mean weights (and range) of obese African subjects

STUDY			Weight (kg) M	F
Olupitan & Adadevoh	(1967)	Lagos	85.2 (70.9—102.3)	88.1 (63.2—116.3)
Bolodeoku, Adadevoh & Palmer	(1972)	Ibadan	87.9 (71.0—102.4)	87.4 (68.3—152.9)
Mngola & Aluoh	(1973)	Nairobi	91.3* (66.5—103)	

* males and females together

metric indices based on known patterns in the normal population.

The African physique varies somewhat amongst the different groups, but obesity in the buttocks is fairly common particularly in the female. Indeed, in her it is recognized as a symbol of beauty (de Rachewiltz, 1964). Also, skinfold thickness measurements suggest that fat distribution in the obese shows an increased preference for the suprailiac and abdominal areas. Whilst in normal Nigerian adults subscapular skinfold and, to a lesser extent, triceps skinfold show correlation with body weight, in obesity this correlation occurs more with triceps and suprailiac skinfolds (Adadevoh, unpublished data; Bolodeoku & Adadevoh, 1974). In Nigerian obese subjects, mean skinfold thicknesses were 3.12 cm (range 1.9—4.84) suprailiac; 4.07 cm (range 1.20—5.56) triceps; 3.86 cm (range 1.50—5.50) infra-scapular (Bolodeoku & Adadevoh, 1974).

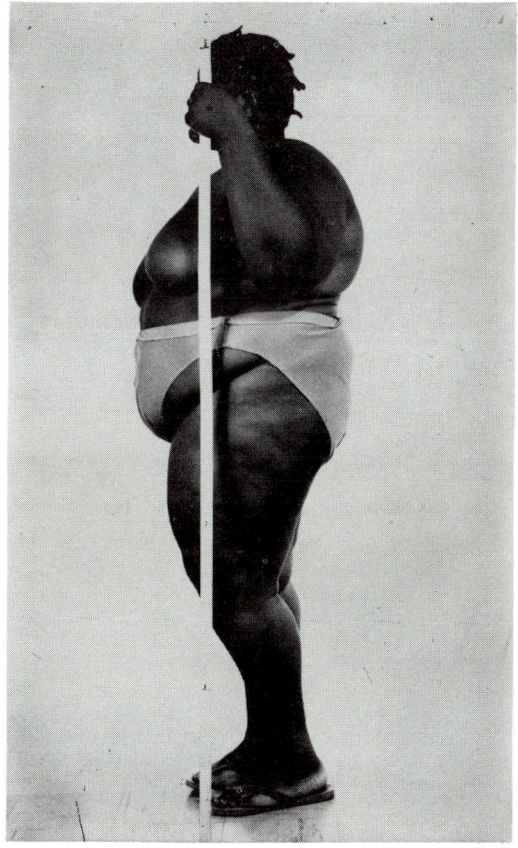

Figure 5.5
Obese Nigerian child aged 11 years.

Childhood obesity is encountered infrequently. Figure 5.5 shows the most obese, of a total of twelve obese children, studied over the last eight years. In all, obesity was due to overeating. The incidence in the population is not reflected by these medical referrals, all of whom were markedly obese. Marginal obesity particularly in adolescents seems acceptable socio-culturally and traditionally but notwithstanding this its prevalence is far less than among Europeans and Americans.

The concept in Europe and America that childhood or adolescent obesity forms a major reservoir for adult obesity is seemingly not the case for Africans. Malnutrition in childhood and retarded growth occur widely. On attaining adulthood, the apparently sudden economic emancipation provides for some an increased intake of energy, fat and protein. More study needs to be made on the effect of these changes on energy and carbohydrate metabolism, on endocrine secretion and patterns of disease.

TREATMENT

Only a few studies are available on the treatment of obesity in the African. Haddock (1969) reported that attempts at weight reduction in Accra were largely unsuccessful and that more was required than dietetic advice, exhortation and outpatient supervision. Mngola & Alouch (1973) stated similarly that in Nairobi a reduction in calorie intake is always difficult as the majority of their population find it difficult to follow a standardized dietary regimen. Owusu (1971) has however reported satisfactory control of all male Accra diabetics treated with diet alone.

In a combined physician-dietitian therapeutic regime, Olupitan and Adadevoh (1967) reported significant weight loss in Nigerian obese subjects on a low calorie diet. The importance of the low calorie diet being based on a number of local staple foods and the rations allowed being described in terms of models and their equivalent monetary value as purchased in the food stalls and markets in towns, were stressed. Improvement in the patients' health on weight reduction encourages him to continue. However 25 per cent of patients defaulted and these were mostly men.

Recently, the effectiveness of treatment with fenfluramine in obese Nigerians and Kenyans has been reported (Bolodeoku *et al*, 1972; Mngola & Alouch, 1973). In both studies satisfactory results were obtained without any restriction of food intake. Experience with other appetite suppressant drugs has not been reported even though their sporadic use, particularly in the cities, is recognized.

Long-term studies elsewhere of the effect of dietary therapy for obesity have often revealed disappointing results. These studies are essentially lacking in the African. Our subjects who have maintained a reduction in weight for many years following therapeutic dietary restriction have invariably been those with diabetes, hypertension and amenorrhoea. The motivation appears to be the improvement in health associated with the weight reduction.

CONCLUSIONS

There are many gaps in the definition and understanding of the pattern of obesity in the African. A host of socio-cultural, economic and nutritional factors which influence the physique of the African also tend to influence the development of obesity and diseases associated with it. The apparent low prevalence of obesity may be contributed to by the absence of appropriate standards of anthropometric indices based on studies in defined 'normal' or 'reference' groups. There is a need for detailed studies in most areas which will include biochemical correlates and the influence of obesity or body functions which is seen mainly in adulthood.

Acknowledgements

I am particularly grateful to Dr. J.F. Harries, Nairobi, for some literature from East Africa; Mrs. E.O. Olusanya and the WACMR (Nigeria) for permission to use data included in Tables 5.1 and 5.2; and the Medical Illustration Unit, University of Ibadan for the figures. Figures 5.3 and 5.4 are from a study undertaken in the Department of Chemical Pathology, University of Ibadan in 1965 and from which the Republic of Nigeria Nutrition Survey 1967 derived.

REFERENCES

ABRAMSON, J.H. & GAMPEL, B. (1960) Observations on the nutritional status of low-paid African labourers in Natal. *S. Afr. Med. J.*, 34, 1050.

ADADEVOH, B.K. (1970) Endocrine patterns in the African: Clinicobiochemical assessment (review article). *Trop. Geogr. Med.*, 22, 125.

ADADEVOH, B.K. (1972) Nutrition problems and agricultural resources. *Nig. Med. J.*, 2, 112.

ADADEVOH, B.K. & LUKANMBI, F.A. (1972) Insulin levels in Nigerian adults, children and pregnant women. *Horm. Metab. Res.*, 4, 136.

ANDERSON, J. (1972) Obesity. *Brit. Med. J.*, 1, 560.

BOLODEOKU, J.O. & ADADEVOH, B.K. (1974) Metabolic and clinical effects of fenfluramine in obese patients. *Nig. Med. J.*, **in press**.

BOLODEOKU, J.O., ADADEVOH, B.K. & PALMER, E.O. (1972) Therapeutic effect of fenfluramine (Ponderax) in obese Nigerians—weight reducing and hypotensive properties. *Nig. Med. J.*, 2, 199.

BUTTERFIELD, W.J.H. (1969) In *Obesity Medical and Scientific Aspects.* Proceedings of the First Symposium of the Obesity Association of Great

Britain. Ed. Baird, I.M. & Howard, A.N. p.5 Edinburgh & London: E & S Livingstone Ltd.

COLES, R.M. (1957) The relation of height and body weight of Uganda African patients. *E. Afr. Med. J.*, 34, 619.

DE RACHEWILTZ, B. (1964) *Black Eros:* The sexual customs of Africa from prehistoric times to the present day. London: George Allen & Unwin Ltd.

DOVLO, R. (1972) In *Environmental Influences on Food Consumption.* Proceedings of the Ghana Working Group on the Environment. Vol. 1. p.95. Accra, November.

East African Conference on Nutrition and Child Feeding (1969) Sponsored by the Republic of Kenya and USAID with participation of FAO, UNICEF & WHO. Nairobi, Kenya, May. Washington D.C. 20402: U.S. Govt. Printing Office.

Editorial, *S. Afr. Med. J.* 43, 1273 (1969). The measurement of obesity.

FLEISCHMANN, V. & ADADEVOH, B.K. (1973) Hyperuricaemia and gout in Nigerians. *Trop. Geogr. Med.*, 25, 255.

HADDOCK, D.R.W. (1969) Obesity in medical out-patients in Accra. *Ghana Med. J.*, 8, 251.

HADDOCK, D.R.W., ALLOTEY, J.B.K. & AKPEBU, E.K. (1972) Some aspects of hypertension in general medical clinic in Accra. *Ghana Med. J.*, 11, 49.

JOHNSON, T.O. (1969) Distribution of arterial blood pressures in a Lagos metropolitan sample survey. *Ghana Med. J.*, 8, 155 (abstract).

JOHNSON, T.O. (1970) Height and weight patterns of an urban African population sample in Nigeria. *Trop. Geogr. Med.*, 22, 65.

McGREGOR, I.A. & SMITH, D.E. (1952) A health, nutrition and parasitological survey in a rural village (Keneba) in West Kiang, Gambia. *Trans. Roy. Soc. Trop. Med. Hyg.*, 46, 403.

MNGOLA, E.N. & ALOUCH, J.A. (1973) Fenfluramine in the treatment of obese Africans. Paper presented at the East African Medical Research Council Annual Meeting, Nairobi, January-February.

MOORE, R. & ROBERTS, A. (1957) An investigation of the pattern of disease prevalent in parts of the Rufiji district. *E. Afr. Med. J.*, 34, 571.

OLUPITAN, R.C. & ADADEVOH, B.K. (1967) Therapeutic effects of a low calorie diet in obesity. *W. Afr. Med. J.*, 16, 141.

OLUSANYA, E.O. & OMOLOLU, A. (1972) Dietary practices and nutrition in West African Council for Medical Research (Nigeria). *Proceedings of the First Medical Research Meeting in Yaba*, February. p. 126. Lagos: Academy Press Ltd.

ORR, J.B. & GILKS, J.L. (1931) The physique and health of two African tribes. *Spec. Rep. Ser. Med. Res. Coun.*, London, No. 155.

OSUNTOKUN, B.O., REDDY, S., AKINKUGBE, F.M., FRANCIS, T.I., OSUNTOKUN, O. & TAYLOR, G.O.L. (1971) Diabetes mellitus in Nigerians: a study of 832 patients. *W. Afr. Med. J. n.s.* 20, 295.

OWUSU, S.K. (1971) Diabetes in Accra. *Ghana Med J.*, 10, 203.

Republic of Nigeria Nutrition Survey 1965 (1967) A report by the Nutrition Section, Office of International Research, N.I.H., Bethesda. U.S. Department of Health and Welfare.

SEFTEL, H.C. (1961) Diabetes mellitus in the urbanized Johannesburg Afican. *S. Afr. Med. J.*, 35, 66.

SLOME, C., GAMPEL, B., ABRAMSON, J.H. & SCOTCH, M. (1960) Weight,

height and skinfold thickness of Zulu adults in Durban. *S. Afr. Med. J.*, **34**, 505.
TAYLOR, G.O. (1971) Studies on serum lipids in Nigerians *Trop. Geogr. Med.*, **23**, 158.
U.S. Department of Health, Education and Welfare (1966) Public Health Service Publication No. 1485. Obesity and Health U.S. Govt. Printing Office.
West African Conference on Nutrition and Child Feeding (1968) Dakar, Senegal, March. Sponsored by the Republic of Senegal and USAID with participation of FAO, UNICEF & WHO. U.S. Govt. Printing Office, Washington, D.C. 20402.

6. The Problem of Obesity in Developing Countries: Its Prevalence and Morbidity

R. RICHARDS and M. deCASSERES

Malnutrition in infancy and early childhood remains one of the most important disorders contributing to infant and childhood mortality in third world countries. The factors contributing to the disorder are protean, but centre mainly around protein-calorie deficiency modified by economic, cultural, religious and educational customs. Again total protein-calorie deficiency leading to an increased susceptibility to disease still plays a major role in the mortality and morbidity of adults in many third world areas. It may appear surprising therefore to find that in the midst of poverty and sub-standard nutrition in developing countries the problem of obesity should manifest itself.

Reports on the prevalence of this problem are scanty, as in these areas attention has been focused mainly on malnutrition. There are a number of reports on height/weight measurements of Africans in Kenya (Orr & Gilks, 1931), Nigeria (Nicol, 1959), Uganda (Coles, 1957) and Jamaica (Ashcroft et al, 1966). Little mention of obesity is made in these reports, except for a comment by Ashcroft and coworkers (1966) on an index of 'stoutness'. The awareness of obesity as a problem in the West Indies began to emerge during the study of the epidemiology of diabetes mellitus which commenced in 1961 and is continuing.

THE PREVALENCE OF OBESITY

A review of the patients attending a diabetic clinic in Jamaica revealed that 80 per cent of the female diabetic patients were obese as defined by the Metropolitan Life Insurance Company Table of Desirable Weight (1948), whereas only 18 per cent of the male patients showed a similar degree of obesity. These figures prompted us to look at obesity in a segment of the population of Jamaica to assess the prevalence and magnitude of the problem.

THE PROBLEM OF OBESITY IN DEVELOPING COUNTRIES

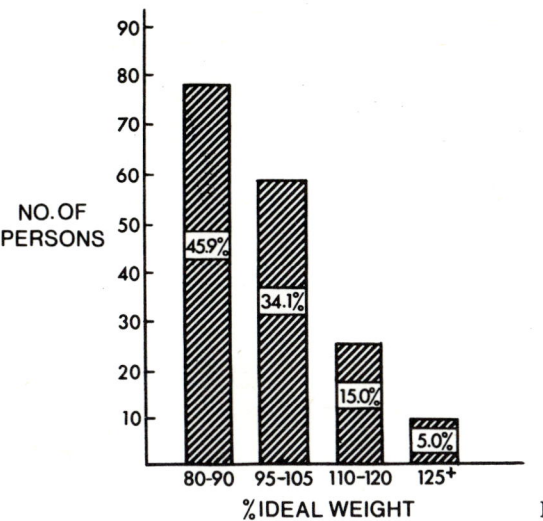

Figure 6.1

While investigating thyroid function in a semi-urban population we undertook anthropometric measurements on 530 randomly selected individuals (360 women and 170 men) between the ages of 16 and 70 years (Goldberg & Richards, 1964).

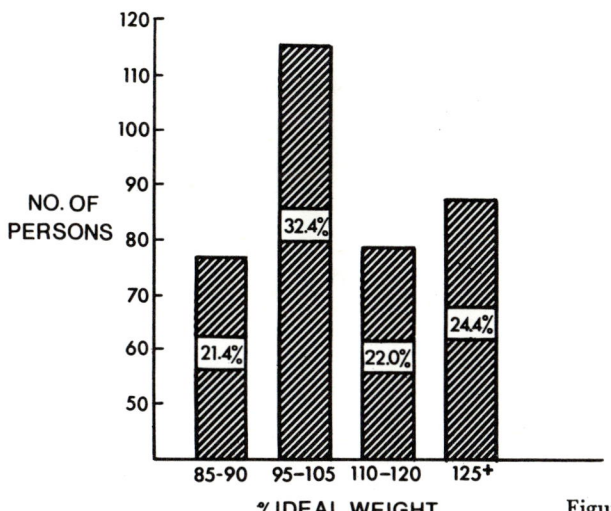

Figure 6.2

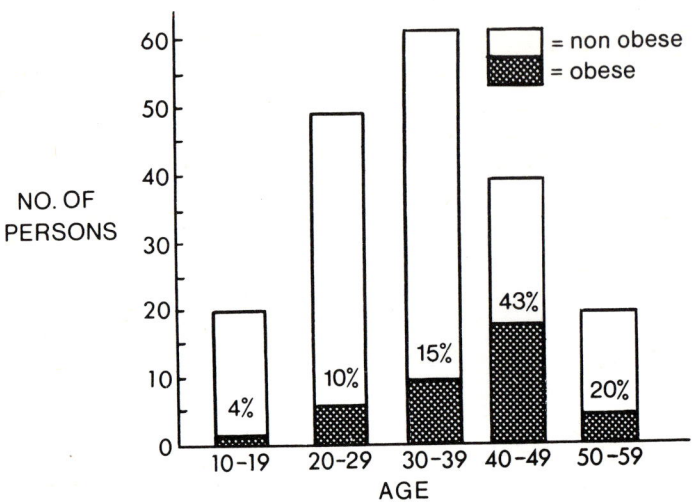

Figure 6.3

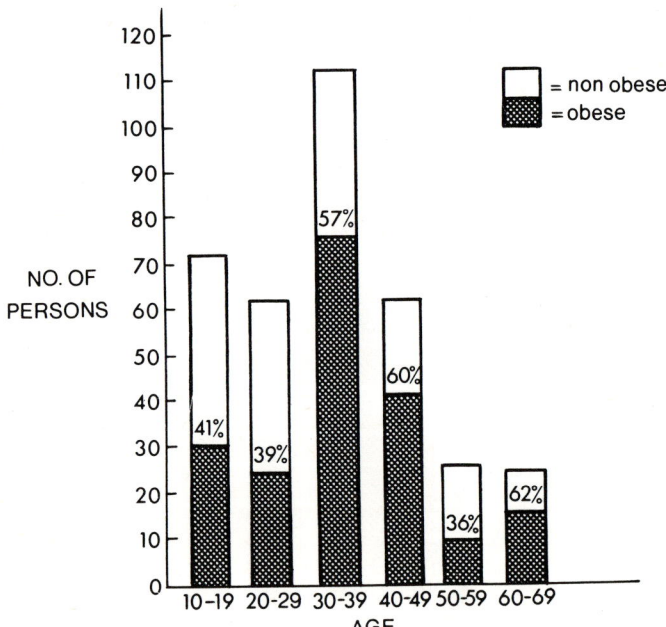

Figure 6.4

THE PROBLEM OF OBESITY IN DEVELOPING COUNTRIES 77

For clinical purposes obesity was considered to be present in individuals who exceeded their ideal body weight by more than 10 per cent. Figures 6.1 and 6.2 show the weight distribution as a percentage of the ideal body weight for men and women in the population sample. It will be seen that 20 per cent of all men are obese but only five per cent are more than 25 per cent overweight. More than 50 per cent of the women studied were obese and 24 per cent were more than 25 per cent overweight.

Figures 6.3 and 6.4 show the prevalence of obesity for the two sexes in the various age groups. Figure 6.3 shows that the greatest prevalence of obesity occurs in the 40–50 year age group for males where it reaches 43 per cent, but it falls to 20 per cent in the over 50 age group. In contrast Figure 6.4 shows that from the second decade obesity occurs in 41 per cent of Jamaican women, reaching a peak of 60 per cent in the 40–50 year age group, and that over the age of 60 years it occurs in 62 per cent of the female population studied. The overall prevalence of obesity for the age group 10–60 years was found to be 20 per cent of the male population and 46.4 per cent of the female population of Jamaica. If a figure of 20 per cent in excess of body weight was used as the index of significant obesity, then obesity in the male population was five per cent and that for the female population 24.4 per cent. A more recent survey in 1973 has shown obesity (more than 20 per cent of ideal body weight) to occur in 9.5 per cent of males and in 62.8 per cent of females (Figure 6.5).

TERRITORY	YEAR	PREVALENCE OF OBESITY > 120% BODY WEIGHT	
		male	female
JAMAICA	1965	5%	24.4%
BARBADOS	1969	7%	31%
GUYANA	1971	13.1%	39.4%
TRINIDAD	1970	12.6%	28%
BARBADOS	1972	2.5%	41%
JAMAICA	1973	9.5%	62.8%

Figure 6.5

The reason for this increase in the occurrence of obesity is not clear, but it is probable that it has coincided with the increased economic wealth of the community. It has also been observed that whereas obesity is four times as common in the lower economic group of women, the converse is true for the male Jamaicans.

A number of height and weight measurements were carried out in some of the other Caribbean territories (Fig. 6.5). These showed that obesity in the female population was between four and 20 times more common than it is in the male populations of the various territories. It is perhaps noteworthy that Trinidad and Guyana both have a higher prevalence of obesity in their male populations than do Barbados and Jamaica. The two former countries have a higher proportion of East Indians (45–50 per cent) in their populations than do Barbados (0.02 per cent) and Jamaica (0.08 per cent). It is conceivable that the Indian male contributes to the frequency of obesity in these territories to a greater degree than his African counterpart (Poon-King *et al*, 1968).

MORBIDITY

Figure 6.6 shows the diseases associated with obesity discovered during the 1973 obesity survey referred to above. Hypertension and diabetes mellitus are probably the two most common non infective diseases seen in the English-speaking West Indian territories. Mor-

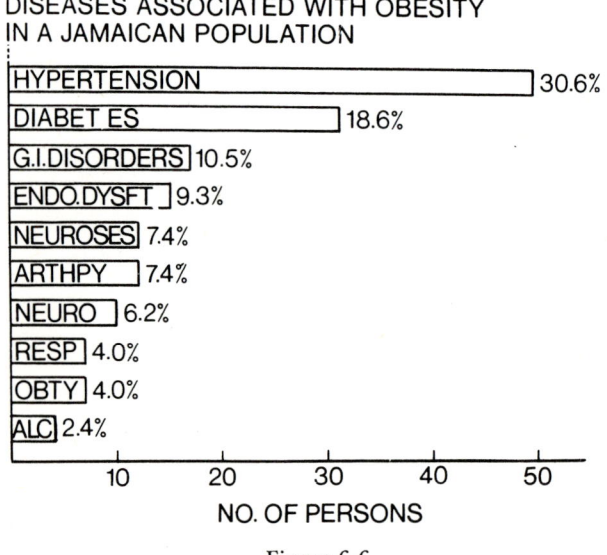

Figure 6.6

bidity and mortality statistics from the Registrar General's office show that hypertension and hypertensive cardiovascular disease is the major cause of death in both sexes in the Caribbean. Diabetes mellitus is the next most common cause of death in these countries, 22.6 per 100,000 in Trinidad and Tobago and 21.8 in Jamaica. When this is compared with 7.9 per 100,000 in the U.S.A. and 6.8 in the U.K. the magnitude of this problem can be seen. The true occurrence of hypertension in the West Indian population has not been accurately calculated but it occurs in approximately 10 per cent of the adult population. It will be seen from Figure 6.6 that in the obese population it occurs almost three times more frequently than in the general population at risk.

Diabetic surveys have been performed by Tulloch (1961, 1962) and Poon-King *et al* (1968) and give a prevalence of 1.26 per cent and 2.4 per cent respectively. More recent unpublished figures suggest that the true figure approximates to six per cent of the adult population in most of the West Indian territories where 1 hour post prandial blood sugar concentrations of 180 mg/100 ml or more are used as the criterion for the diagnosis of diabetes mellitus. The prevalence of diabetes in the obese population is 18.6 per cent or about three times that reported in the general population. The 10 most common diseases affecting the obese population in Jamaica are shown in Figure 6.6. All these diseases are from three times to as much as 20 times as common in the obese West Indian population as in the population at risk. These complications of obesity are strikingly similar to those reported in the literature for the more developed American and European countries.

It is difficult to explain the high frequency of obesity seen in a relatively impecunious society such as exists in the West Indies, when compared to the standard of living enjoyed in the more developed countries. Malnutrition and subnutrition are common disorders in the first two years of life in these areas, and account for almost 25 per cent of all admissions to paediatric wards in Jamaica. Subnutrition continues in early childhood to the early teens. Obesity begins to manifest itself in the female population from the 25th year of life and reaches enormous proportions from the age of 30 onwards. It is not surprising, therefore, that diabetes mellitus occurs most frequently in the 30–50 year age group in the female population and is almost four times more frequent than in the male population of the same age group. Most third world countries have a high carbohydrate intake as their economic dependence is predominantly agricultural, with a heavy dependence on non-dairy products. It is conceivable that the ready availability of starch in preference to animal protein, contributing as it must the main calorie requirements of these populations, leads to increased lipogenesis and the development of obesity.

The prevalence of diabetes mellitus and hypertension and its complications places a heavy strain on the somewhat limited medical resources of communities such as ours, with a heavy economic toll in terms of morbidity and drug therapy for such diseases.

Re-education and nutritional counselling should go a long way towards a reduction in the frequency with which this disorder presents in such communities.

REFERENCES

ASHCROFT, M.J., LING, L., LOVELL, H.G. & MIALL, W.E. (1966) Heights and weights of adults in rural and urban areas of Jamaica. *Brit. J. Soc. Prevent. Med.*, 20, 22.

COLES, R.M. (1957) The relation of height and body weight of Ugandan African patients. *E. Afr. Med. J.*, 34, 619.

GOLDBERG, I.J.L., RICHARDS, R., McFARLANE, H. & HARLAND, W.H. (1964) Thyroid uptake of radioiodine in normal subjects in Jamaica. *J. Clin. Endocrin.*, 24, 1178.

NICOL, B.M. (1959) The protein requirements of Nigerian peasant farmers. *Brit. J. Nutr.*, 13, 307.

ORR, J.B. & GILKS, J.L. (1931) The physique and health of two African tribes. *Med. Res. Coun.*, 155, London: H.M.S.O.

POON-KING, T. & HENRY, M.V. (1968) Prevalence and natural history of diabetes in Trinidad. *Lancet*, 1, 155.

TULLOCH, J.A. (1961) The prevalence of diabetes mellitus in Jamaica. *Diabetes*, 10, 286.

TULLOCH, J.A. (1962) in *Diabetes Mellitus in the Tropics*, p. 8. London: E.S. Livingstone.

DISCUSSION

Dr. Widdowson. The belief now in this country is that overfeeding during the first year of life predisposes to obesity later, and in the adult. The obesity in Nigeria and Jamaica occurs in women who were not presumably overnourished, in fact probably undernourished during their first year of life. Certainly, this is more likely to have been true 20 or 30 years ago when these women were babies than it is among babies now. What is the truth about this? Have any studies been made on fat cell numbers in African or West Indian populations, and what are we to believe about the effect of underfeeding or overfeeding early in life on later obesity?

Dr. Richards. Perhaps I can answer this in two ways. The patterns of malnutrition, as seen in the West Indies, are of two types. First there is the classical protein-calorie malnutrition, which we call marasmus and, secondly, there is protein malnutrition, in which there is adequate calorie intake, in terms of carbohydrate, but not of protein—this is classical kwashiorkor which is by far the commoner form of infantile malnutrition. These children tend to present as pot-bellied, obese and oedematous, with abnormal hepatic and renal function. It is conceivable that this second group, because of their high calorie and carbohydrate intake, adhere to the patterns seen in European countries, whereas the marasmic group would be likely not to have an increase in numbers of adipocytes. However, there is no preponderance of malnutrition in the female infant, as compared to the male infant, yet the pattern of obesity in adult life is totally different in the two sexes. It cannot be entirely a matter of infant feeding history.

Dr. Craddock. I was interested in Dr. Richard's comment that the increased incidence of diabetes in the population of Indian-origin in the West Indies probably had a genetic background. Of course, this has been shown in South Africa too. However, it is interesting that amongst the Indians living in India, diabetes is extremely rare. There is a similar low prevalence of hypertension, peptic ulcer and many other diseases of civilization. The few cases which occur are in those who come from the South of India and who have been eating mainly refined sugar and refined carbohydrates in general. This confirms the worldwide epidemiological evidence that it is the eating of refined carbohydrate, and sugar in particular, which gives rise to the incidence of all these common disorders.

Professor Yudkin. Has Professor Adadevoh any more information about the disorders associated with obesity—or does he consider it worth obtaining? I was interested because his associations appear, in many respects, different from those we find in Western European countries and North America. Following Dr. Richards' statement that only 4 per cent of his very obese patients presented for treatment of their obesity, I wondered whether any studies had been carried out on the sociological or psychological aspects of this enormous prevalence of obesity amongst adult women? What sort of attitudes do these people have towards their obesity? They do not seem to be very concerned—certainly not sufficiently to seek advice. On the other hand, I was interested to discover that there is beginning to be popular discussion about the disadvantages of obesity, and its treatment. Is it entirely true that the high prevalence of obesity is due to socio-economic advances? Certainly, from Dr. Richards' statements, it seems that the improved economic situation in Jamaica has led to a considerable increase in its prevalence; but there was a high prevalence previously, and there is still a high prevalence in some of the poorer parts of Africa, so there are clearly other social or psychological factors that make for this very high prevalence of obesity in these countries.

Professor Adadevoh. Diseases such as hypertension, diabetes, osteoarthritis, gout, etc. have been recorded in association with obesity, but a wider epidemiological survey needs to be undertaken in our African communities in order to assess specifically the prevalence of obesity and of associated diseases. A few of the reports which I included in my chapter have attempted to do this, but it is my opinion that they only offer indications that these diseases occur. With regard to the attitude of the female to obesity, I think that it remains an acceptable phenomenon in the African. Few come forward for treatment, and unless there is associated disease which troubles them, treatment is unlikely to succeed. The attire worn by the market women looks much better on the Nigerian women when they are fat than when they are slim. A round neck is looked upon as a sign of beauty. It is the younger, sophisticated girl who reads newspapers and magazines who does not accept obesity. With regards to socio-economic factors, we are beginning to see obesity in the male, particularly in those who have become executives with expense accounts.

Dr. Richards. Like some of the European countries, we find that the prevalence of obesity in women in the higher socio-economic groups is far less than in the lower socio-economic groups. Perhaps the same factors apply and they are making a conscious effort to remain slim whereas, in the lower socio-economic groups, women from the age of 22 or 23 onwards, with five, six or seven children, are house-bound looking after the family and have an exremely curtailed social existence.

Dr. Ashwell. Professor Adadevoh has said that the obese Nigerian has an unusual fat distribution compared with Europeans and Americans. It is predominantly in the buttock. Could you summarize any other differences between obese Nigerians and, say, obese Londoners?

Professor Adadevoh. The obesity in the buttocks which I described makes them completely out of proportion. We have made some skinfold thickness measurements in which we gained the impression that this type of obesity is more common in our environment.

Professor Keen. Dangers are encountered when we try to extrapolate from obesity in one population to obesity in another. The degree of selection which various populations have undergone differs greatly. Although it is just a matter of a few hundred years, child survival and adult survival in Europe show a very different pattern from that in the African continent. Perhaps we are looking at people who would have died otherwise, and who would not have been available for the study. At our peril do we make direct comparisons without regard to such factors. I should like to ask Professor Adadevoh about the extremely high degree of correlation between the serum cholesterol level and the diastolic blood pressure in his population, and the absence of any correlation at all between the serum cholesterol and the systolic pressure.

Professor Adadevoh. The population we studied were soldiers and were the only measurements to show any correlation. I should like to see some studies in females of the same age and to compare them.

Dr. Brook. It is possible that the physiological accumulation of adipose tissue in the African may be quite different from that in the European. With regards to the adipose cell model referred to in Chapter 7 no one has attempted to connect the growth of the adipose cell with nutritional status. However, I should like to commend Dr. Richards' remarks because it seems to me that with marasmus and kwashiorkor there is a ready-made model which may shed some light on these two aspects and their inter-relationship, if any.

Dr. Richards. Do you have any ideas on the reason for the difference in prevalence of diabetes in our two populations, Professor Adadevoh?

Professor Adadevoh. Diabetes is reported more in males than in females in West Africa. It may be that the male goes to the hospital more often than the female. In South Africa it is more varied; some communities report more in the females, and others more in males.

Dr. Curtis-Prior. Professor Adadevoh suggested that obesity begins in Nigerian women soon after their first pregnancy. On the basis that their infants are breast-fed, could he comment on the fact that in Britain obesity following pregnancy appears to be associated with an increasing use of bottle feeding?

Professor Adadevoh. I cannot state what factors are responsible; I have given one possibility, namely their indulgence in food-fads. Inactivity has also been suggested.

Dr. Durnin. May I make a plea for very careful assessment of the medical implications of obesity, as opposed to the sociological implications? We should be extremely careful that discrimination is made between men and women. Not only sociologically, but probably medically also, the disadvantages of what we call obesity for a woman are quite different from those for a man. I should like to reinforce Professor Keen's remark that populations differ markedly. It is extraordinary that we still use Metropolitan Life standards to apply to African populations, Asian populations, etc. We ought, at least, to use skinfold measurements. At least they represent subcutaneous fat. It is possible that they also represent total body fat. When the effects of obesity are being compared, I hope that an assessment of fat will be made generally, and not an assessment of overweight. It is worth pointing out that the skinfold measurements quoted by Professor Adadevoh are less than those described for Europeans. This may indicate that he is presenting a normal population and that he should not make comparisons with Europeans and North Americans.

Professor Adadevoh. Most of the information from which my conclusions were drawn came from Nigeria, Ghana, East Africa and South Africa where many are extremely fat. Even for the very fat ones amongst them, the figures I quoted are relatively low. Comparisons have to be made with the European figures.

Dr. Stowers. Professor Adadevoh mentioned the Masai who are known to have the remarkable ability to stabilize their serum cholesterol independent of dietary influences. Do they have any other deviations in how they deal with an excess of calories, particularly of fat? Are they hard gainers or are they comparable to other races?

Professor Adadevoh. I do not know. However, insulin concentrations amongst the Masai are comparable to those in Londoners, whereas in other groups we have studied with high carbohydrate intake, the insulin concentrations are extremely high. The Masai are difficult to study; they live in a very closed environment.

7. Critical Periods in Childhood Obesity

C. G. D. BROOK

Obesity is a disorder of the adipose organ which results in an increase in its size. It is a condition which causes serious emotional and physical disability in childhood and carries considerable morbidity and mortality in adult life. Treatment of the condition is difficult and expensive in time, money and manpower and, at least in childhood, is frequently not successful. The current emphasis in this field should therefore be on preventitive measures.

Although it is manifestly possible to become obese through the excessive laying down of fat at any age, the object of this chapter is to suggest that there are certain ages at which preventitive measures taken in childhood are likely to be most effective in reducing the prevalence of obesity in adult life.

GROWTH OF THE ADIPOSE ORGAN

Body fat can be regarded as an organ and can be measured by a number of sophisticated techniques. I shall confine myself to the measurement of its increase by the use of skinfold measurements. These correlate well with total body fat measured by other methods both in adults (Durnin & Rahaman, 1967) and in children over a wide range of age and shape (Brook, 1971a; Pařísková & Roth, 1972). The latter authors showed that the accuracy of measurement is not greatly increased by measuring a large number of skinfolds and that a combination of the measurements of triceps and subscapular skinfold thicknesses, which are representative of limb and body fat, gives a good indication of total body fat.

In the fetus fat, that is white adipose tissue, appears late in gestation at about 30 weeks. Figure 7.1 shows what happens to body fat in both sexes during childhood and adolescence. These data are the results of cross sectional measurements of children and the figure

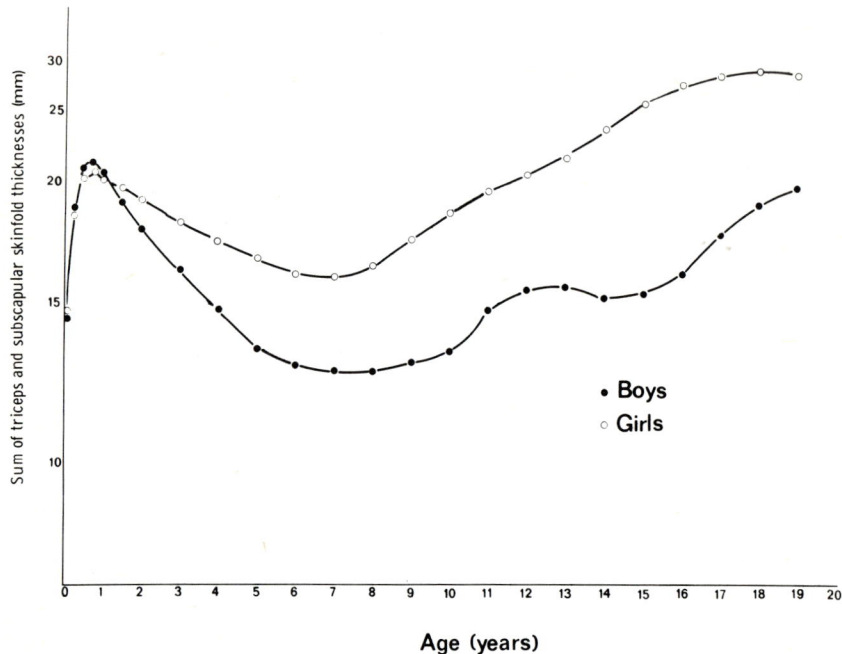

Figure 7.1
Growth of total body fat in childhood.

shows the sum of the 50th centile measurements of triceps and subscapular skinfold thicknesses in millimetres taken at the various chronological ages. By using cross sectional data and also by using the sum of the measurements the changes shown are minimized but do show how fat accumulates in normal subjects.

After a very rapid increase in body fat over the first nine months of life, which occurs slightly earlier and is slightly greater in males than females, fat is lost in both sexes during the early years of childhood. This loss is less in girls than in boys. From the age of eight, when the earliest maturing girls will be starting puberty, there is a gradual increase in body fat which continues throughout puberty. In males there is the interesting phenomenon of a pre-adolescent fat spurt from the ages of 10 to 12 and then a further considerable increase during puberty proper. My contention is that each of these periods of rapid increase in total body fat are periods when it is extremely easy for an exaggeration of the normal physiological process to carry an individual over into clinical obesity, a state from which it is much less easy to withdraw. These then are the critical periods at which efforts at prevention are likely to be most successful and it makes economic sense, therefore, to confine our efforts in the first instance to these periods.

CELLULAR GROWTH

The growth of an organ proceeds by a combination of cell multiplication and enlargement. The extent of the contribution made by each of these processes probably differs from organ to organ as does the age at which different events take place. Body fat is unique as an organ in man in that it is relatively easy to measure and extremely easy to sample (Hirsch & Goldrick, 1964). From a sample of adipose tissue it is possible to measure the mean weight of lipid per cell,

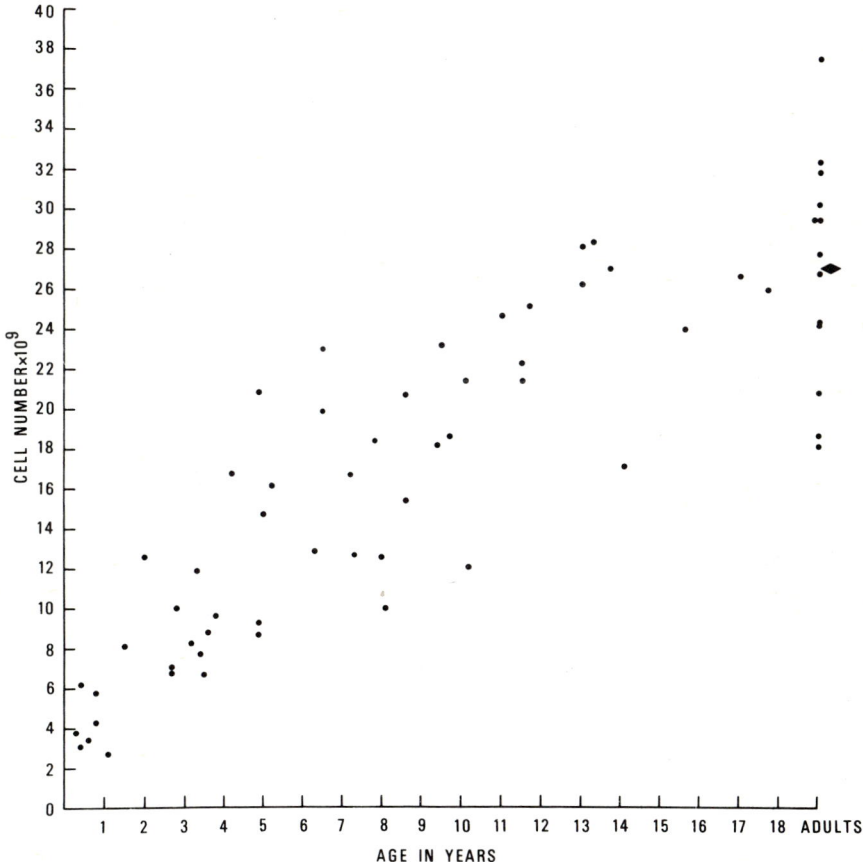

Figure 7.2
Increase in the number of adipose cells with age in normal subjects.

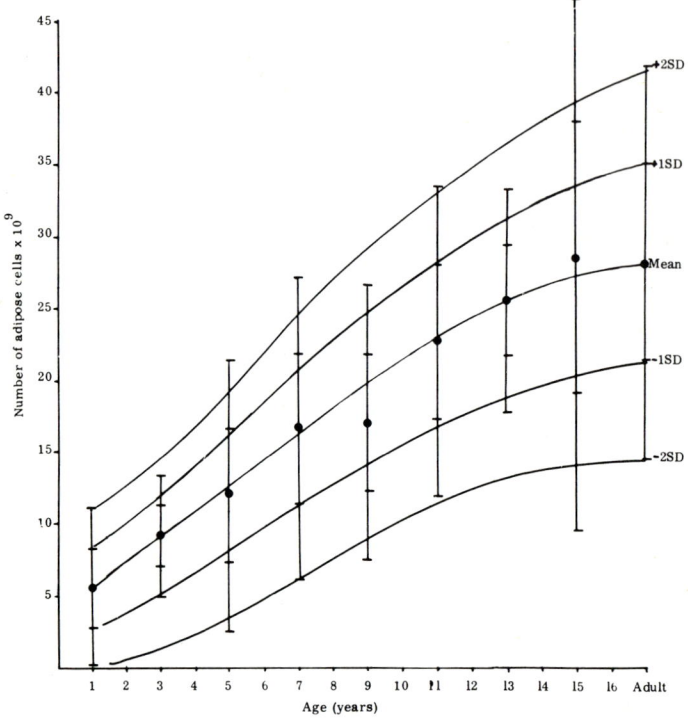

Figure 7.3

Mean values (± 2 SD) of total number of adipose cells in control children and adults.

which is a measure of its size, by estimating the lipid content of the sample, for example by gas-liquid chromatography, and by counting the number of cells per wet weight of adipose tissue after fixation of the tissue in osmium tetroxide in a cell counter (Hirsch & Gallian, 1968). This is a repeatable measurement with a coefficient of variation of 10.8 per cent (Brook, 1972a).

If the total amount of body fat is measured, for example from skinfold measurements, it is possible to calculate the total number of adipose cells in the body if the assumption is made that all adipose cells contain the same mean amount of fat. This is not strictly true for adipose cells from deep sites, which contain less lipid than cells from subcutaneous sites, but is true for adipose cells taken from different subcutaneous sites in the same subject (Brook, 1971b). As most adipose tissue in normal subjects is subcutaneous, the calculation based on sampling from this site probably gives a reasonable estimate. Certainly the results reported by different workers using the same techniqes are in remarkable agreement.

Growth of the adipose organ in childhood appears to be largely due to cell multiplication; both in Knittle's (1971) data and in my own (Brook, 1972a) there is very little discernable pattern between the age of a child and the size of his adipose cells. Figure 7.2, however, shows the increase in the number of adipose cells with age in 64 children (46 boys and 18 girls) and 17 adults (11 men and six women) who were undergoing elective surgery but who were otherwise healthy and had weights and skinfold thicknesses within the normal ranges. The number of cells increased up to puberty but no differences were found between adolescent and adult values. No sex

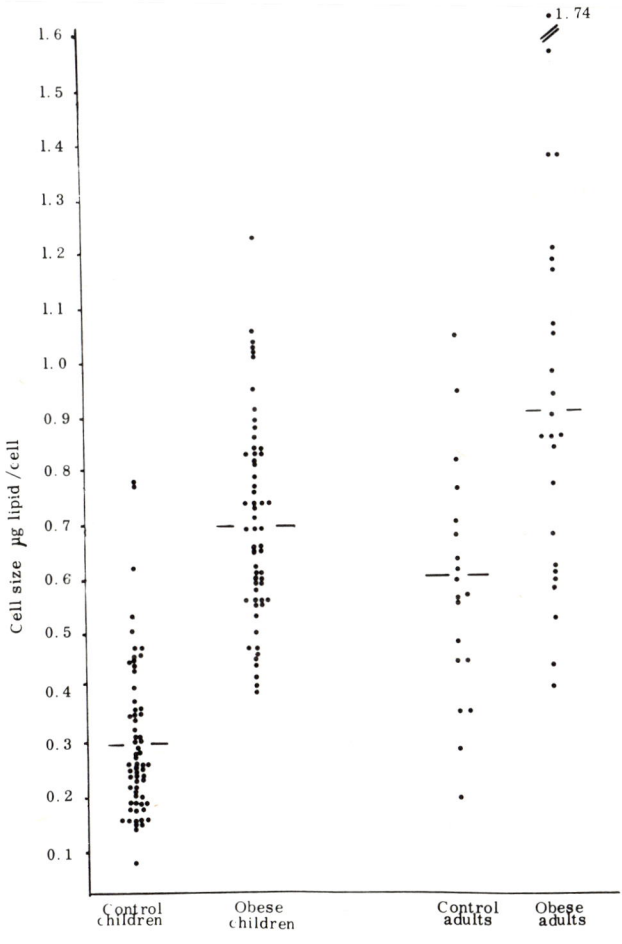

Figure 7.4
Adipose cell size in normal and obese subjects.

differences were found, probably because the number of subjects was too small and the methods too inaccurate, but it appears that the major differences in body composition between adult men and women are accounted for by differences in adipose cell size and not cell number.

The control population was split into two-year age groups and, after confirming that the distribution in each group was not obviously different from gaussian, the means and standard deviations were calculated for each group. These values were then plotted and curves fitted by eye (Fig. 7.3). From this graph it is possible to draw distribution histograms of adipose cell number in various groups of children.

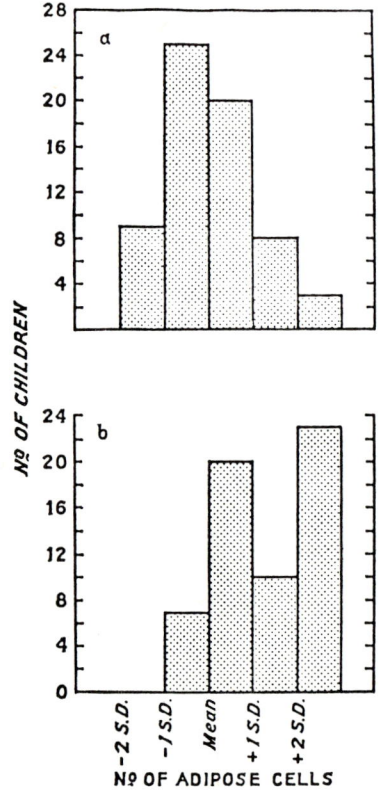

Figure 7.5
Total number of adipose cells.
a) Control children
b) Obese children

ADIPOSE CELLS AND OBESITY

Data were obtained from 52 obese children (18 boys and 34 girls) and 25 obese adults (4 men and 21 women). All the subjects were considerably obese by any criterion. Figure 7.4 shows the size of the adipose cells in these individuals compared to controls. Although in both adults and children the means were significantly higher in the obese groups, the overlap was considerable. Figure 7.5 shows the data for the number of adipose cells in the obese children. The distribution is skewed in the obese group.

The age of onset of obesity in the children was determined by objective criteria (Brooks *et al*, 1972) and allocation was made into two groups according to whether or not the children had gained weight excessively in the first year of life. Twenty nine had done so (early-obese, Group E) and 23 had not (late-obese, Group L). The age of onset in the adult patients was unfortunately ascertained by

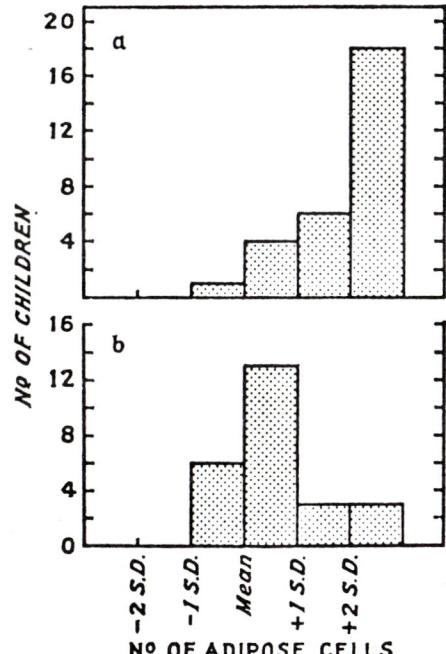

Figure 7.6
Effect of age at onset of obesity on the number of adipose cells in obese children.
a) Early-obese children
b) Late-obese children

92 OBESITY SYMPOSIUM

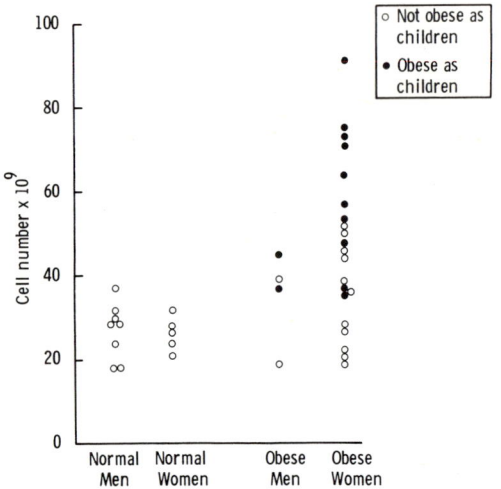

Figure 7.7
Total number of adipose cells in control and obese adults.

history alone, as it proved impossible to obtain objective records.

The effect of age at onset of obesity on the number of adipose cells in obese children and adults is shown in Figures 7.6 and 7.7. The histogram method was not employed for the adults because of the small numbers of subjects. The figures show that in children increased numbers of adipose cells were found in those who had gained weight excessively in the first year of life; the number of adipose cells in the L group children did not differ significantly from the controls. In adults an increased number of adipose cells was associated with a history of obesity dating from childhood. This finding is in agreement with the data of Hirsch & Knittle (1970) who showed that the increase in the number of adipose cells in obese adults was greatest in those who dated the onset of their obesity to childhood.

In 14 children, adipose tissue sampling was repeated after a period of weight loss and this showed that fat cells once laid down cannot be lost (Figure 7.8). Others have shown this in the rat (Hollenberg & Vost, 1968) and in adult man (Sims *et al*, 1968).

As well as the changes in adipose tissue cellularity the E group of obese children showed other somatic differences: they were taller and had more advanced bone ages than normal children, while the L group children were identical with controls (Brook, 1973). There was however, no difference in fatness between the two groups and the increase in adipose cell number, unlike the increase in height, could not be explained purely on the basis of growth acceleration (advanced bone age). There was no difference either in the degree of fatness of the two groups of obese adults.

From these data it appears that overnutrition in the early months of life has lasting consequences on the number of adipose cells laid down in man. Data from low birthweight children and from children deficient in growth hormone (Brook, 1972b) confirm that for the adipose organ there is a period of determination when the cell complement is established. In this period the organ is sensitive to external circumstances so that changes in nutrition and other influences, e.g. growth hormone, are reflected in changes in adipose tissue cellularity either by increasing or decreasing the number of adipose cells. At the end of this sensitive period, which probably extends from the intrauterine period to the first nine months of life, the organ seems to become more or less immune to external circumstances and cell multiplication proceeds uniformly from the basic complement (Fig. 7.9).

Two further questions relating to adipose tissue cellularity and obesity remain to be answered. The first is whether it is in fact true that all adults with an increased number of adipose cells had gained weight excessively in the first year of life; the second is whether it matters that an individual has an increased number of adipose cells. There are no informed answers to either of these questions. Unless the theory of a sensitive period finishing in infancy is wrong it does

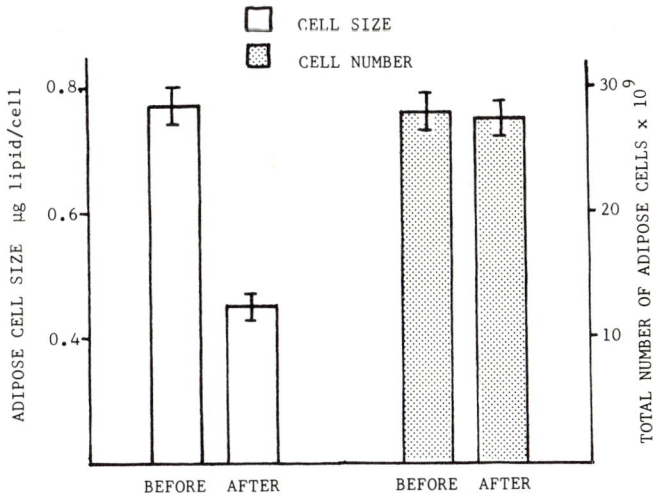

Figure 7.8
Mean (± SEM) values of adipose cell size and number before and after weight loss in 14 obese children.

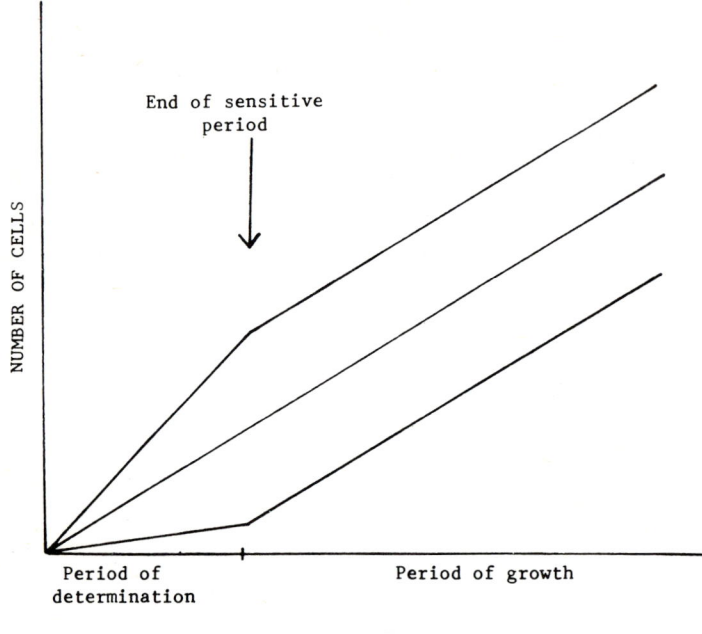

Figure 7.9
Model for the cellular growth of an organ.

seem remarkable how many adults were obese as babies! The alternative is that there is a period later in life when the adipose organ becomes sensitive again. My data are quite insufficient to show it but it seems quite likely that adipose cell multiplication follows the curve for total body fat described in Figure 7.1. Unfortunately it would take a very large volume of cross-sectional data or a longitudinal study to prove this hypothesis but if it were right then it would be quite reasonable to think that in the later periods of childhood adipose cells start to rapidly multiply again. At such times it is likely that the organ might again become sensitive to external influences rather in the same way as rapidly dividing cells elsewhere are preferentially sensitive to chemical inhibition, a principle made use of in the chemotherapy of cancer. Thus the pubescent girl who gains weight rapidly may be in the same position as the rapidly gaining baby.

Whether the changes in adipose tissue cellularity matter is not known. The circumstantial evidence points strongly to the suggestion that obesity and fat cell number are related and if the hypothesis outlined above is correct this would reinforce the argument that periods of rapid increase in body fat are the times to prevent obesity.

PRACTICAL IMPLICATIONS

As children grow so they should put on weight but the rate at which they do both these things should be the same. A departure from normal weight velocity (Tanner et al, 1966) should be a signal to look for a cause. If such a departure is due to the laying down of excessive amounts of fat, which can be easily detected by the use of skinfold caliper, the response of the attending physician or adviser should be immediate. The calorie intake should be adjusted to restore the equilibrium and this will usually be effected by a reduction in carbohydrate ingestion, though it should be remembered that fat has twice as much calorific value per unit weight. When dealing with children it should be emphasized that there are certain nutrients which are essential for growth and the advice of a dietitian may need to be sought if the calorie intake has to be drastically reduced.

If headway is to be made in clinical obesity these steps need to be taken at any age when weight gain is excessive, but they are probably likely to have most impact when they are employed at the times of rapid increase in body fat. These times are in the first year of life and in puberty. Health education focusing attention on these periods is likely to be repaid in the reduction of the adult incidence of obesity.

I am grateful to Professor J.M. Tanner and Mr. R.H. Whitehouse for permission to use their as yet unpublished 1970 British skinfold standards for the calculations of total body fat in children.

REFERENCES

BROOK, C.G.D. (1971a) Determination of body composition of children from skinfold measurements. *Arch. Dis. Childh.* **46**, 182.
BROOK, C.G.D. (1971b) Composition of human adipose tissue from deep and subcutaneous sites. *Brit. J. Nutr.*, **25**, 377.
BROOK, C.G.D. (1972a) Obesity in childhood. M.D. Thesis, University of Cambridge.
BROOK, C.G.D. (1972b) Evidence for a sensitive period in adipose cell replication in man. *Lancet*, **2**, 624.
BROOK, C.G.D. (1973) Fat Children. *Brit. J. Hosp. Med.*, **10**, 30.
BROOK, C.G.D., LLOYD, J.K. & WOLFF, O.H. (1972) Relation between age at onset of obesity and size and number of adipose cells. *Brit. Med. J.*, **2**, 25.
DURNIN, J.V.G. & RAHAMAN, M.M. (1967) The assessment of the amount of fat in the human body from measurements of skinfold thickness. *Brit. J. Nutr.*, **21**, 681.
HIRSCH, J. & GALLIAN, E. (1968) Methods for the determination of adipose cell size in man and animals. *J. Lipid. Res.*, **9**, 110.

HIRSCH, J. & GOLDRICK, R.B. (1964) Serial studies on the metabolism of human adipose tissue. *J. Clin. Invest.*, **43**, 1776.
HIRSCH, J. & KNITTLE, J.L. (1970) Cellularity of obese and non-obese human adipose tissue. *Fed. Proc.*, **29**, 1516.
HOLLENBERG, C.H. & VOST, A. (1968) Regulation of DNA synthesis in fat cells and stromal elements from rat adipose tissue. *J. Clin. Invest.*, 47, 2485.
KNITTLE, J.L. (1971) Childhood obesity. *Bull. N.Y. Acad. Med.*, 47, 579.
PAŘÍSKOVÁ, J. & ROTH, Z. (1972) The assessment of depot fat in children from skinfold thickness measurements by Holtain Caliper. *Human Biol.*, **44**, 613.
SIMS, E.A.H., GOLDMAN, R.F., GLUCK, C.M., HORTON, E.S., KELLEHER, P.C. & ROW, D.W. (1968) Experimental obesity in man. *Trans. Ass. Amer. Phys.*, **81**, 153.
TANNER, J.M., WHITEHOUSE, R.H. & TAKAISHI, M. (1966) Standards from birth to maturity for height, weight, height velocity and weight velocity: British children 1965. *Arch. Dis. Childh.*, 41, 454 & 613.

DISCUSSION

Dr. Dwyer. Dr. Brook, have you looked at the data on cellularity in relation to physiological age rather than chronological age? By physiological age I mean, for instance, menarche in girls or pubertal signs in boys.

Dr. Brook. Menarche is about the only constant feature in the growth of girls. Recently it has been shown that there is very little correlation between pubertal growth and the development of pubertal signs and, for example, bone age. This has destroyed much of our thinking. I have looked at the obesity data in relation to bone age. This showed that children who gained weight rapidly in the early months of life tend to be children who are tall and also have compensatory advance in bone age. The differences that I showed still, however, remain.

Dr. Garrow. Despite Dr. Brook's great care not to assign too great an importance to the subject of fat cell number, there are two factors which do not fit in with the idea of a critical period of cell development. First, as he has mentioned, there is the rather poor correlation between the fat cell number in adults and their earlier history of obesity. Secondly, there is a Swedish study by Mellbin & Virille (1973) in which a correlation between velocity of weight gain during the first year and obesity at seven years was not observed. I should like then to suggest, rather than there being a critical period of fat cell development, that it takes a long time to change fat cell number, whereas fat cell size can be changed quite quickly. The children who became obese earlier would have had a longer time in which to replicate their fat cells. This would seem to meet both the objections to the theory of there being a specifically critical period in the first year.

Dr. Brook. That is reasonable. We took a retrospective look at our obese children and found that there was not that much difference between those who had clearly put on weight rapidly from the age of three, and those who had gained weight very early. As for adults, your arguments are not particularly relevant because there are few adults who can recollect what occurred during their early life, i.e. during the sensitive periods. When most people talk about 'juvenile onset of obesity' they are referring to obesity dating from childhood. I refer to that very much earlier period which most adults do not remember too well, and very few have records.

Dr. Ashwell. Do you have any views on how the cell number is increased at any of these times? In other words, does cell division take place, or is recruitment of new cells occurring?

Dr. Brook. I do not know.

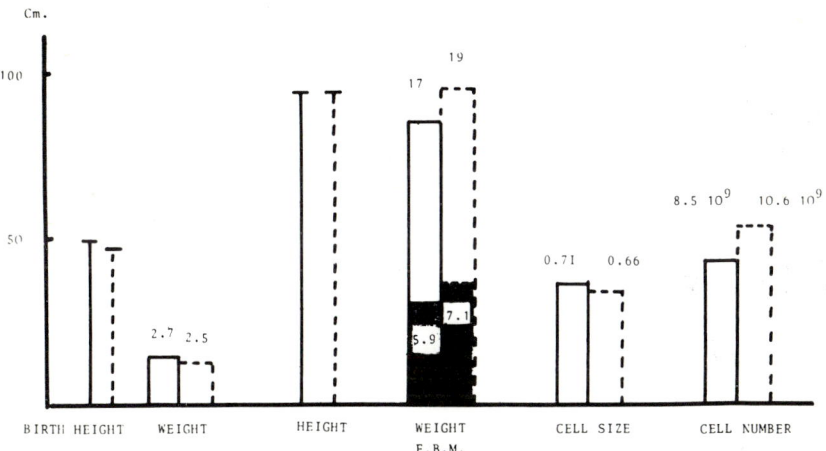

ADIPOSE TISSUE CELLULARITY IN TWO OBESE IDENTICAL TWINS 4Y.2M.OLD
Figure 7.10

Professor Guy-Grand. In a similar study in obese children we have confirmed Dr. Brook's data. Figure 7.10 shows the adipose tissue cellularity in identical twin girls, with different feeding patterns during their early childhood. The twin on the left was slightly longer and heavier at birth. Subsequently, both were overfed, but the smaller twin to a greater extent. Four years later both were obese. The one who was initially the smaller had become the heavier and the fatter. Fat body mass (FBM) is shown as the black area. This twin had the same cell size as her sister, but an increased cell number. A low birth weight may exert some protection against the hyperplastic effect of early over-nutrition.

Dr. Stowers. Dr. Brook has shown that there was an increase of fat cell number just prior to puberty—mainly in boys—could that be due to the so-called 'adrenarche', the increase in adrenal steroid activity before puberty? Or is it some independent mechanism?

Dr. Brook. I doubt it, as the changes I describe occur at about the age of nine to ten, which is some time before 'adrenarche'.

Dr. Stowers. The peak occurs at about 11 years. Your start was about seven years, but was rising steeply by 11, and there was another peak about the age of 13.

Dr. Brook. It is possible then.

Dr. Widdowson. First, I want to put in a good word for the adipose organ because if we did not possess it, we should all be dead; it is the means of storing the excess energy which is taken in, over and above our requirements. In this respect, I am extremely interested in this increase in the amount of fat in the body in the first nine months or so of life. I gather that Dr. Brook's figure 7.1 shows the absolute measurement of the thickness of the subcutaneous tissue in the children. This suggests that the child of nine months has a much thicker layer—in absolute terms—of adipose tissue than a boy of eight or nine. If the deposition of fat is an index of energy intake exceeding energy expenditure, it is interesting that it seems physiological for this to happen in the first nine months, and then for energy intake to be less than expenditure later.

Dr. Salans. I would like to add some of our own data and some of our own experience with over 200 patients, to the data presented by Dr. Brook. Our data may extend some of his hypothetical considerations a little further, and may add some caution to the interpretation of his findings.

We have observed that when the cellular character of the adipose tissue is considered retrospectively (by historical means and, as often as possible, by documenting history with medical records or photographs), a very good relationship is seen between the adult cell number and the age in life at which obesity begins. In general, obesity which begins early in life is much more likely to be associated with hypercellularity of the adipose tissue, than obesity beginning later in life.

This early onset hypercellular obesity is apparently one which can occur at any time until the age of 20 years, at least in our population. None of our patients whose obesity began after that age showed hypercellularity. In fact, when we looked at those individuals with adult onset obesity occurring after the age of 20, who had had obesity for more than 20 years, we were unable to demonstrate a relationship between the duration of obesity and the cellular character of the tissue.

I want to stress that hypercellularity seemed to occur within two specific periods: first, within the first year or so of life and, secondly, just before puberty. In our studies, this was particularly true of the male, as opposed to the female population in the schools. We saw hypercellularity occurring in individuals whose obesity began between the age of eight and 13 years and this was more often the case in males than females.

Dr. Bray. Dr. Brook has measured subcutaneous fat to estimate total body fat. Do you know whether the skinfold measurements used are a real reflection of total body fat rather than just a subcutaneous portion? Is it fair to say that the adipose tissue is a single organ, rather than several separately functioning organs; that is, do subcutaneous fat and deep fat, such as mesenteric fat, function in the same way? Is there sufficient information available to indicate that mother should be encouraged to modify the infants' feeding pattern in the first year or so of life, as this seems to be a critical period for the development of adipose cellularity?

Dr. Brook. First, the measurement of total body fat is a difficult exercise in children; under-water weighing is not feasible and invasive techniques are unpopular. The skinfold equations which I used were based on the work of Dr. Durnin, and were validated by the measurement of total body water, using deuterium oxide.

In answer to whether the adipose organ is one or more organs, I have some data which relate to the difference in size of cells of subcutaneous adipose tissue and of adipose tissue taken from a deep site. These data suggest that there are differences.

There are relatively few data on the proportion of the body fat which is subcutaneous in man, but it seems likely that it is the major part.

When one is talking about the total number of adipose cells, enormous extrapolations and assumptions are being made in the calculations. Too much stress should not be laid on absolute numbers. I would only say that it is a never-ceasing source of surprise to me that so many workers in so many parts of the world come up with the same answers. I do not think that we have sufficient evidence to modify feeding habits as far as adipose cells are concerned. With regard to the general health of children, the answer is that we should be careful of the way in which the infants are fed. I do not necessarily think that it has anything to do with how their adipose tissue cells grow.

Professor Adadevoh. My comments are directed to Dr. Brook's model, and how it is related to states of low nutrition. Do you feel that starvation, or under-nutrition in early life, are critical factors in adipose cell growth, and does the genesis of obesity occur less in a community with low nutrition? Secondly, could you comment on intrauterine nutritional states and their effects on adipose cell growth at birth and later in life? I suppose the former can only be measured by birth weight, or perhaps skinfold measurement can be made on newborn babies.

Dr. Brook. I have no data relating to malnutrition in post-natal life, as it is rare in this country. Our series of low birthweight children, I should stress, are a pre-selected group because the parents came to consult us as the infants were of low birthweight and had failed to grow. These children had a low number of adipose cells. However, at least two of the children in this group, by any other criterion would have been regarded as obese. This re-emphasizes the fact that we should not talk too much about the number of adipose cells and the nutritional status. At the same time, I looked at a series of children who were deficient in growth hormone. These children had a rather decreased complement of adipose cells, but not as few as the low birthweight children. This suggests that the 'insult' to adipose cell replication came later in the period of development than in the other group.

Dr. Galton. Is it not somewhat misleading to use the term 'critical period' in the development of the adipose organ? I thought that critical periods of development were when cells were laid down, final numbers were established and no further change could then occur. Surely, hypercellularity at different stages in development is not the same as critical periods; for instance, during liver development there will be hypercellularity as the liver forms but, at any stage during adult life, the liver can be regenerated and new liver cells made. Is the adipose organ not more like this, in that at any stage in adult life fibroblasts can be recruited to form adipocytes? In fact, it is true to say that there is no one period when the adipose organ is being laid down.

Dr. Brook. You may well be right. There are many opinions. Dr. Salans' data do not suggest that this is true but I do not think it is an 'open and shut' case. I do not agree with your interpretation of the meaning of 'critical period', but this is a semantic argument, rather than an actual medical difference of opinion.

Dr. Craddock. As a family doctor I am convinced that the best place at which to start the prevention of obesity is during the ante-natal period. In my own experience well over half of ante-natal patients have needed modification of their diet to prevent excessive weight gain during pregnancy. This is the time to inculcate good eating habits in the mothers, who will then inculcate good eating habits in their children.

Dr. Brook. Did you find that an excessive weight gain in pregnancy makes any difference to the birthweight and adiposity of the infants born?

Dr. Craddock. There has been some difference of opinion about this in the literature. I think it is accepted generally now that an excessive weight-gain in pregnancy leads to a heavier child in developed countries.

Dr. Brook. The published information is poor.

Dr. Björntorp. Figure 7.11 shows data from two groups of obese subjects; we have called them hypertrophic and hyperplastic obesity, using rather arbitrary limits. We measured average fat cell size in the abdominal, femoral and gluteal regions of subjects who were matched for age, sex and body fat. The hypertrophic obese patients showed an increase of fat cell size in all three regions. In the hyperplastic subjects, however, there was an increase in the abdominal region only. Thus, there is a difference in size and metabolism in different regions in different groups as well as large variations in individuals as Dr. Salans has pointed out.

Dr. Lloyd. There seems to be a general feeling that it is extremely dangerous to be a fat baby; this may be true, but we do not have very much data to support this. Work in Sheffield has been quoted to show that a fat baby becomes a fat child. We have already heard that

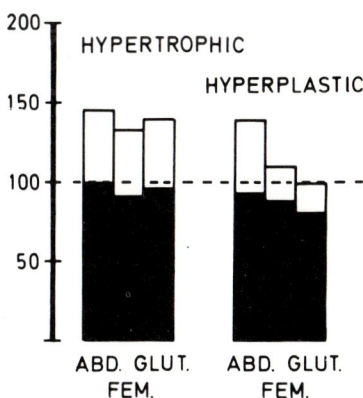

Figure 7.11

the Scandinavian data do not support this. However, if the Sheffield information is read carefully, the facts are that the majority (80 per cent) of fat babies are not apparently fat at school entry. I use the word 'fat' with some hesitation because all this is based on weight data and I am uneasy about talking in terms of weight alone. Only 20 per cent of fat babies become fat children. This is in keeping with the prevalence data, suggesting that in Britain today perhaps 20 to 25 per cent of babies are too fat but, in the school years, before the pubertal spurt is reached, the figures are about two to five per cent. A quick sum shows that this fits rather well. It is known that, after puberty and in adult life, the prevalence of fatness increases to over 20 per cent. We do not know, however, whether it is the fat babies who have thinned, who become fat later. Perhaps we could spend our time more profitably considering what it is about these thin children, who were fat as babies, which enables them to become thin during the childhood years. We may learn more about the total problem of prevention of obesity from a study of this group than from the fat child who is a very unrewarding subject for study.

Dr. Stowers. Relating to Dr. Lloyd's remarks, I should like to give some data in connection with the implications of birthweight. We have been testing for diabetes in pregnancy in Aberdeen, using obesity of the mother as an indication for test. Our data go back 30 years and we have looked at the birthweights of these same mothers. We find that six out of seven of the mothers who had a birthweight above the 85th centile became diabetic during pregnancy, whereas only one in over 20 of those of normal birth weight developed diabetes when pregnant.

Professor Yudkin. I suppose that we are back to the question whether a high birthweight is an index of obesity.

Dr. Quaade. I know from my own studies that there can be no doubt that obese children were very often heavy at birth. A birthweight of over 4 kg correlated highly with obesity in childhood. Overweight in children also correlates highly with obesity in parents. It is safe to assume that a lot of adipose tissue is laid down in intrauterine life and, in my opinion, adipose cells may be laid down for reasons of thermal regularity in early life.

Dr. Ashwell. I have noticed that many women, when interviewed, say that they gained weight when pregnant. Is it possible that pregnancy is one of these critical periods when hypercellularity occurs?

Dr. Brook. I do not think we know.

Dr. Lemonnier. We have carried out experiments in which a high fat diet was given to adult rats *ad libitum*. The diet was started at

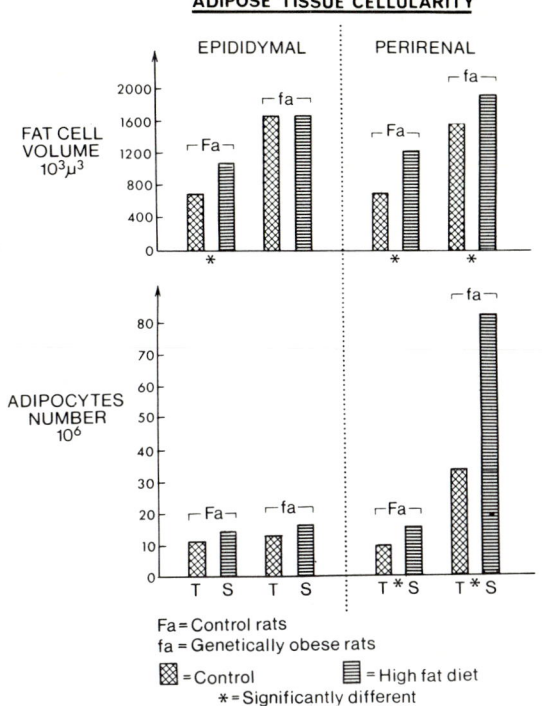

Figure 7.12

five months of age and continued for a further seven months. At one year of age we investigated the cellularity of these animals. Figure 7.12 shows the cell size and cell number of the control group of animals. When this group was fed a high fat diet there was an increase in cell size but no change in cell number. Investigation of the perianal adipose tissue of the same animals showed an increase in cell size and also in cell number. This experiment suggested that fat cells may increase in adult animals when a high fat diet is given. The second group, shown in the figure, represents genetically obese animals. Feeding this group a high fat diet produced an increase in cell size and no change in cell number in the epidermal site. In the perianal adipose tissue, as Dr. Bray has shown in subcutaneous tissue, there is an increase in cell size and an increased cell number. This suggests that genetically obese animals are very much influenced by a high fat diet. The influence of genetics and diet on fat cell number is strikingly different at different sites.

REFERENCE

MELLBIN, T. & VIRILLE, J-C. (1973) Physical development of children 7 years of age in relation to velocity of weight gain in infancy with special reference to incidence of overweight. *Brit. J. Preventive & Soc. Med.*, 27 (4), 225.

8. Psychological and Social Factors in the Pathogenesis of Obesity

J. T. SILVERSTONE

'If the increase of wealth and the refinement of modern times have tended to banish plague and pestilence from our cities, they have probably introduced the whole train of nervous disorders and increased the frequency of corpulence' (Wadd, 1816).

Thus the concept that obesity is related to psychological and social factors is by no means new. It is only in recent years however that these ideas have been taken up with any enthusiasm. In the 1930's it was usual to attribute obesity to disturbance of the endocrine glands, although such disturbance was very rarely found. It was the absence of any detectable endocrine abnormality which led clinicians dealing with the problem in the 1940's and 50's to follow a more psychological approach. Unfortunately in many cases their enthusiasm got the better of them: all obesity was explained on the basis of emotional disturbance. As this took place in the heyday of psychoanalytic theorizing most of the formulations presented were couched in the idiosyncratic language of the Freudian analyst. For example: 'Neurotic obesity in women is an autoplastic manifestation of various unconscious impulses and egodefenses. Among the former we find derivatives of oral drives aiming at partial incorporation and retention of both maternal and paternal love-objects' (Byochowski, 1950). While it would be foolish to deny the importance of emotional factors in many cases, we must guard against accepting these as the sole explanation.

During the last decade or so, experimental psychologists and epidemiologists have begun to make their own contributions; these question psychodynamic perturbations being the only, or even the most frequent, factors in the pathogenesis of obesity. As we shall see, social and perceptual aspects of the problem also play a very large part.

Emotional aspects of the problem will, however, be discussed before consideration is given to some of the more recent psychological and sociological findings.

EMOTIONAL FACTORS

The present position of those who hold the view that emotional factors are all-important in the aetiology of obesity has recently been summarized by Kiell (1973) in his introduction to a series of papers on the psychology of obesity: 'However obesity may be defined, there is now general agreement that persistence in overeating has its basis in unresolved emotional problems and that the overeating serves as a substitute for other satisfactions . . . a more enlightened outlook perceives the adipose person as the victim of social and unconscious forces which compel him to persist in a repetitive, self-destructive pattern'.

If neurotic conflicts were the basic pathogenic factor in obesity, we might reasonably expect to find that the obese were generally more emotionally reactive (neurotic) than non-obese. This is not the case; neuroticism was found to be no higher among obese subjects than among those of normal weight (Silverstone, 1968). That is not to say that a proportion of obese people do not overeat in response to stress; what it means is that it is only a proportion of the obese who do this. We do not know why some people turn to eating when they get upset, while others turn to alcohol, or to smoking, or to their general practitioners for tranquillizers. Hilde Bruch (1957) suggested that certain households are highly preoccupied with the subject of food. Not only is food proferred in abundance; food, particularly sweets, is seen as a short-term panacea for all emotional distress and minor physical trauma. One can almost hear the over-concerned, over-protective mother urging her child: 'Here, have a sweet, you'll feel better!'. Bruch suggested that such situations breed obesity because the child learns to use food as an anxiety reducer. In addition to food being proferred in times of stress, refusal of food can cause disappointment, even resentment in the person offering the food, usually a mother; this will in turn set up feelings of guilt in the reluctant recipient. Thus a particular pattern of learned reactions towards eating is set up in the mind of the child brought up in an atmosphere in which food is given such importance.

Highly emotionally reactive individuals (commonly referred to as 'neurotic') will feel under emotional strain a great deal of the time; if they are also people who have learned to turn to food whenever they become anxious or upset then they will be prone to seek solace in food very frequently; they will consequently eat more than they physiologically require, and they will become fat. This type of obese patient presents considerable problems in management, for not only do they have to exert the self-denial required of all dieters, they have to do this in the face of repeated stresses which they are no longer able to relieve by food. Probably as a consequence of these difficulties neurotic obese patients tend to do less well in weight reducing programmes than non-neurotic patients (Silverstone & Cooper, 1972; Stunkard & Solomon, 1965).

PERCEPTUAL DISTURBANCES

In most people eating occurs as a response to, and is modified by, the sensation of hunger. Furthermore, it has been clearly established that at a given meal the hungrier the person feels the more he eats (Silverstone, 1967). Thus the time of eating, and the quantity eaten, are largely determined by the degree of hunger present; this in turn would appear to be a reflection of certain underlying physiological mechanisms including gastric motility, arterio-venous glucose levels and skin temperature, all influencing the activity of the hypothalamic feeding and satiety centres. While this close relationship between hunger and eating can at times be over-ruled by psychological and social factors, such as the insistence by a hostess to consume yet more of the food she has prepared, or the rapid adaptation in eating patterns which can occur when changing from one time zone to another (Silverstone, 1972), it generally holds true most of the time for the majority of the people.

In contrast, there are certain fat individuals who do not seem to relate eating to physiological hunger. Their eating, instead of being influenced by internal bodily events, occurs entirely in response to external sensory cues—they have an abnormality of perception in that they do not perceive hunger in response to the same signals as do normal subjects. As a consequence of their lack of experience in linking physiological signals to hunger these fat people are not very good at judging how much they have eaten (Bruch, 1961, 1964), nor do they associate feeling hungry with the onset of fasting gastric motility in the same way as normal subjects (Stunkard, 1959). Thus the signalling mechanisms which normally initiate both the cessation of eating and the onset of eating become blunted. In a series of ingenious experiments, Schachter (1968, 1971) examined further the relationship between eating and food cues in obese and in normal subjects. In one experiment he recorded how many crackers his subjects consumed when ostensibly taking part in a 'taste' experiment. He included two experimental conditions: in one the subjects were given roast beef sandwiches beforehand, in the other condition they were not. While the normal weight students ate fewer crackers after they had been fed, the obese subjects ate just the same amount in both conditions. In another experiment subjects were asked to help themselves to roast beef sandwiches while supposedly waiting for some other investigation to take place (the true investigation was related to eating, and the only measurement taken was the number of sandwiches eaten). Again, there were two conditions; in one there were three sandwiches on the plate, in the other only one sandwich. In both situations the subjects were told that there were more sandwiches in the refrigerator and that they were free to help themselves. The normal weight subjects ate an average of just under two sandwiches whatever the number on their plates, the obese subjects on the other hand ate almost twice as much when they had three sandwiches in front of them than when they had one. Schachter's conclusions from these findings are as follows: 'Eating by the obese seems unrelated to any internal, visceral state, but is determined by external, food relevant areas such as the sight, smell and taste of food ... for normals these external factors clearly interact with internal state'. While Schachter's experiments are of considerable interest, not least for the deviousness of their design, the results can be applied with any confidence only to the population of obese people he actually studied; they were University students in New York City. To generalize from this highly selected group to the whole spectrum of obesity is, I believe, unwarranted. Schachter has also speculated, on the basis of similarities noted between his obese subjects and those reported as occurring in rats which have become obese as a result of hypothalamic lesions, that distorted eating behaviour may be due to brain lesions of some kind (Schachter, 1971). Confirmation or otherwise of these provocative ideas must wait more detailed analysis of hypothalamic function in obese humans. While it could well emerge that certain fat people do have an underlying disturbance in their central nervous system, I think it highly unlikely that this will explain the majority of cases of obesity, particularly in those whose obesity comes on after the age of 30, but this will be discussed later. Furthermore, recent experiments have cast some doubt on the postulated differential abilities of normal and obese subjects to detect internal cues; neither were able to tell high calories from low calorie liquid meals (Wooley *et al,* 1972).

SOCIAL FACTORS

Although most experimental psychologists have concentrated on the younger obese subjects, and certainly they are the most emotionally affected by their overweight, obesity is in fact much commoner among those over 30, and even more so among those over 40. In a recent epidemiological survey undertaken in the London Borough of Richmond the prevalence of significant obesity in the population was three times greater among those over 30 than those under 30 (21 per cent: 7 per cent) (Baird *et al,* 1974). This finding is in broad agreement with other epidemiological studies undertaken both in London (Silverstone *et al,* 1969) and in New York (Goldblatt *et al,* 1965).

The prevalence of obesity also varies with social class; obesity is found twice as often among those of lower socio-economic status and the difference is particularly marked in the case of women. What emerges from these epidemiological data is the finding that within urban communities in the United States and in Britain (and probably in the rest of Europe) obesity is most common among middle-aged working class women, and far less common among younger women, and among those from the upper social classes, whatever their age. A similar pattern is emerging in the case of children; the less privileged are more likely to be fat (Howard *et al,* 1971; Whitelaw, 1971).

These variations in the prevalence of obesity between different social classes are more likely to reflect general social pressures than individual metabolic disorders or psychological disturbances. One explanation of these findings incorporates the notion that, while we all tend to put on weight as we grow older, more people in the upper social classes care enough about such weight gain to do something about it. In other words it is not the tendency to become fat, but the concern with being overweight, which distinguishes women of the upper socio-economic classes from their less advantaged contemporaries. There is some evidence to support this view; McKenzie (1967) showed that at a given time twice as many English women in the upper social classes (22 per cent) were actively dieting to lose weight as were doing so in the lower social classes (11 per cent); the same holds true for American women (Dwyer *et al,* 1970). This differential response to overweight probably not only implies a greater understanding by social classes I and II that obesity is a health risk, but also reflects a differential set of social expectations. While, as Hilde Bruch remarked, in our society at the present time 'Slenderness is next to Godliness', this is not true for other cultures. Where we, or at least our fashion photographers, require even more stick-like women, other cultures demand the opposite. Certain East African tribes started to fatten their girls up from the age of eight, the king's harem containing the fattest women in the tribe (Powdermaker, 1960). Such cultural patterns are likely to reflect economic as well as aesthetic differences between one society and another. Where famine is frequent, and mere subsistence the rule, corpulence is a sign of wealth and status; and until recently it was a sign of relative health, or at least a reassurance that pulmonary tuberculosis, an ever prevalent danger, had not set in. Both food and health were until very recently bound up with wealth and status in our society; it is likely that those in the lower socio-economic groups remember, more vividly than the better off, the privations of poverty and the ravages of tuberculosis; they are thus less likely to feel so impelled to emulate the current standards of slimness.

These epidemiological observations assume some importance when we come to the treatment of obesity. It is very unlikely that a plump, middle-aged woman whose family say they prefer her that way and who cannot believe that she is in any way at risk, will accept with any enthusiasm advice to lose weight. Until it is socially unacceptable to be overweight amongst older women of social classes IV and V, the differences in prevalence of obesity will remain, and despite exhortation from their doctors, such women will resist attempts to get them to reduce their weight. This differential attitude is reflected in success rates among dieters from different social classes: those from social classes IV and V do less well than those from classes I and II (Brereton, 1967).

CONCLUSION

Although obesity is the most common nutritional disorder in our society, its pattern of distribution within that society is far from uniform. Therefore when coming to formulate general principles we must take care to remember that any one explanation is unlikely to suffice for all cases.

I would suggest that, rather than try to establish one all-embracing theory, we should seek out the differences which distinguish one type of obesity from another. On the basis of our findings we may then begin to refine our classification of the condition to the point where we have sufficient understanding of each type to point to the pathogenic factors underlying it. This in turn will allow a more rational approach to treatment, with a greater chance of success than has been possible up till now.

REFERENCES

BAIRD, I.McL., SILVERSTONE, J.T., GRIMSHAW, J.J. & ASHWELL, M. (1974) The prevalence of obesity in a London borough. *Practitioner*. 212, 706.

BRERETON, P.J. (1967) Some observations on obese patients. Paper read to *British Dietetic Association's Symposium on Obesity*. London.

BRUCH, H. (1957) In *The Importance of Overweight* New York: Norton.

BRUCH, H. (1961) Conceptual confusion in eating disorders. *J. Nerv. Ment. Dis.* 133, 46.

BRUCH, H. (1964) Psychological aspects of overeating and obesity. *Psychosomatics*, 5, 269.

BYCHOWSKI, G. (1970) On neurotic obesity. *Psychoanalyst. Rev.*, 27, 301.

DWYER, J.T., FELDMAN, J.J. & MAYER, J. (1970) The social psychology of dieting. *J.Hlth. Soc. Behav.*, 11, 269.

GOLDBLATT, P.B., MOORE, M.E. & STUNKARD, A.J. (1965) Social factors in obesity. *J. Amer. Med. Ass.*, 192, 1039.

HOWARD, A.N., DUB, I. & McMAHON, M. (1971) The incidence, cause and treatment of obesity in Leicester schoolchildren. *Practitioner*, 207, 662.

KIELL, N. (1973) In The *Psychology of Obesity*, Springfield: Thomas.

McKENZIE, J.C. (1967) Profile on slimmers. *Commentary*, 9, 77.

POWDERMAKER, H. (1960) An anthropological approach to the problem of obesity. *Bull. N.Y. Acad. Med.*, 36, 285.

SHACHTER, S. (1968) Obesity and eating. *Science*, 161, 751.

SCHACHTER, S. (1971) Some extraordinary facts about obese humans and rats. *Amer. Psychologist*, 26, 129.

SILVERSTONE, J.T. (1967) The measurement of hunger in relation to food intake. *Proc. 7th Int. Congr. Nutr., Hamburg*, Oxford: Pergammon.

SILVERSTONE, J.T. (1968) Psycho-social aspects of obesity. *Proc. Roy. Soc. Med.*, 61, 371.

SILVERSTONE, J.T. (1972) Psychology of appetite. *Acta. Diabet. Latina*, 9, supple. 1.

SILVERSTONE, J.T. & COOPER, R.M. (1972) Short-term weight loss in refractory obesity. *J. Psychosom. Res.*, 16, 123.

SILVERSTONE, J.T., STUNKARD, A.J. & GORDON, R.P. (1969) Social factors in obesity in London. *Practitioner*, 202, 682.

STUNKARD, A. (1959) Obesity and denial of hunger. *Psychosom. Med.*, 21, 281.

STUNKARD, A. & SOLOMON, J. (1965) Psychiatric and somatic factors in the treatment of obesity. *J. Psychosom. Res.*, 9, 249.

WADD, W. (1816) In *Cursory Remarks on Corpulence*, London.

WHITELAW, A.G.L. (1971) The association of social class and sibling number with skinfold thickness in London schoolboys. *Human Biol.*, 43, 414.

WOOLEY, O.W., WOOLEY, S.C. & DUNHAM, R.B. (1972) Can calories be perceived and do they affect hunger in obese and non-obese humans? *J. Comp. Physiol. Psychol.*, 80, 250.

DISCUSSION

Professor Adadevoh. I am a little concerned about the lack of reference to parity and to the pattern of obesity. We have already commented that there is a need to prevent obesity in the ante-natal clinics and that there is an increase in weight in women during pregnancy.

Dr. Silverstone. In our society parity tends to be higher in lower social class women, and this may be a factor although we have not examined it.

Dr. Bray. Dr. Silverstone, could you expand a little on Dr. Schachter's work? He has been very provocative in his thesis which suggests that environmental factors may be more important than internal factors in the regulation of food intake in obese humans. This work has had a practical application in Richard Stuart's use of behavioural modification for the treatment of obesity. You seem to imply that there is evidence now that Schachter's hypothesis may not be correct, that lean people may be just as sensitive as fat people to environmental cues. There is certainly data to support that. If that is so, where does that leave behaviour modification as an approach to treatment?

Dr. Silverstone. Thin people are just as insensitive to food cues, or to measuring their own calorie intake, as fat people. I do not think it necessarily leaves behaviour modification out on a limb. It may apply to some but not to all fat people. Schachter explains all obesity in this way and, in my opinion, this is where he is wrong. Behaviour modification, as practised by Stuart, is a mixture of commonsense, Pavlovian conditioning and operant conditioning. As such, it helps some people. I do not think it is based on Schachter's work entirely, in fact, it arose before Schachter had published his work. It arose from work in Nuremberg where it was stated that the behaviour which should be controlled is eating, so this is where we should attack. It was a swing away from the psychodynamic formulation of psychiatrists which says that eating is only a symptom of an underlying unconscious conflict. It is known that animals' behaviour can be affected, by shaping, by reward, by punishment; so why not try this with man? This was done with some moderate success. Stuart took up this with great enthusiasm and published eleven cases, all of whom did remarkably well with this amalgam of various approaches, which he says are based on scientific learning principles.

Dr. Galton. Do you think that you have underestimated the role of neuroticism in this case? In an obesity clinic, one receives the impression that many of the people attending are neurotic. We use the Eysenck personality inventory, which, I assume, is similar to the Cornell Medical Index, in order to assess neuroticism. It seems to me that the questionnaire asks the wrong questions, the questions related to the growth of sociability, rather than exploring localized areas of neuroticism in relation to food, feeding behaviour and eating. Does the Cornell Medical Index remedy this deficit?

Dr. Silverstone. The Cornell Medical Index is concerned mainly with emotional-type symptoms, such as sweating, etc. Like the

Eysenck Scale, it measures two things. It measures not only neuroticism but also extraversion and intraversion, or, if you like, sociability. The end score is picked out by concerning yourself with certain questions only; this is the whole point of Eysenck's Scale. Another point is that people who go to hospital, for whatever cause, are rated as more highly neurotic than people who do not. Some years ago, McCance from Aberdeen studied outpatients at St. Thomas's Hospital and showed that those attending the obesity clinic were no more neurotic than those attending the general medical clinics. However, they were much more neurotic than a random sample of the population. Thus, hospital attenders, in this sense, tend to be classified as more neurotic.

Dr. Durnin. One generally assumes that if neuroses are a strong component in the development of obesity, this leads to over-eating. The assessment of over-eating worries me because I do not think that over-eating can be dissociated from energy balance. It is possible to over-eat, yet to eat relatively small amounts of food. We have recently finished an analysis of two studies. These were cross-sectional studies of 611 adolescents; 200 were measured seven years ago and 400 about one year ago. We measured the food intake of all of these children over seven days, by means of a weighing technique, and we also measured their body fat. There were some rather surprising results. There are gross differences between boys and girls. The boys showed quite confusing results in almost all parameters, as compared to the girls. However, the fattest girls had food intakes which were very much less than those who were lean. If the fattest 10 per cent were compared to the 10 per cent who were least fat, it was found that the thinnest girls ate about 2,200 Kcal/day and the fattest girls about 1,700 Kcal/day. This just does not fit in with the general theory that many of these girls might be neurotic, and might be over-eating.

Dr. Silverstone. One of the points I tried to make was that neuroticism is by no means the major cogent factor. I think it is a factor in some adults who say that they put on weight when they are upset. Other adults say the opposite. There is this sub-group which puts on weight when upset and it is they who have the greatest difficulty in losing weight because, if they get upset continually, they turn to food almost without reference to their total energy needs at that moment.

Dr. Anand. Dr. Silverstone mentioned that the external and internal monitoring systems play an important role. To my mind, there are three systems which play an important role in the adjustment of our feeding behaviour. We have an external environmental system which gives us information that food is available; this is one of the primary factors which will determine our feeding behaviour. There is also the internal monitoring system, the hypothalamic and other mechanisms. These systems, however, only play a basic role in producing the subjective feeling of hunger, which is the drive to eat.

In addition, the higher nervous mechanisms, especially the limbic system, have a very marked influence on modulation. Both psychological conditioning and social conditioning, as well as neocortical conditioning, habit formation, etc, will all influence the feeding behaviour pattern greatly. If these become abnormal they will change this modulation system. The limbic effects are mediated ultimately through the hypothalamic region and are bound to affect feeding behaviour. We know that the emotional disturbance of conditioning will not only increase food intake, but sometimes decreases food intake, such as in cases of anorexia nervosa. The internal monitoring system only gives us monitoring in terms of the homoeostatic needs, but this is not the final answer. Human beings are not like rats and other animals, and do not just eat for calories; we have a much higher encephalization. Men may be hungry and still may not eat, or may not be hungry and go on eating. We have a different type of modulation from the higher nervous activity. We have to consider the whole behaviour; external conditioning, internal monitoring and higher conditioning, to give us the total behaviour.

You showed some extremely interesting results about the effect of stomach contractions and blood glucose. I should like to add a few points which fit in well with your findings. It can be shown experimentally in animals that the hunger contractions in the stomach will occur, not only when the stomach is empty, but when there is no triggering of the satiety centre by increased glucose utilization. If the satiety centre is destroyed, increased glucose utilization will not stop the hunger contractions; these will only cease if the satiety centre is being triggered by glucose utilization. When glucose utilization is low, and the stomach is empty, there are two factors, the subjective feeling from the feeding centre and the objective feeling of hunger coming from the contractions from the stomach. This gives the feeling of maximal hunger because of their additive effect. Insulin will only produce an effect by its action on glucose utilization. As long as there is sufficient glucose, then the administration of insulin will increase glucose utilization, and hunger actually decreases. It is only later on that the hunger is increased.

Dr. Silverstone. I agree that it is an extremely complex machine.

Dr. Baird. What percentage of women who are more than 30 per cent above their average weight show either depression or phobic anxiety states?

Secondly, do some very fat subjects become psychologically worse on weight reduction, and is there any way to predict this?

Dr. Silverstone. I do not know the answer to the first question. On the whole, using these questionnaires as a guide, the disturbances do not seem any different from the norm. Nor do I know the answer in relation to very fat people. For moderately fat people, we have some evidence to show that dieting does not seem to increase depression. Following this up for 12 weeks showed no increase in emotional disturbance.

9. Neurological Mechanisms Regulating Appetite

B. K. ANAND

Innate feeding behaviour is gentically determined and is characteristic of the species. The motivated behaviour of feeding depends upon the 'drives' of hunger and satiety which are elicited and reduced directly by changes in the internal environment and are thus homoeostatic in nature. Most basic motivational forces depend upon central nervous regulation which result in drives arising from some physiological needs and these would be true for feeding behaviour also (Anand, 1968, 1970).

Feeding is essential for meeting the energy requirements of the body. Energy balance is brought about by adjustment of four important variables—food intake, stored energy, work and heat production. In maintaining an appropriate equilibrium food intake has to be matched with the other three variables. Ordinarily the energy stored in the fat depots of the body does not change appreciably over long periods and body temperature is maintained at normal levels by adjusting heat loss to heat production. In such situations food intake (energy intake) is adjusted mainly to the metabolic activity of the body (energy utilization) which results in work and heat production (Anand, 1967).

Previously, hunger, appetite and satiety, which one associates with food intake, were often regarded as problems in the domain of the physiology of digestion. Certain theories were put forward to explain adjustment of feeding behaviour either from changes in peripheral blood composition, or from sensory information coming from the alimentary tract. Recent experimental studies, however, have shown that regulation of feeding behaviour is very much a phenomenon operating through the central nervous system (Anand, 1961). Further, it has been shown that essentially the central nervous mechanisms which regulate food intake also obtain precise information about the other three adjustments for energy balance, which are also brought about through the adjoining areas in the central nervous system. Experimental evidence now exists to show that information about both energy intake and energy utilization is provided to the central nervous mechanisms which maintain energy balance and is influenced through feed-back of information about energy utilization and further modulated from needs of the body for maintenance of body temperature.

HISTORICAL

Food intake depends considerably on the sensation of hunger. At the beginning of this century it was not clear whether the sensation of hunger originated at the periphery or was of central origin. The proponents of the 'peripheral' theory speculated that activities of some peripheral structures, probably the stomach, were the prime sources for the feelings and phenomenon of hunger. On the other hand, the proponents of the 'central' theory suggested that the feeling of hunger was mainly due to a certain state of activity of some of the areas of the brain (Anand, 1961).

Peripheral theory

It was observed that the feeling of hunger-pangs was accompanied by rhythmic contractions of the stomach, and that hunger contractions of the stomach were inhibited by intravenous injection of glucose and were strengthened by injections of insulin which lowered blood glucose. On the basis of these observations it was considered that the whole hunger-satiety complex was determined by the presence or absence of activity in gastric musculature.

However, other observations did not fit in with this theory. Nearly complete removal of the stomach, or partial or almost total denervation of the stomach either by vagotomy or splanchnectomy, which eliminate hunger contractions, did not modify hunger sensations, appetite or feeding. Further, physiological variations of blood glucose in man did not closely relate to periods of hunger sensation.

Central theory

Initial theories for effects of the central nervous system on food intake and body weight came from clinical observations on patients with hypophyseal tumours. It was not clear then whether changes in the body weight were due to endocrine disturbances, as a result of pressure effects of tumours on the base of the brain.

With the development of experimental stereotactic techniques, studies on the hypothalamus could be made with greater accuracy.

Hetherington & Ranson (1940) were the first to show that lesions of the medial hypothalamus, independent of the state of the hypophysis, caused obesity in rats. These observations were confirmed by many other workers who further observed that obesity was due to a voracious increase in eating, or hyperphagia. It was only in 1951 that Anand & Brobeck (1951a,b) described for the first time that lesions in the lateral hypothalamus, irrespective of the state of the medial hypothalamus, resulted in a complete cessation of eating, or aphagia, resulting in death from starvation. Thus it became clear that the basic mechanisms which regulate food intake were located centrally, in the medial and lateral areas of the hypothalamus.

EXPERIMENTAL OBSERVATIONS ON ANATOMICAL SUBSTRATES

HYPOTHALAMIC MECHANISMS RELATED TO FEEDING

Anand & Brobeck (1951a,b) found that localized lesions made bilaterally in the extreme lateral hypothalamus at the rostro-caudal plane of the ventromedial nucleus caused complete cessation of feeding or aphagia in rats (Fig.9.1). Thus the lateral hypothalamic area was considered an important locus for providing drives for feeding behaviour and was, therefore, designated as the *feeding*

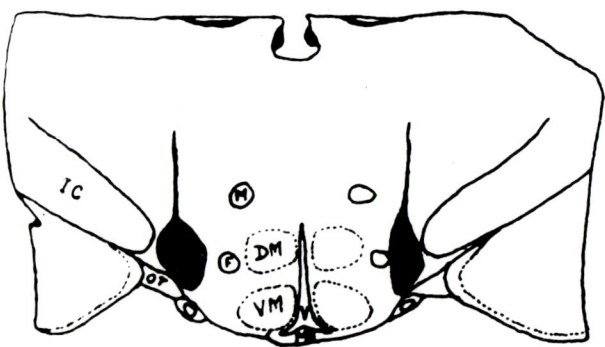

Figure 9.1

Diagram representing a section through rat brain passing through the hypothalamus in the tuberal region (ventromedial nucleus), rostral to the pituitary stalk and caudal to the optic tract. The heavy shaded areas represent bilateral lesions in the lateral hypothalamus (lateral to the fornix and medial to the internal capsule), resulting in complete aphagia and death of the rat due to starvation. The areas of the lateral hypothalamus were, therefore, designated as the 'feeding centres'.
(From Anand & Brobeck, 1951a).

centre. Hetherington & Ranson (1940) had previously shown that lesions of the ventromedial nuclei of the hypothalamus caused obesity in the rat. This was confirmed by Anand & Brobeck (1951a,b) who further observed that lesions restricted to regions lateral to the ventromedial nuclei, but sparing lateral hypothalamic areas as well as the ventromedial nuclei, were enough to cause obesity

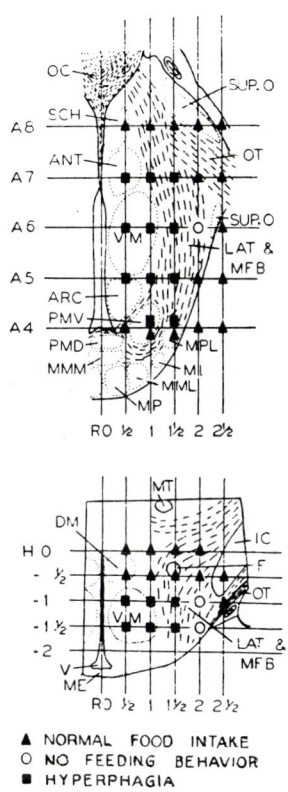

Figure 9.2
Diagram representing the right side of rat hypothalamus in the horizontal plane (upper diagram) and in cross section (lower diagram) at the level of the ventromedial nucleus. Horsley-Clarke coordinates are superimposed. Feeding behaviour of rats with small bilaterally symmetrical lesions in each area is indicated. Lesions in the lateral hypothalamus (LAT) resulted in aphagia, whereas lesions in the ventromedial nucleus (VM) and between VM and LAT resulted in increased food intake and obesity. Lesions in other areas did not produce any changes in food intake. Thus LAT is designated as the 'feeding centre' and VM as the 'satiety centre'
(From Anand & Brobeck, 1951b)

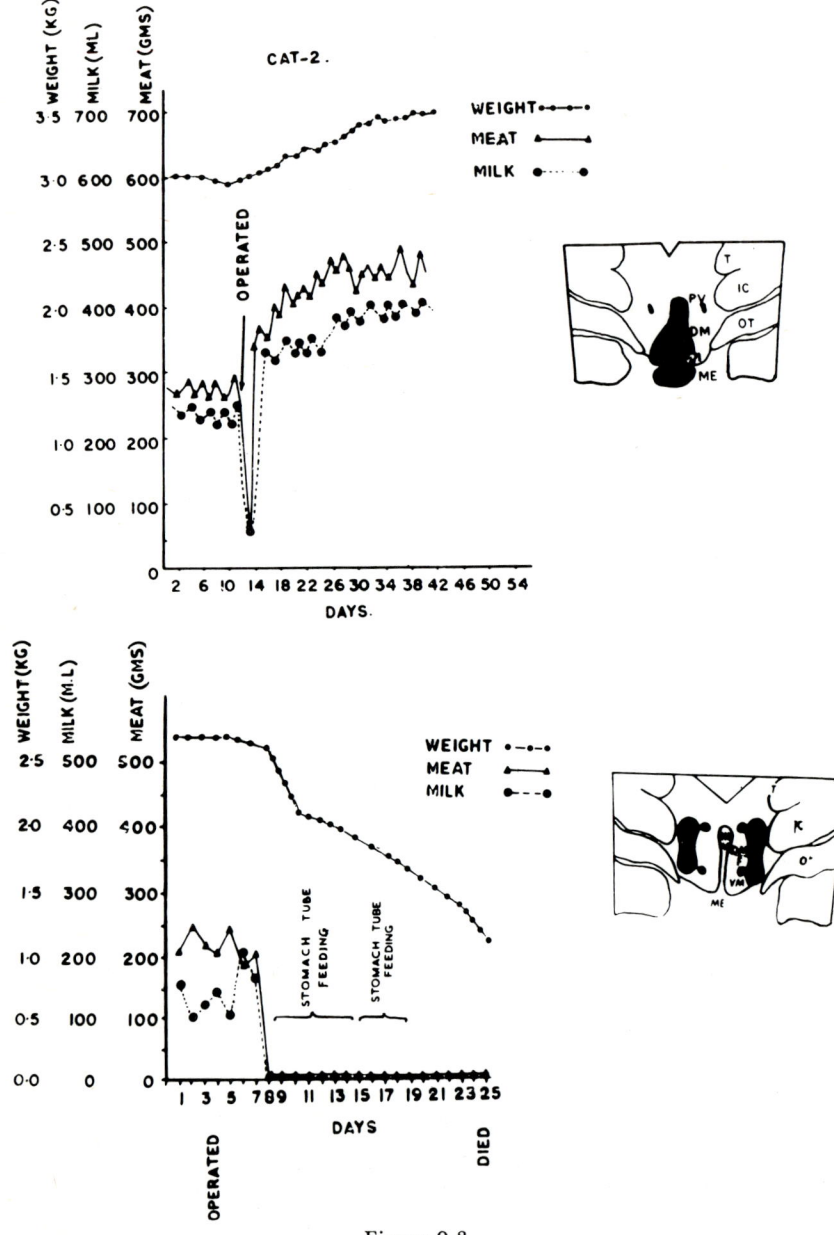

Figure 9.3
Spontaneous food intake and body weights of cats before and after hypothalamic lesions of satiety (upper diagram) and feeding (lower diagram) centres, which resulted in hyperphagia and aphagia, respectively.
(From Anand et al, 1955).

and hyperphagia (Fig. 9.2). It was, therefore, suggested that axons projecting from the ventromedial nucleus to the lateral hypothalamic area were probably interrupted by such lesions. They also found that obese and hyperphagic rats, after lesions of their ventromedial nuclei or their projections, could be made completely aphagic by additional lesions of the lateral hypothalamic area. Thus they established the concept that the lateral hypothalamus or feeding centre is an important area facilitating feeding behaviour and that the ventromedial hypothalamus or *satiety centre* exerts an inhibitory effect on the feeding centre to modulate the drives of feeding behaviour according to the state of energy balance in the body.

Starting with this information, further experimental studies were undertaken which confirmed the existence of the feeding and satiety centres in the hypothalamus of the rat and other mammals such as the cat, dog, rabbit and monkey (Anand *et al*, 1955) (Fig. 9.3).

Opposite effects were observed when these areas were electrically stimulated each day in conscious unanaesthetized animals through chronically implanted electrodes (Anand & Dua, 1955; Delgado & Anand, 1953) (Fig. 9.4). Stimulation of the ventromedial hypo-

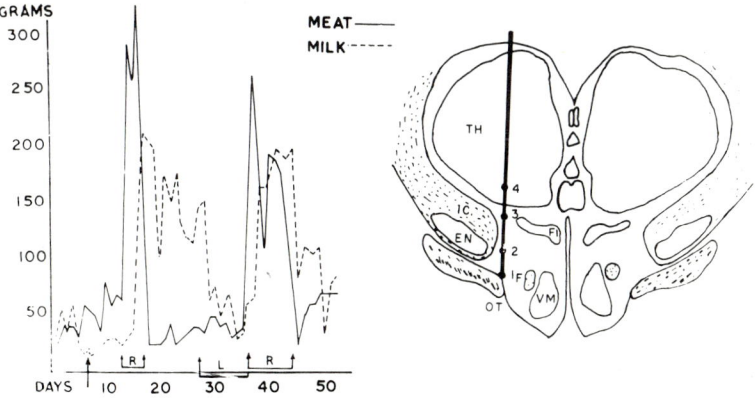

Figure 9.4

Food intake of an unanaesthetized conscious cat with and without electrical stimulation of hypothalamic points through chronically implanted electrodes. On the days the right 'feeding centre' (represented in the diagram on the left) was stimulated for one hour, it resulted in a marked increase in the intake of both meat and milk (represented as R on food intake chart). After cessation of stimulation there was a lag period before food intake returned to the pre-stimulation level. Stimulation of a control point in the left hypothalamus (represented as L on food intake chart) did not result in any change in feeding behaviour.
(From Delgado & Anand, 1953).

thalamus resulted in decreased daily food intake while stimulation of the lateral hypothalamus produced a marked increase in daily food intake. Such results have also been confirmed by several other workers in goats, chickens, rats, cats, etc. Observations in some clinical syndromes such as anorexia nervosa (Singh et al, 1958) and neoplasia provide further evidence that such hypothalamic mechanisms also operate in man.

Additional correlation between hypothalamic feeding centres and feeding behaviour in animals was also observed by recording electrical activities from the regions of feeding and satiety centres during states of hunger and satiation. During the hunger state (starving animal) the EEG activity of the feeding centre is high while that of the satiety centre decreases. Such EEG alterations during hunger and satiety are observed only in the hypothalamic centres and not in the other areas of hypothalamus or other regions of the brain (Anand, 1959, 1960).

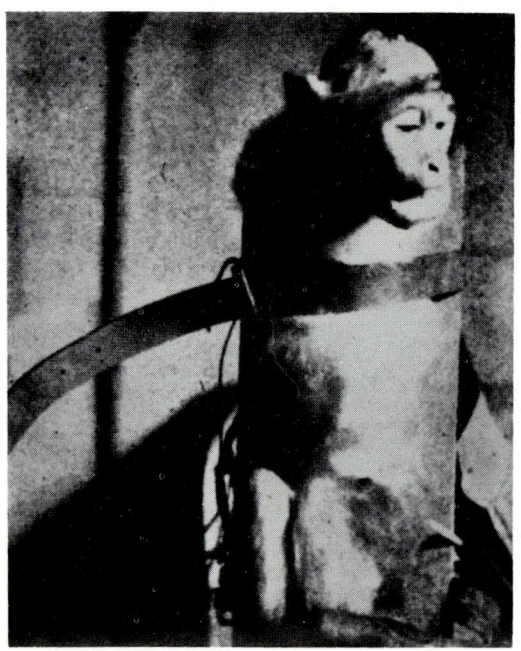

Figure 9.5
Monkey showing protrusion of tongue ('eating automatism') as a result of electrical stimulation of the amygdala.
(From Anand & Dua, 1956).

Limbic Status and Feeding Behaviour

Experimental evidence for the participation of the limbic system in the activity of eating has also been provided. Electrical stimulation of various limbic lobe structures produces eating automatisms: chewing, licking and salivation (Anand & Dua, 1956) (Fig. 9.5).

Lesions of the amygdala cause temporary aphagia for a few days, followed by hyperphagia. The effects of amygdalar lesions are more marked in monkeys than in cats, but these effects last only for a few days, after which food intake returns to normal. Extensive lesions of the temporal lobe are more effective in altering food intake than lesions of the amygdala alone (Anand & Brobeck, 1952; Anand et al, 1958).

Similarly, frontal lobe lesions produce temporary changes in food intake, both hypo- and hyperphagia. Besides being temporary, the quantitative changes in food intake with limbic lesions are less pronounced than those observed with hypothalamic lesions. However, after temporal lobe lesions animals, especially monkeys, show a marked loss in their capacity to discriminate between edible and non-edible objects. These observations imply that limbic areas of the brain modify feeding behaviour through a mechanism based on their capacity to discriminate between edible and non-edible objects, as well as food preferences.

Reticular Formation and Food Intake

Lesions in certain areas of the reticular formation in monkeys also affect food intake (Subberwal & Anand, 1965). Lesions in the region of the red nucleus and surrounding pigmented structures, as well as in the region of the substantia nigra, cause an increase in food intake. Lesions in the caudal reticular areas and medulla however result in a decrease in food intake. Electrical stimulation of rostral medullary regions produces an increase in the daily food intake. Stimulation in the midline areas of the midbrain reticular formation and in lateral areas of the pons cause a decrease in daily food intake.

REGULATION OF ACTIVITIES OF CENTRAL NERVOUS MECHANISMS RELATED TO FEEDING

Signals for the hypothalamic regulating system

I have already stressed that adjustment of food intake to energy expenditure is a hypothalamic function. As a result of feeding, certain changes are produced in the body which directly or indirectly stimulate the activity of the hypothalamic satiety centre and possibly also the higher cerebral regions (Anand, 1962, 1963). The satiety centre, by suppressing the activity of the feeding centre, brings about the state of satiation. Subsequently, when the food eaten is disposed of through conversion to heat, work or some form of stored energy, activation of the satiety centre ceases and the feeding centre becomes more active, leading again to the state of hunger. This concept that satiety is regulated rather than hunger, is further substantiated by the fact that after destruction of the satiety centre the rate of feeding in the feeding period is not much affected, but the animals no longer show a normal satiety period. In spite of great variations in energy expenditure constancy of body weight and reserves indicate the existence of regulatory mechanisms adjusting food intake to energy expenditure (Anand, 1961).

This regulation can be subdivided into two components working within biometrically defined limits. The first, and possibly the more important, regulation is the short-term regulation; the other, operating over a longer period, may correct the errors of the short-term regulation.

SHORT-TERM REGULATION

Various suggestions have been put forward regarding the nature of the change, or changes, produced as a result of feeding, which signal to the regulating system that further feeding should be stopped. Experimental evidence suggests that the principal mechanisms for short-term regulation include, first of all, the afferent nerves coming from the gastrointestinal tract which provide information about the acts of eating, swallowing and the presence of food in the stomach and intestine. Later changes in the internal environment produced as a result of eating provide information about energy balance. Because considerable delay is involved before precise information is supplied through the latter channel, the sensory information from the alimentary tract plays an important role for adjustment of the feeding behaviour as the changes introduced in the *milieu interieur* (Anand, 1962, 1967).

Signals During Intake of Meals

Sensory information from the alimentary tract for adjusting the activity of hypothalamic feeding centres

1. Oropharyngeal afferents

The electrical activity recorded from hypothalamic centres through implanted electrodes before, during and after the act of taking food and its passage through the oropharyngeal region, shows an increase in the hypothalamic satiety centre (Anand, 1961). This suggests that hypothalamic centres are influenced, to some extent at least, by afferent signals coming from the oropharyngeal region. Satiety is probably brought about by signals of oropharyngeal receptors associated with taste, chewing, swallowing, etc.

2. Gastric afferents

The role of gastric nerves in the act of feeding has been a matter of speculation for a long time, and experiments were designed to elicit their role in adjusting the activity of hypothalamic feeding centres. Activity of gastric nerves was evoked experimentally in cats either by electical stimulation or by inflating a balloon within the stomach.

Gastric afferents were activated by the distension of the balloon and the EEG activity of the hypothalamic satiety and feeding centres recorded through stereo-taxically implanted electrodes (Sharma *et al*, 1961). In other experiments the discharge rate of single neurones (units) in these hypothalamic centres were recorded on an oscilloscope (Anand & Pillai, 1967). Gastric distension led to the production of high voltage regular waves and occasional spikes in the EEG

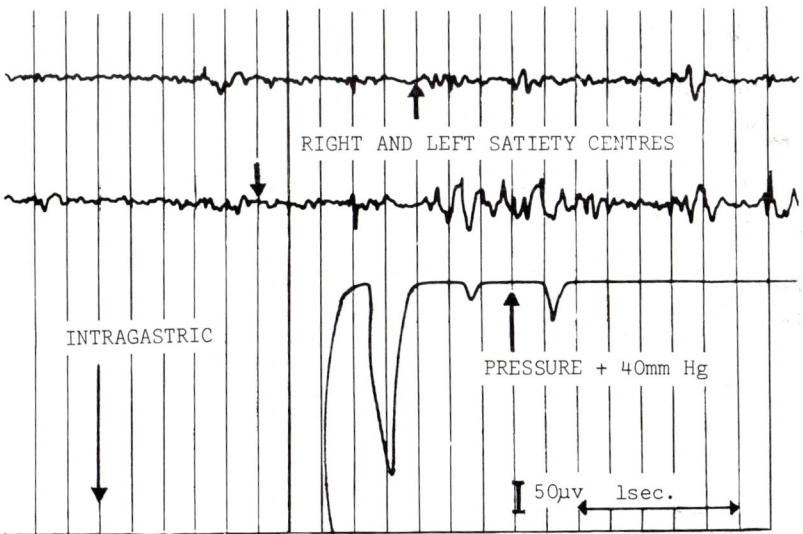

Figure 9.6
Bipolar recording, through chronically implanted electrodes, of EEG activity of left and right satiety centres of a cat. The intragastric pressure was recorded through a water-filled balloon. On raising intragastric pressure to +40 mm Hg, high voltage irregular waves appeared in the EEG of the satiety centres indicating their activation.
(From Sharma *et al*, 1961).

activity of the satiety centre (Fig. 9.6). Similarly, distension of the stomach, or the electrical stimulation of the gastric vagal nerves, resulted in a significant increase in the frequency of discharge of the satiety centre neurones with a simultaneous decrease in the activity of feeding centre neurones (Fig. 9.7 & 9.8). Control procedures involving distension of the peritoneum or stimulation of other afferent nerves did not change the activities of the satiety or feeding centre neurones. Nor did distension of the stomach after cutting the gastric vagal nerves affect the activity of hypothalamic centres. These results indicate that gastric distension brings about satiation through sensory information routed through vagal afferent nerves. Distension of the stomach by means other than food is as effective in bringing about a cessation of eating through activation of the satiety mechanism. However, when the source of such signals is permanently

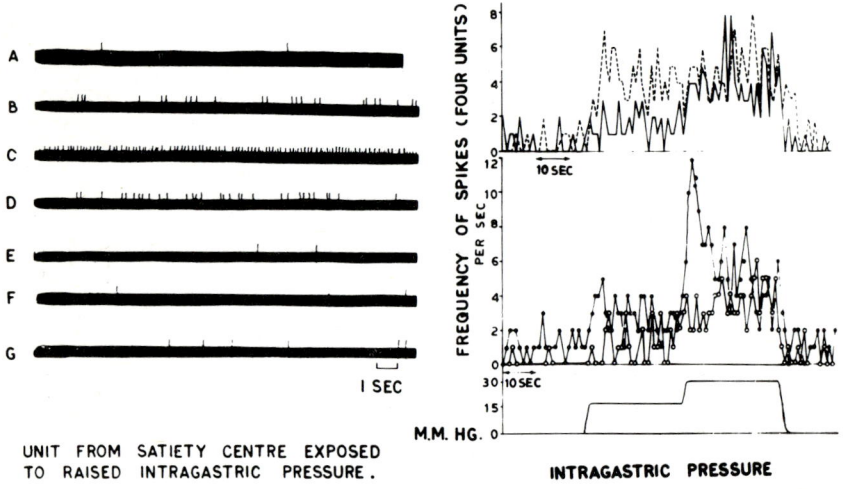

Figure 9.7
Spontaneous unit activity recorded from a neurone in the satiety centre of a starving cat (left diagram) showing effects of gastric distension by intragastric balloon. (A) control; (B) immediately after raising the intragastric pressure to 15 mm Hg; (C) to 30 mm Hg; (D) 5 min after raising intragastric pressure to 30 mm Hg; (E) after deflation of the intragastric balloon; (F) after raising the pressure in the intraperitoneal balloon (control) to 30 mm Hg and (G) on raising the pressure in the intragastric balloon after severing the gastric vagal nerve.
On the right can be seen the spike frequencies of four units from the satiety centre of different cats, correlated with changes of pressure in the intragastric balloon. The approximate linear relationship between the increased spike frequency of the satiety neurones and the intragastric pressure is demonstrated. (From Anand & Pillai, 1967).

interrupted by denervation normal feeding proceeds, indicating that some adaptive mechanism may still be operating.

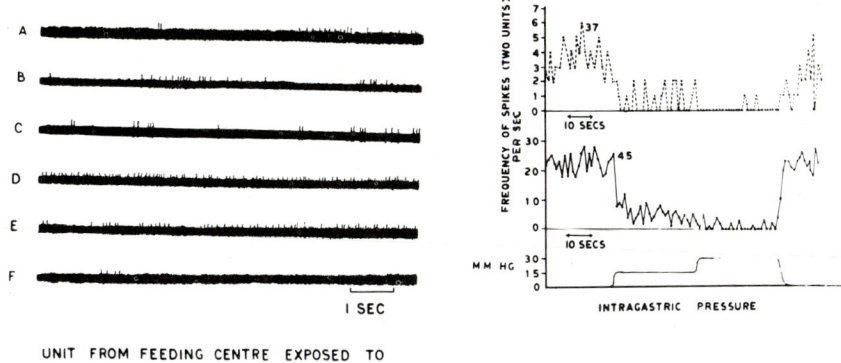

UNIT FROM FEEDING CENTRE EXPOSED TO
RAISED INTRAGASTRIC PRESSURE

Figure 9.8
Spontaneous unit activity recorded from a neurone in the feeding centre of a starving cat (left diagram), showing the effects of gastric distension. (A) control; (B) immediately after raising the intragastric pressure to 15 mm Hg; (C) to 30 mm Hg; (D) after deflation of the intragastric balloon; (E) after raising the pressure in the intraperitoneal balloon (control) to 30 mm Hg and (F) on raising the pressure in the intragastric balloon after severing the gastric vagal nerve. On the right can be seen spike frequencies of two feeding centre neurones, correlated with changes in intragastric pressure. Decreased activity of the feeding centre neurones is related to increased intragastric pressure.
(From Anand & Pillai, 1967).

The relationship between gastric hunger contractions and the electrical activity of the hypothalamic feeding centres was also investigated and it was observed that gastric contractions did not produce any change in the electrical activity of either the feeding or the satiety centre (Sharma *et al*, 1961). On the other hand, increasing the activity of the satiety centre by increasing glucose utilization (see below), by increasing blood glucose or by the use of glucagon resulted in the inhibition of gastric hunger contractions. Injections of glucagon administered after producing lesions in the satiety centre did not inhibit gastric hunger contractions although the blood glucose remained elevated. These experimental studies illustrate the fact that distension of the stomach results in increased activation of the satiety centre, which in turn suppresses the activity of the feeding centre and removes the drive or urge for further eating.

Thus immediately after taking a meal distension of the stomach initiates the mechanism of satiety. This state of satiety is further maintained by digestion and absorption (see below) of food products and their utilization. After some hours when the absorbed materials are disposed of, activation of the satiety centre ceases and the feeding centre becomes active resulting in a subjective feeling of hunger. At this stage, the empty stomach gives hunger contractions, which provide a further objective basis for the feeling of hunger.

Some evidence has also been obtained for the effects of gastrointestinal activity on the electrical activity of areas of brain subserving conscious feelings. It was observed that increasing the pressure inside the gastrointestinal tract produced high voltage slow waves in the orbitofrontal cortex, and low voltage fast activity in the caudate and other areas of the limbic system, simulating awakening responses.

3. Intestinal afferent nerves

The role of intestinal afferent nerves in adjusting feeding behaviour has also been investigated. It is possible that distension of the intestine with food, as well as the products of digestion, may provide signals through baro- and chemoreceptor afferents to the hypothalamic centres. Information is available to suggest that such afferent discharges occur when food is being digested in the intestine, but it is not known what role the signals play in adjusting hypothalamic activity. Evoked electrical responses were recorded from the hypothalamus (Anand *et al* 1970) and other regions of brain during electrical stimulation of intestinal mesenteric nerves (Fig. 9.9). Potentials evoked by stimulation showed regional peculiarities and reciprocal relationship in the negative and positive phases of response from the satiety and feeding centres of the hypothalamus. In the periphery of the satiety centre, potentials were negative-positive and in the remaining parts of the satiety centre they were monophasic negative. Short latency responses were also evoked in extrahypothalamic areas like cortex, thalamus and brainstem by stimulation of mesenteric nerves. These data indicate that sensory information routed via intestinal afferent nerves also influences the activity of the hypothalamic feeding centres.

Infusion of certain products of the digestion of carbohydrates and proteins through intestinal loops resulted in increased discharges through mesenteric nerves. This suggests that some chemosensitive receptors in the intestine sensitive to products of digestion bring about satiation through sensory afferents and thus provide the activating mechanism during the period when gastric distension is complete but when products of digestion have still not been **absorbed.**

BETWEEN-MEAL INFORMATION TO HYPOTHALAMIC FEEDING CENTRES

CHEMOSENSITIVE AND THERMOSENSITIVE MECHANISMS

In response to the absorption of the products of digestion changes are introduced in the internal environment which provide specific information to the hypothalamic feeding centre (Anand, 1962, 1963, 1967, 1972). The ingestion of a single meal is accompanied by a number of changes in the body, both chemical and thermal, and more than one such change may be acting as a signal to the nervous regulating mechanism. Available experimental evidence however suggests that such a regulation is chemostatic and more particularly glucostatic.

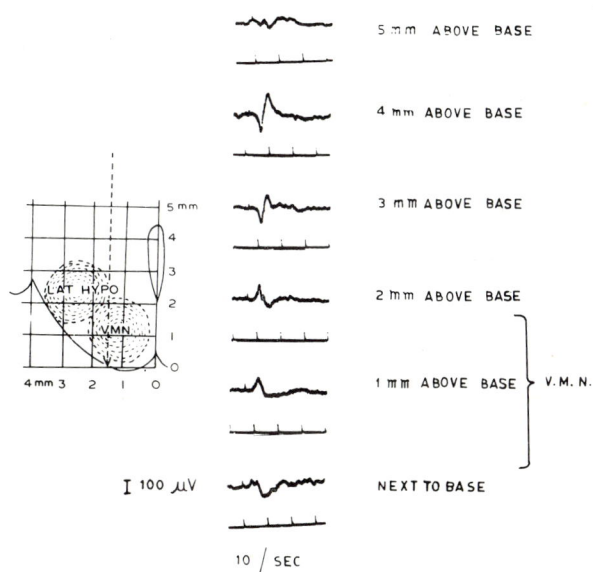

Figure 9.9
Electrical potentials evoked in the hypothalamus during stimulation of the intestinal mesenteric nerve in a cat. The evoked potentials were predominantly of negative polarity in the ventromedial nucleus (VMN) and were negative-positive at the periphery of VMN suggesting projection of mesenteric afferents into satiety centre
(From Anand et al, 1970).

Chemosensitive mechanisms

The hypothalamic centres contain sensitive neurones capable of responding to the chemical signals of the circulating blood, and among the important signals proposed are availability or utilization of glucose, concentration of metabolites related to the size of body fat reserves, the concentration of amino acids and water concentration or shifts among the compartments of the body.

Glucostatic or gluco-sensitive mechanisms. Glucose appears to be an essential, if not the only, source of energy to the nervous system. Animals are hungry where blood glucose concentrations are low and they are satiated by injections of glucose. Raising blood glucose also abolished gastric hunger contractions. During intervals between meals the body content of fats and proteins, which are proportionately enormous, decrease insignificantly, whereas the body's stores of carbohydrate decrease proportionately more. Injections of gold thioglucose into mice cause degeneration of nerve cells in the ventromedial hypothalamus suggesting the presence of cells which concentrate glucose preferentially. From this and other indirect evidence, it appeared that some neurones in the hypothalamus may act as gluco-receptors which sense blood glucose levels and adjust food intake through mechanisms of hunger and satiety.

Electroencephalographic activity has been recorded in unanaesthetized animals through electrodes chronically implanted in the hypothalamic feeding centre and other areas of the brain. Recordings were made at varying intervals after normal feeding and starvation for different periods (Anand *et al,* 1961d). Simultaneously arterial and venous blood glucose concentrations were estimated. It was observed that the EEG activity of the satiety centre increased after feeding, while the activity of the feeding centre simultaneously decreased. On the other hand during hunger there was a significant decrease in the activity of the satiety centre, while that of the feeding centre reverted to normal. Electrical activity of other areas of brain did not show any significant changes during hunger or satiation. It was also seen that changes in the electrical activity of the hypothalamic centre correlated closely with changes in the arteriovenous glucose differences i.e. the degree of glucose utilization, rather than with arterial blood glucose values. Thus, feeding behaviour is related more to the degree of glucose utilization in the body rather than to absolute concentrations of glucose in the circulating blood.

This was confirmed in another series of experiments in which blood glucose concentrations were altered experimentally and the effect on the EEG activity of the hypothalamic centre was studied

(Anand et al, 1961b). Hyperglycaemia produced higher frequency discharges in the EEG activity of the satiety centre whereas the activity recorded from the feeding centre showed a drop in voltage. Conversely, hypoglycaemia slowed the EEG activity of the satiety centre, while the activity of the feeding centre was slightly increased. The EEG activity of other hypothalamic areas or of cortical regions was not altered by these changes of blood glucose. In these experiments also the changes in the electrical activity of the hypothalamic centres were closely correlated with the changes in arteriovenous glucose differences. It was therefore hypothesized that the hypothalamic centres have some specific mechanisms which are sensitive to the level of glucose utilization in the body.

Experiments were also conducted to study the responses to electrical discharges of single neurones belonging to these centres, by the use of stereotactically guided microelectrodes (Anand et al, 1962). Changes in the frequencies of these unit discharges provide

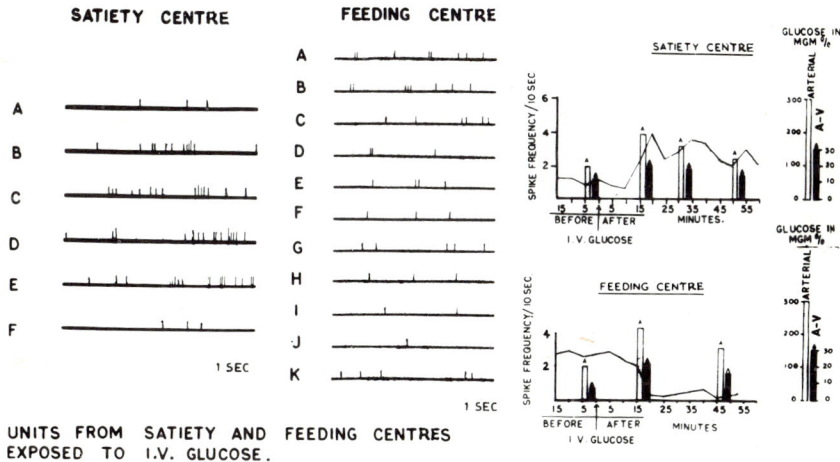

Figure 9.10

The effects of intravenous glucose infusion on single neurone activity of the hypothalamic satiety and feeding centres. On the left are recorded the unit activities from a neurone in the satiety centre and a neurone in the feeding centre, before glucose (A) and at frequent intervals after intravenous glucose infusion (B to K). The activity of the satiety centre unit increased and that of the feeding centre unit decreased, with the rise of blood glucose, but tended to return to pre-infusion levels within an hour. On the right the spike frequencies of a unit from the satiety centre and a unit from the feeding centre are correlated with changes in arterial blood glucose and arteriovenous glucose difference, produced by intravenous infusion of glucose. These also show the inverse relationship between the activities of satiety and feeding centres.
(From Anand et al, 1964).

specific evidence for changes in the functional activity of neurones constituting these hypothalamic centres. Single unit (neurone) potentials were recorded in normal animals in states of hunger and satiety. It was observed that in animals which are not fed for 12 to 24 hours, the unit activity of satiety centre neurones was much higher while that of the feeding centre neurones was simultaneously decreased. These results show a reciprocal functioning of feeding and satiety centre neurones dependent upon the state of hunger or satiation.

Further studies on the discharge rate of single neurones of the hypothalamic centres were carried out when these were exposed to changes in blood glucose and glucose utilization produced by intravenous glucose infusion, or insulin injections, or combinations of both (Anand *et al*, 1964). Discharge rates of these units at different periods were correlated with the estimations of arterial and venous glucose concentrations. After intravenous glucose infusions the frequency of spikes recorded from satiety centre neurones increased and that of feeding centre neurones decreased significantly

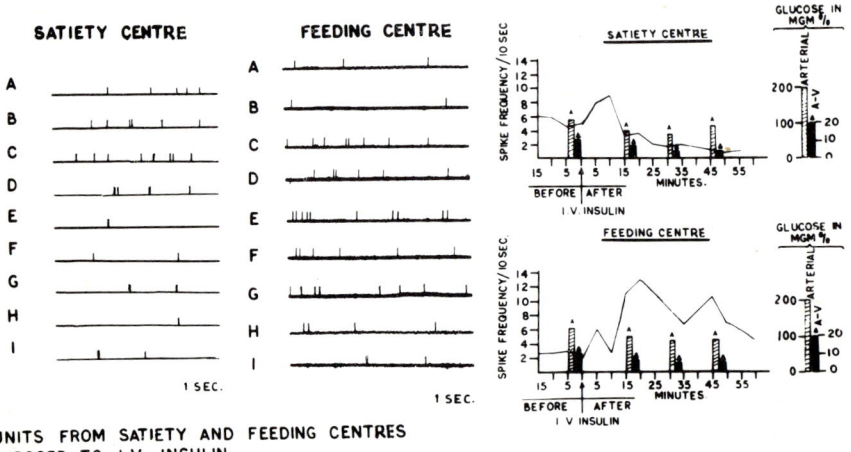

Figure 9.11

The effects of an injection of insulin on single unit activity of the hypothalamic satiety and feeding centres. On the left unit activities from satiety and feeding centre neurones are recorded before insulin (A) and at frequent intervals after insulin (B to I). On the right the spike frequencies of units from the satiety and feeding centre neurones are correlated with changes in blood glucose and arteriovenous glucose difference resulting from the injection of insulin. Insulin hypoglycaemia resulted in increased unit activity of the feeding centre and decreased unit activity of the satiety centre neurones. It should be noted that this effect was produced after 10 to 15 min.
(From Anand *et al*, 1964).

(Figs. 9.10 & 9.11). The changes in the frequency of spike activity occurred within five to 15 minutes after infusion and were sustained for a period of up to one hour and then gradually declined. After intravenous injections of insulin, the spike activity of satiety centre neurones increased initially during the first five to 30 minutes and then decreased. The initial increase of spike activity after an injection of insulin was considered to be due to the insulin facilitating glucose utilization. The subsequent and prolonged decrease of spike activity in the satiety centre after insulin correlated with hypoglycaemia. Unit activity of feeding centre neurones showed an increase after insulin and combined glucose and insulin infusions also produced the expected responses. No significant changes were observed in the unit activity recorded from other hypothalamic and cortical regions. The changes in the unit activity of hypothalamic centres correlate closely with the magnitude of arteriovenous glucose differences. This is demonstrated by the fact that changes in spike frequency of the hypothalamic centres occur five to 15 minutes after injection and not immediately after raising blood glucose.

As estimations of arteriovenous glucose differences provide a measure of glucose utilization in the body but not specifically in the brain, these studies could not differentiate between changes in the activity of hypothalamic centres due to changes of glucose utilization in the neurones themselves or those due to sensory information coming from glucosensitive mechanisms at the periphery. In further experiments the brains of the animals were deafferented by making mid-collicular cuts through the brainstem (Chhina et al, 1971b). The results obtained were exactly the same as with intact nervous system, i.e. increased glucose utilization activated the satiety neurones (Fig. 9.12) and simultaneously inhibited feeding neurones. These results, therefore, indicate that the basis for alteration of the activities of feeding and satiety centres is not dependent on peripheral nervous influences but is the direct result of changes in glucose utilization within the central nervous system. These experiments, however, still do not specifically indicate that the responses may be directly due to changes of glucose utilization in the satiety and feeding neurones themselves.

It was not clear from these experiments whether the inhibition of feeding neurones was in response to activation of satiety neurones which send lateral inhibitory projections to feeding neurones, or whether it was due to the direct effect of glucose utilization on the feeding neurones. Studies were, therefore, conducted in rats in which longitudinal cuts were made stereotactically between the medial (satiety) and lateral (feeding) hypothalamus, and unit discharges of satiety and feeding neurones studied in response to changes in blood glucose and glucose utilization. As the satiety centre was still activated and the feeding centre inhibited to some extent by increased glucose utilization, this indicates that changes in glucose utilization do directly affect the activity of both satiety and feeding centres.

As the above results suggest differences in the level of glucose utilization in hypothalamic feeding and satiety centres during states of hunger and satiety, it was considered important to investigate biochemically whether such a mechanism can be detected. Small pieces of hypothalamic feeding and satiety centre areas of hypothalamus were dissected from monkeys kept in states of hunger and satiety. The brains were frozen in liquid air and processed under hypothermia. The oxygen and glucose uptake of these centres, as

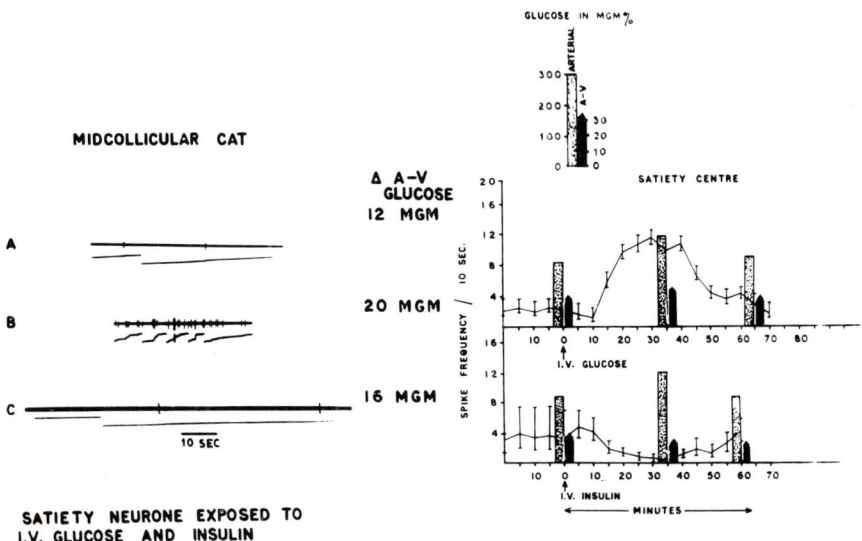

Figure 9.12
The effects of intravenous glucose and insulin on the unit activity of a satiety centre neurone in a deafferented cat. On the left are records of unit activity from a satiety centre neurone before giving glucose (A), 30 min after i.v. glucose infusion (B) and 30 min after i.v. insulin (C). On the right spike frequencies of a satiety centre neurone are correlated with changes in blood glucose and arterio-venous glucose difference resulting from administration of glucose and insulin. The results indicate that responses after deafferentation are similar to those obtained in the intact animal, suggesting that glucose utilization produces its effects directly on the brain and not through peripheral chemosensitive mechanisms.
(From Chhina *et al*, 1971).

well as tissues from other hypothalamic areas, were estimated using the Warburg technique (Anand *et al*, 1961c). The results were expressed per unit of DNA to allow for differences due to variations in cell counts. It was observed that in the fed monkeys uptake of both oxygen and glucose by the satiety centre area was greater than that of the feeding centre area, while in starving monkeys both the glucose and oxygen uptakes were higher in the feeding centre area. These results provide additional confirmation for the presence of gluco-receptor mechanisms in the hypothalamic centres.

The different types of experimental evidence presented above all clearly indicate that there is some kind of chemosensitive mechanism in the satiety centre, which is responsible for increasing the activity of these neurones at the time of increased glucose utilization in the body (Anand, 1967). This also further confirms the hypothesis that energy (food) intake has to be adjusted to caloric requirements and the best information about caloric balance in the body at any time is provided by the level of glucose utilization.

Lipostatic mechanisms. It has been suggested by some workers that the hypothalamic mechanisms are concerned only in the prevention of an overall surplus of energy intake over expenditure which would cause deposition of fat in depots, and that this lipostasis is achieved through sensitivity of hypothalamic centres to varying concentrations of circulating unspecified metabolites related to the size of body fat reserves. To test this, EEG and single neurone recordings from the hypothalamic satiety and feeding centres were carried out and the effects of intravenous infusions of fat emulsion (Lipomul) studied (personal observations). No direct sensitivity of hypothalamic feeding centres to circulating fat contents was demonstrated. However, it has been reported that in subjects consuming adequate carbohydrate NEFA (non-esterified fatty acid) concentrations correlate inversely with glucose utilization and thus are related to the feeling of satiety-hunger.

Mechanisms sensitive to amino acids. As a reciprocal relationship has been suggested by some workers between the serum amino acid concentrations and appetite, studies were also conducted to test the effect of infusions of protein hydrolysate on the EEG as well as single neurone unit activities of feeding and satiety centres (Anand *et al*, 1965). Increasing the amino acid content of circulating blood did not produce any specific change in the EEG or unit activity of the hypothalamic feeding centres. Some increase in the firing rate of anterior hypothalamic osmo-sensitive neurones was observed due to osmotic changes produced by the protein hydrolysate. These electrophysiological studies suggest that the amino acid content of blood does not provide any signals for adjusting the activities of satiety and feeding centres.

Adrenergic sensitive mechanisms. It has been reported that local administration of cholinergic drugs induces drinking while similar treatment with adrenergic substances results in feeding. Experiments were, therefore, performed to study the effects of administration of small quantities of adrenaline crystals into the hypothalamic feeding and satiety centres. It was observed that adrenaline administered to the satiety centre or to the midlateral hypothalamic areas produced a fall in the one hour and 24 hour food intake (Suri *et al,* personal communication). On the other hand, adrenaline administered to the lateral hypothalamic feeding centre area led to a significant increase in food intake. Similar chemical stimulation in other areas of the hypothalamus produced no significant changes. The results suggest that the mechanisms influencing food intake are probably adrenergically mediated.

Thermosensitive mechanisms

Some workers have proposed the concept of a thermostatic or thermosensitive regulation of food intake. They suggest that animals eat to keep warm and stop eating to prevent hyperthermia. This regulation is achieved through small changes in body temperature produced by the specific dynamic action (SDA) of the food eaten, and this extra heat possibly signals to the hypothalamic mechanisms. We performed experiments to record single spike activity from the satiety and feeding centres when they were exposed to localized heat of $0.5°-1°C$ (Anand *et al,* 1966). The data obtained showed that the spontaneous activity of neurones in these centres is not affected in any way by small local changes of temperature. On the other hand, localized heating of anterior hypothalamic neurones increased their firing rates (temperature regulating mechanisms). Similarly, it has been shown that direct local cooling of the anterior hypothalamus results in eating, whereas warming the same area inhibits eating. Thus, the relationship that exists between the specific dynamic action of the ration and the amount of food eaten is probably operating indirectly through the anterior hypothalamic temperature sensitive mechanisms. This demonstrates the integration between the thermosensitive anterior hypothalamic region and the feeding centres in the middle hypothalamus.

It appears then that the hypothalamic mechanisms related to feeding are ordinarily directly influenced through information provided to them about the energy balance through changes in the level of glucose utilization, but that in those circumstances where temperature regulation is upset the heat regulating centres would also influence the nervous mechanisms for feeding.

LONG-TERM REGULATION OF FEEDING BEHAVIOUR

Long-term regulation corrects errors introduced over a period of time through short term mechanisms. That such errors occur is a common observation. Very often, especially in higher mammals including man, food intake does not correspond to energy output and this alters the reserve stores of energy in the body. At the same time, it is well known that most adult men and animals maintain their body weight at the same level, sometimes for years. This indicates that long-term regulation must also be playing an important and precise role. Very little experimental work is available to suggest mechanisms to explain long-term regulation, but it must be based on information provided to the nervous mechanisms from body energy stores, presumably the fat depots. Some experimental evidence has shown that animals may mobilize a quantity of fat each day dependent on, and increasing with, the total fat content of the body.

DRUGS INFLUENCING APPETITE AND FEEDING BEHAVIOUR

A number of pharmacological preparations are used clinically to control weight, or to modify appetite and food intake. Experimental studies were conducted to find out whether these drugs act by directly influencing the activities of hypothalamic feeding centres.

Phenmetrazine

It has been reported that amphetamine depresses appetite. Studies were conducted with phenmetrazine hydrochloride, an analogue of amphetamine, to test its effects on the electical activity of the hypothalamic feeding centres in cats (Anand *et al,* 1961c). Following administration the frequency and amplitude of the electrical activity of the hypothalamic satiety centres was increased. These experimental observations suggest that amphetamine derivatives depress appetite possibly through the activation of hypothalamic satiety centres.

Fenfluramine

This compound has a strong appetite depressing action, without producing any increase in sympathomimetic activity. Its action on the electical activity of hypothalamic feeding centres and food intake was studied in male rhesus monkeys. Fenfluramine in intravenous doses of 1.5 mg/kg body weight produced a gradual increase in the slow wave EEG activity of the feeding centres (Chhina *et al*, 1971a). The effect became more pronounced after subsequent injections and coincided with anorexia and a decrease in food intake. The EEG activity of the satiety centre changed to a low voltage fast response, especially in starving animals. Arteriovenous glucose estimations suggested that the effects of fenfluramine were due to an increase in the level of glucose utilization in the body. Injections in doses of 3 mg/kg body weight produced drowsiness.

Similarly, experiments were conducted to record the effects of infusions containing 1.5 mg/kg on electrical activity of single neurones of hypothalamic satiety and feeding centres and other adjacent

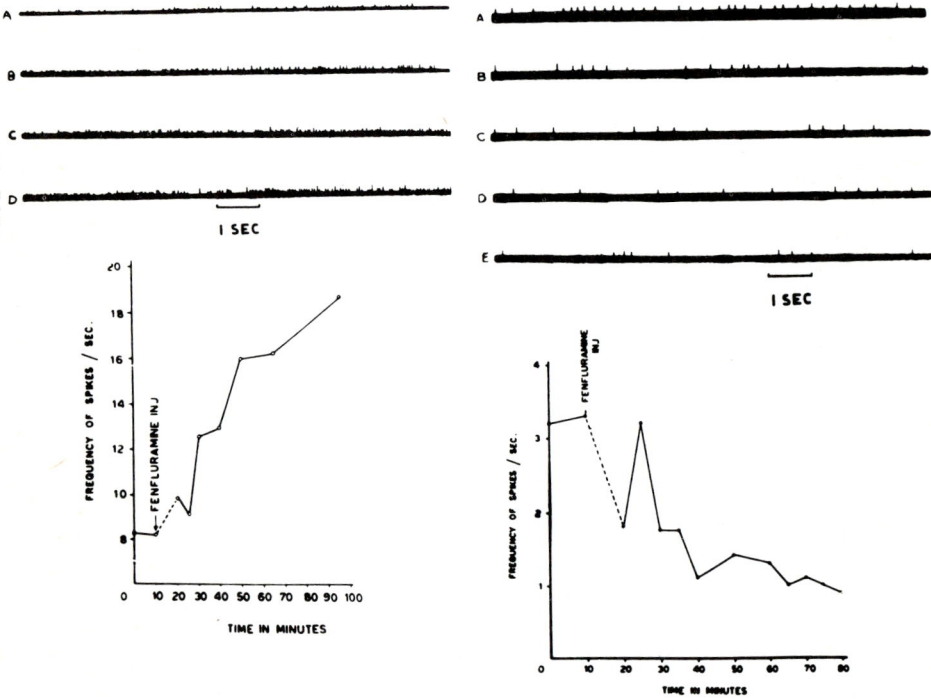

Figure 9.13
The effects of an intravenous infusion of fenfluramine on the unit activity of satiety and feeding centre neurones. On the left are records of unit activity from a satiety centre neurone, before giving fenfluramine (A) and 15 min (B), 30 min (C), 60 min (D) after infusion of fenfluramine. On the right are records of unit activity from a feeding centre neurone, before giving fenfluramine (A) and 10 min (B), 20 min (C), 45 min (D), 60 min (E) after fenfluramine infusion. The lower graph shows average frequencies of these units before and after fenfluramine infusion.
(From Khanna *et al*, 1972).

areas (Khanna *et al*, 1972). The spike frequency of satiety centre units increased while that of feeding centre units decreased. Other hypothalamic units did not show any changes (Fig. 9.13). Simultaneously, the A-V glucose difference also increased indicating an increased level of glucose utilization. Thus, the study demonstrated that fenfluramine may bring about changes in food intake by affecting the hypothalamic centres through change in glucose utilization.

780 SE

This is related to fenfluramine and is an appetite depressing drug. In doses of 7 mg/kg body weight daily it produced similar results on the hypothalamic activities as fenfluramine.

Reserpine

Sympathomimetic drugs also produce alterations of food intake. Clinical observations with reserpine also suggest it has some effect on food intake. Studies were undertaken to find out the effects of this drug on the hypothalamic centres (Anand *et al*, 1961c). No selective effect on the electrical activity of hypothalamic satiety and feeding centres was demonstrated.

Nialamide

Experiments with rats showed that this monoamine oxidase inhibitor when administered in doses of 16 mg/100 g body weight produced a generalized increase in food intake as well as water intake. It did not show any specific effect on the activity of hypothalamic centres.

Tolbutamide

As the hypothalamic centres are strongly influenced by glucose metabolism, the effect of oral antidiabetic drugs on the electrical activity of the hypothalamic areas was also studied. Tolbutamide was injected into the carotid artery of cats and the EEG activity of the hypothalamic feeding and satiety centres recorded (Anand *et al*, 1961c). There was no change in the hypothalamic electrical activity immediately after injection, but when the blood sugar concentration fell there was a selective decrease of the activity of the satiety centre, and a significant increase in the electrical activity of the feeding centre.

Glucagon

This hormone raises blood sugar concentrations. Administration of glucagon to starved animals also decreases gastric hunger contractions. There was no change in the EEG activity of the hypothalamic centres immediately after injection (Sharma et al, 1961). After an hour an increase in the activity of the hypothalamic satiety centres was observed, accompanied by a rise in the blood sugar and arteriovenous glucose difference. I have indicated that glucagon inhibits gastric hunger contractions through activation of the satiety centre and not by acting directly on the stomach.

Cyproheptadine

This antiallergic drug has been found to increase body weight in children. Injections of 2 to 3 mg/kg daily for a week produced increases both in arterial and venous glucose concentrations as well as a decrease in the level of glucose utilization. The EEG activity recorded from the feeding centres showed an increase in frequency of wave amplitude (Chakrabarty et al, 1967). These changes appeared within five to 10 minutes of giving the injections and persisted for about two hours. The change in frequency and amplitude of the EEG became more pronounced on successive days of treatment indicating a cumulative effect of the drug. Increased activity of the feeding centre was eliminated if the animal was allowed to feed.

2-Deoxy-D-Glucose

2-deoxy-D-glucose (2-DG) inhibits glucose metabolism and intracellular glucose utilization, probably by competing with glucose for the hexokinase substrate. Its effect on neurones that are intimately dependent on glucose utilization is therefore likely to be highly pronounced. 2-DG, 100-200 mg/kg body weight, was administered to cats by slow infusion through the carotid artery so that the chemical was available first to the brain. At this dose generalized alterations of blood sugar do not occur. Single unit activity of hypothalamic neurones was simultaneously recorded (Desiraju et al, 1968). These experiments revealed a clear decrease of the electrical activity of the neurones of the satiety centre following administration of 2-DG, and a simultaneous increase of the electrical activity of neurones of the feeding centre. These results confirm that alterations of glucose utilization produce alterations of activity in the hypothalamic satiety and feeding mechanisms specifically, while the activities of other areas of brain are not altered. This also explains the findings of others who have recently shown that administration of 2-DG into the hypothalamic centres produces a marked increase in food intake.

From the various experimental findings presented it appears that most of the pharmacological preparations used to modify food intake produce some of their effects through alterations of glucose utilization in the body, thereby altering the activity of hypothalamic feeding behaviour.

CONCLUSIONS

Experimental data provide evidence for a specific anatomical and functional system for the regulation of food intake located in the hypothalamus. The primary and basic hunger mechanism, located in the feeding centre, provides the drive to eat, i.e. a mechanism of motivation for feeding. Its uninhibited activity results in hunger. Its activity is, however, modulated and influenced from the satiety centre through its lateral projections. The satiety centre acts as an inhibitory 'brake' over the feeding centre. Thus, without the activation of the satiety centre the normal activity of the feeding centre results in a hunger drive. When the satiety centre is activated in response to eating it inhibits the feeding centre, thus eliminating the hunger drive and resulting in the state of satiation.

The limbic and neocortical areas provide a psychosomatic mechanism of modulation on the hypothalamic feeding centres through various anatomical interconnections and functional integrations with the hypothalamic centres. The limbic and neocortical influences provide the innate and conditioned modulations underlying conscious mechanisms of appetite or discrimination and selection of foods for eating. The cortical influences vary according to the evolutionary encephalization of the species.

The hypothalamic and the diencephalic areas act through the lower brainstem and spinal reflex centre to orient the individual for the act of feeding, procurement and preferences of food, as well as in termination of feeding. The influences of brainstem and spinal reflexes in feeding behaviour are vital.

Although lesions of the feeding centre cause an immediate interruption of feeding behaviour, the animal can gradually recover after the initial shock and new nervous mechanisms are established. Rats with feeding centre lesions initially become aphagic and adipsic. However, if such rats are protected from starvation by tube feeding, they recover their eating behaviour, but first prefer to take liquid. Similarly, rats with lesions of their satiety centre also stabilize their food intake after initial hyperphagia. Animals with hypothalamic lesions can still eat because of feeding reflexes operating through the spinal cord and brainstem. These are activated by sensory stimuli which make the animal aware of the presence of food. In fact, the basic feeding responses in the animal can be observed even after complete decerebration. However, for integrated normal feeding behaviour and energy balance, hypothalamic and other diencephalic areas seem to be necessary.

Energy balance in the body is maintained through adjustments of four variables—food intake, work, heat production and stored energy. In maintaining proper equilibrium food intake has to be matched with the other three variables. As energy stored in the fat depots of the body does not change appreciably over long periods and the body temperature is maintained at normal levels, food (energy) intake is mainly adjusted to the metabolic activity of the body (energy utilization).

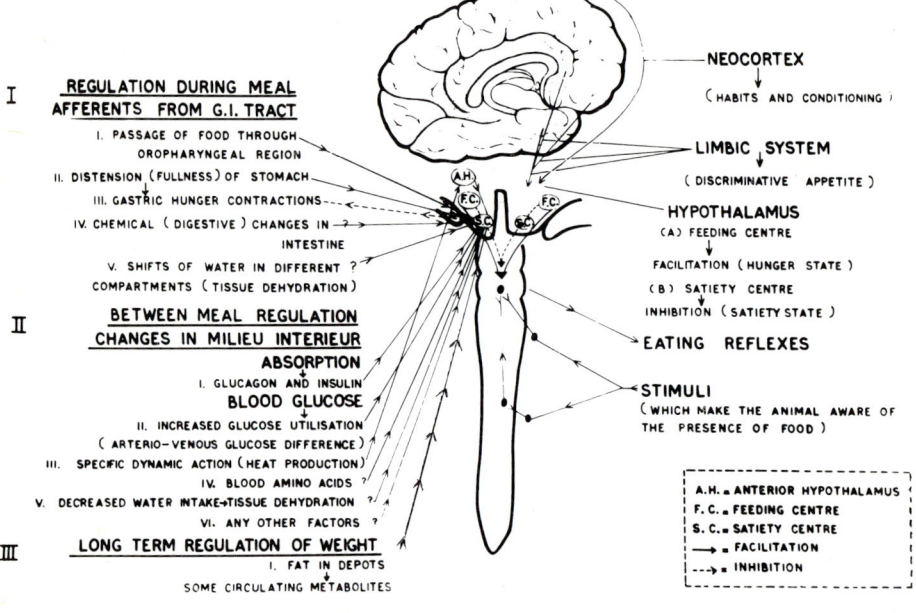

Figure 9.14
Diagrammatic representation of the nervous regulation of feeding behaviour.

Information about both energy intake and energy utilization is relayed to those hypothalamic centres related to feeding (Fig. 9.14). During the food intake, signals pass through afferent nerves coming from the gastrointestinal tract. Food absorption further suppresses feeding in response to chemical changes, mainly the increase in glucose utilization, by activating the satiety mechanisms. It may be that increased heat production in response to SDA and changes in blood amino acid and fatty acid concentrations also trigger the satiety mechanisms, although direct evidence in support is lacking. As these changes disappear, the animal becomes hungry again.

Possibly some long-term regulatory mechanisms are operating to keep the body weight constant over long periods. These mechanisms come into operation whenever stored energy changes.

When body temperature changes food intake is adjusted. This may create situations where demands for increased energy intake may be sacrificed in order to prevent hyperthermia; for example, physical exercise in a hot environment may not result in an increase in food intake to the same extent as such exercise in a cold environment. This calls for integration of the central mechanisms regulating body temperature and those regulating food intake.

Finally, it has been stressed that in spite of the requirements for food intake in response to energy expenditure, feeding is very closely correlated with water exchanges in the body.

It thus appears that the central nervous mechanisms related to feeding are influenced not only by sensory afferent pathways from the alimentary canal and by chemical and thermal changes produced in the body as a result of eating, but also by many other external and internal environmental changes, and thus integrate with other regulating mechanisms in maintaining homoeostasis. These are further influenced from higher nervous mechanisms.

As long as all these mechanisms are in equilibrium energy balance in the body is maintained. On the other hand, when this equilibrium is disturbed either by alteration of nervous mechanisms by metabolic changes or by psychological stresses (higher nervous modulating influences), the resulting energy balance leads to obesity or cachexia.

REFERENCES

ANAND, B.K. (1959) Higher nervous control over food intake. *Proc. XXI Int. Cong. Physiol. Soc.*, 196.

ANAND, B.K. (1960) Nervous regulation of food intake. *Am. J. Clin. Nutr.*, 8, 529.

ANAND, B.K. (1961) Nervous regulation of food intake. *Physiol. Rev.*, 41, 677.

ANAND, B.K. (1962) Influence of metabolic changes on the nervous regulation of food intake. *Proc. XXII Int. Cong. Physiol. Soc.*, 680.

ANAND, B.K. (1963) Influence of the internal environment on the nervous regulation of alimentary behaviour. In *Brain & Behaviour*, p.43, Ed. Brazier, M.A.B. Washington: Am. Inst. Biol. Sci.

ANAND, B.K. (1967) Central chemosensitive mechanisms related to feeding. In *Hand Book of Physiology, Alimentary Canal*, p.249. Washington: Am. Physiol. Soc.

ANAND, B.K. (1968) Limbic system in innate animal behaviour. *Proc XXIV Int. Cong. Physiol. Soc.*, 288.

ANAND, B.K. (1970) Regulation of visceral activities by the central nervous system. *Ciba Foundation Symposium on Central Processes in Multicellular Organism*, p.356, Ed. Wolstenholme, G.E.W. & Knight, J. London: J & A Churchill Ltd.

ANAND, B.K. (1972) Experimental observations on anorexia. *Advances in Psychosomatic Medicine*, 7, 243.

ANAND, B.K., BANERJEE, M.G. & CHHINA, G.S. (1965) Activity of single neurones in the hypothalamic feeding centres: effect of protein hydrolysate. *Ind. J. Med. Res.*, 53, 1172.

ANAND, B.K., BANERJEE, M.G. & CHHINA, G.S. (1966) Single neurone activity of hypothalamic feeding centres: effect of local heating. *Brain Res.*, 1, 269.

ANAND, B.K. & BROBECK, J.R. (1951a) Localization of a feeding centre in the hypothalamus of the rat. *Proc. Soc. Expt. Biol. Med.*, 77, 323.

ANAND, B.K. & BROBECK, J.R. (1951b) Hypothalamic control of food intake in rats and cats. *Yale J. Biol. Med.*, 24, 123.

ANAND, B.K. & BROBECK, J.R. (1952) Food intake and spontaneous activity of rats with lesions in the amygdaloid nuclei. *J. Neurophysiol.*, 15, 421.

ANAND, B.K., CHHINA, G.S., SHARMA, K.N., DUA, S. & SINGH, B. (1964) Activity of single neurones in the hypothalamic feeding centres: effect of glucose. *Am. J. Physiol.*, 207, 1146.

ANAND, B.K., CHHINA, G.S. & SINGH, B. (1962) Effect of glucose on the activity of hypothalamic 'Feeding Centres'. *Science*, 138, 597.

ANAND, B.K. & DUA, S. (1955) Feeding responses induced by electrical stimulation of hypothalamus in cat. *Ind. J. Med. Res.*, 43, 113.

ANAND, B.K. & DUA, S. (1956) Electrical stimulation of the limbic system of brain (visceral brain) in the waking animal. *Ind. J. Med. Res.*, 44, 107.

ANAND, B.K. & DUA, S. (1958) Hypothalamic control over water consumption in the rat. *Ind. J. Med. Res.*, 46, 277.

ANAND, B.K., DUA, S. & CHHINA, G.S. (1958) Higher nervous control over food intake. *Ind. J. Med. Res.*, 46, 277.

ANAND, B.K., DUA, S. & CHHINA, G.S. (1961a) Effect of neocortical lesions over food intake. *Ind. J. Med. Res.*, 49, 491.

ANAND, B.K., DUA, S. & SHOENBERG, K. (1955) Hypothalamic control of food intake in rats and monkeys. *J. Physiol. (Lond)*, 127, 143.

ANAND, B.K., DUA, S. & SINGH, B. (1961b) Electrical activity of feeding centres under the effect of changes in blood chemistry. *E.E.G. Clin. Neurophysiol.*, 13, 54.

ANAND, B.K., KUMAR, M. & CHHINA, G.S. (1970) Evoked responses from hypothalamus in response to stimulation of mesenteric nerves. *Ind. J. Physiol. Pharmacol.*, 14, 27.

ANAND, B.K. MALHOTRA, C.L., DUA, S. & SINGH, B. (1961c) Electrical activity of hypothalamic feeding centres under the effect of Reserpine, Rastinon and Preludin. *Ind. J. Med. Res.*, 49, 152.

ANAND, B.K. & PILLAI, R.V. (1967) Activity of single neurones in the hypothalamic feeding centres: effect of gastric distension. *J. Physiol. (Lond).*, 192, 63.

ANAND, B.K. SUBBERWAL, U., MANCHANDA, S.K. & SINGH, B. (1961d) Glucoreceptor mechanism in the hypothalamic feeding centres. *Ind. J. Med. Res.*, 49, 717.

ANAND, B.K., TALWAR, G.P., DUA, S. & MHATRE, R.M. (1961e) Glucose and oxygen consumption of hypothalamic feeding centres. *Ind. J. Med. Res.*, 49, 725.

CHAKRABARTY, A.S. PILLAI, R.V., ANAND, B.K. & SINGH, B.(1967) Effect of Cyproheptadine on the electrical activity of the hypothalamic feeding centres. *Brain Res.,* 6, 561.

CHHINA, G.S. KANG, H.K., SINGH, B. & ANAND, B.K. (1971a) Effect of fenfluramine on the electrical activity of the hypothalamic feeding centres. *Physiol. Behaviour.,* 7, 433.

CHHINA, G.S., SINGH, B., RAO, P.S. & ANAND, B.K. (1971b) Effect of glucose on the hypothalamic feeding centres in deafferented animals. *Am. J. Physiol.,* 221, 662.

DELGADO, J.M.R. & ANAND, B.K. (1953) Increase of food intake induced by electrical stimulation of the lateral hypothalamus. *Am. J. Physiol.,* 172, 162.

DESIRAJU, T., BANERJEE, M.G. & ANAND, B.K. (1968) Activity of single neurones in the hypothalamic feeding centres: effect of 2-deoxy-D-glucose. *Physiol. Behaviour,* 3, 757.

HETHERINGTON, A.W. & RANSON, S.W. (1940) Hypothalamic lesions and adiposity in the rat. *Anat. Rec.,* 78, 149.

KHANNA, S., NAYAR, U. & ANAND, B.K. (1972) Effect of fenfluramine on the single neurone activities of the hypothalamic feeding centres. *Physiol. Behaviour,* 8, 453.

SHARMA, K.N., ANAND, B.K., DUA, S. & SINGH, B. (1961) Role of stomach in the regulation of activities of the hypothalamic feeding centres. *Am. J. Physiol.,* 201, 593.

SINGH, B., ANAND, B.K., MALHOTRA, C.L. & DUA, S. (1958) Stress as an aetiological factor in the causation of anorexia nervosa. *Neurology,* 6, 50.

SUBBERWAL, U. & ANAND, B.K. (1965) Role of reticular formation of brainstem in regulation of food intake. *Ind. J. Med. Res.,* 53, 440.

10. Insulin Requirements for Satiety Centre Activity

A. F. DEBONS and I. KRIMSKY

In this chapter we wish to review the evidence for the involvement of insulin in the activity of the ventromedial region of the hypothalamus as a regulator of food intake. The ventromedial hypothalamus, sometimes referred to as the satiety centre, has been shown to be concerned with the adjustment of food intake to variations in energy expenditure (Stevenson, 1969). Normal functioning of this part of the brain is necessary for maintaining the weight of the mature animal within the narrow limits usually observed. This point has been made clearly in the words of Passmore and Draper (1964), 'The food intake of most of us amounts to about 3 lb a day or more. A little arithmetic will show the reader that it has not taken him very long to get outside a ton of food. Yet during this period his weight has probably varied no more than 1 or 2 kg. Obviously this large intake has been somehow 'metered' very accurately so as to supply his needs. A very small error in the 'metering' would soon lead to obesity (an excess of only 3 per cent would lead to a gain in weight of about 14 lb in one year). Even in very fat people the offset of the regulatory system need only be very small'.

The concept of insulin involvement in the regulation of food intake came as an extension of the 'glucostat' hypothesis (Mayer & Thomas, 1967). Mayer had postulated that the level of glucose in the blood determined whether the animal was hungry or satiated, that is, low blood glucose resulting from a period of fasting led to food intake which ended when blood glucose rose to a critical level. This idea was of course not consistent with the situation in diabetes, where hunger, to the point of hyperphagia, persists in spite of hyperglycaemia. Mayer therefore modified the glucostat hypothesis

This work was supported in part by United States Public Health grant AM 12479 and by a contract with the Atomic Energy Commission.

to include the idea that utilization of glucose by special cells of the ventromedial hypothalamus which control food intake was insulin dependent.

Experimental evidence for an effect of insulin on the activity of cells of the satiety centre came from the laboratory of Anand (Anand et al, 1964). These workers investigated the effects of intravenous infusions of glucose or insulin on the electrical activity of single neurones in the hypothalamus. It was shown that in starved animals the electrical activity of the satiety centre neurones was slower than that of feeding centre neurones. The activity of satiety centre neurones increased and that of feeding centre neurones decreased significantly after glucose was given intravenously. Insulin provoked an immediate increase in the neuronal activity of the satiety centre followed by a long-lasting decrease. We agree with these authors that this may have been due to an initial transient increase in glucose utilization by the cells of the satiety centre after insulin injection, followed by an insulin-induced hypoglycaemia and a decrease in availability of glucose. Thus, the firing rate of satiety centre neurones appears to be closely correlated with utilization of glucose, and further this utilization is increased by insulin. The increase in firing rate of satiety centre neurones induced by glucose did not occur immediately, as it did after insulin, but rather began 5-10 minutes after glucose infusion. This is consistent with a more gradual increase in blood insulin levels after glucose infusion. Substantially the same results on the effects of glucose and insulin on the electrical activity of the satiety centre and feeding centre neurones were obtained by Bach and his co-workers (1964).

We have found the glucose analogue, gold thioglucose, to be a useful tool for investigating satiety centre activity. The compound has been shown to induce hyperphagia and obesity in mice (Brecher & Waxler, 1949) and Marshall et al (1955) reported that it causes necrosis of the satiety centre of the hypothalamus in these animals. Further investigations by Mayer (1960) demonstrated that gold thioglucose alone, among a number of structurally related gold thio-compounds, caused necrosis of the satiety centre and resulted in obesity. Mayer suggested that because of the affinity of these cells for the glucose component of the molecule the toxic gold moiety of gold thioglucose accumulated in and destroyed specific glucoreceptor cells of the ventromedial region. In support of this interpretation we found that the inhibitor of glucose uptake, 2-deoxyglucose, prevented induction of hyperphagia and obesity by gold thioglucose (Likuski et al, 1967). Furthermore when 2-deoxyglucose was given alone, it produced extreme hyperphagia for a short period.

Another known inhibitor of glucose transport, phlorizin, has been investigated with respect to its action on food intake and on the prevention of gold thioglucose necrosis of the satiety centre. Glick and Mayer (1968) found that infusion of phlorizin into the lateral cerebral ventricle of the rat produced a pronounced and sustained hyperphagia and resulted in weight gain. An even greater amount of phlorizin administered intraperitoneally had no effect. The question arose whether the phlorizin-induced hyperphagia might be mediated by the satiety centre. We therefore investigated the effect of injecting phlorizin into the ventromedial hypothalamus on the sensitivity of the area to intraperitoneally administered gold thioglucose. We found that injection of phlorizin prevented the usual gold thioglucose-induced necrosis. In another type of experiment, we found that after intravenous injection of ^{3}H-phlorizin, radioactivity (visualized autoradiographically) was confined to a particular cell type in the ventromedial hypothalamus; these cells were situated in the area where gold thioglucose necrosis begins (Figs. 10.1, 10.2, and 10.3).

Figure 10.1 is transverse section through the hypothalamus at the level of the infundibular recess (200X). Numerous labelled cells are present in the lateral portion of the arcuate nucleus and in the adjacent cell-poor area between the arcuate and ventromedial nuclei.

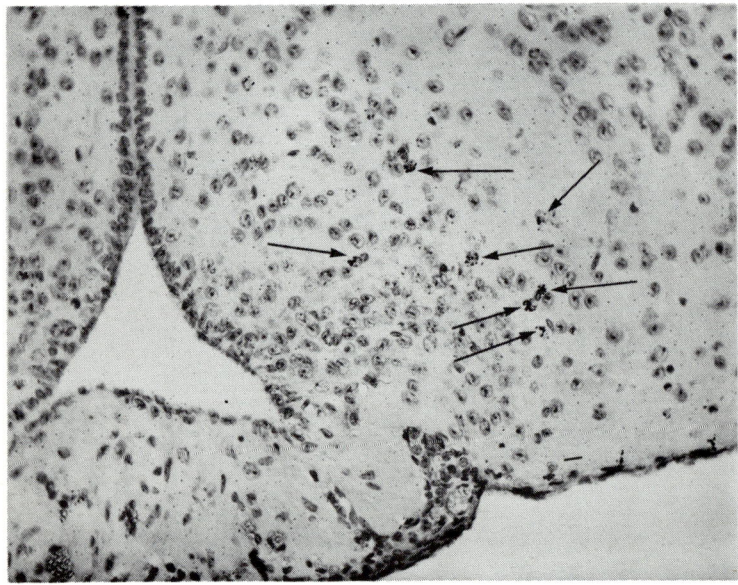

Figure 10.1
Transverse section through the hypothalamus of a mouse after radioactive phlorizin injection

INSULIN REQUIREMENTS FOR SATIETY CENTRE ACTIVITY 149

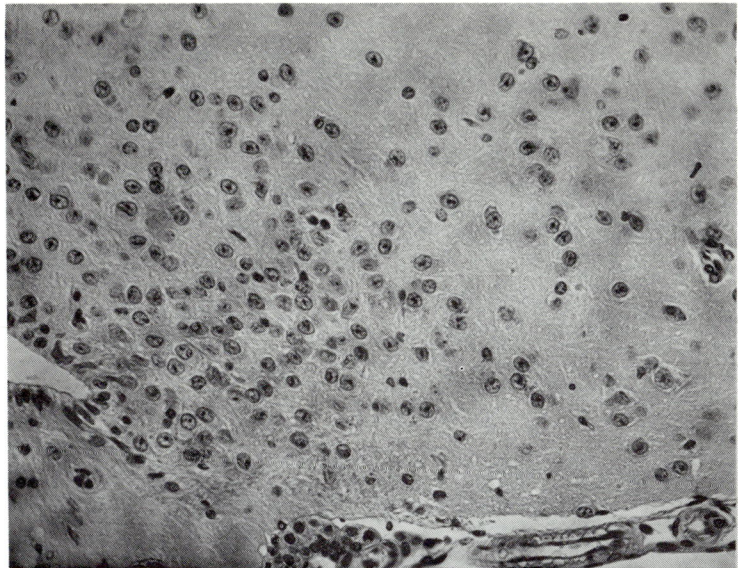

Figure 10.2
Transverse section through the hypothalamus of an untreated mouse.

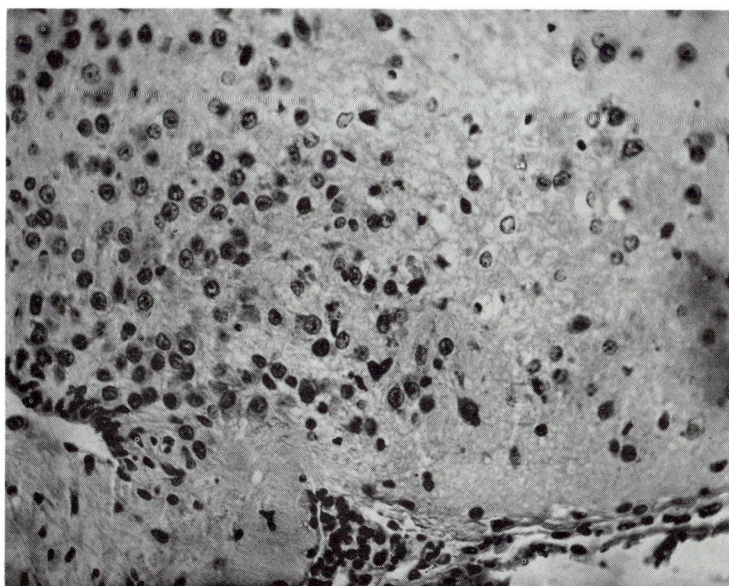

Figure 10.3
Transverse section through the hypothalamus of a mouse treated with gold thioglucose and injected nine hours later with radioactive phlorizin.

Figure 10.2 is a similar section through the hypothalamus of an untreated animal. This is to be compared with Figure 10.3, which is a section through the corresponding area of an animal which had been injected nine hours earlier with gold thioglucose. Pyknotic nuclei and sponginess due to dissolution of the neuropil are to be seen. The coincidence of the area of phlorizin binding cells with the area of initial gold thioglucose-induced pathology is consistent with the view that the phlorizin binding cells are the specific glucoreceptor cells of the satiety centre. In view of the selectivity of phlorizin the presence of a phlorizin-reactive cell type in the ventromedial hypothalamus provides further support for the existence of special glucoreceptor cells in this area involved in the regulation of food intake (Debons *et al.* 1974).

Using sensitivity to gold thioglucose as an indicator of satiety centre activity, we obtained evidence that insulin participates in the activity of the satiety centre. We found that diabetes produced by alloxan or by anti-insulin serum prevented gold thioglucose damage to the satiety centre (Debons *et al*, 1968). If the diabetes was terminated by cessation of anti-insulin serum administration, sensitivity to gold thioglucose returned and the mice then developed hyperphagia and obesity (Debons *et al*, 1969). Similarly, administra-

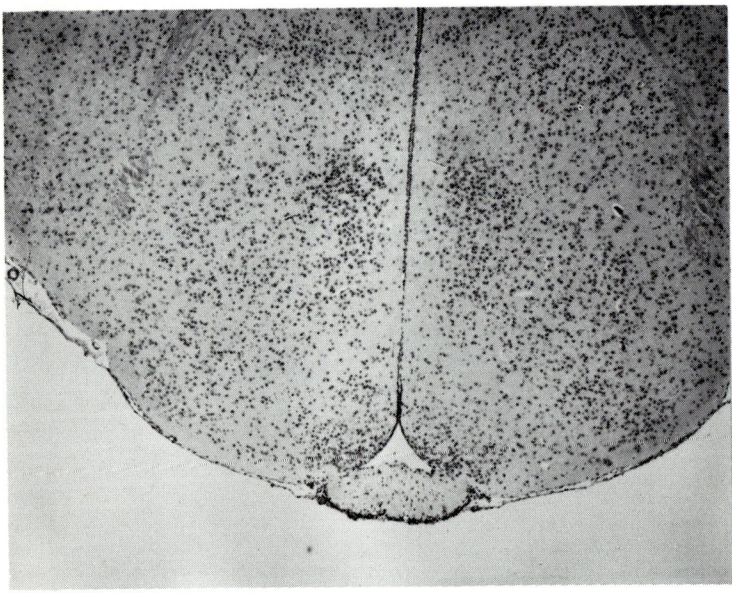

Figure 10.4

Transverse section through the hypothalamus, at the level of the median eminence, of an alloxan-diabetic mouse given gold thioglucose.

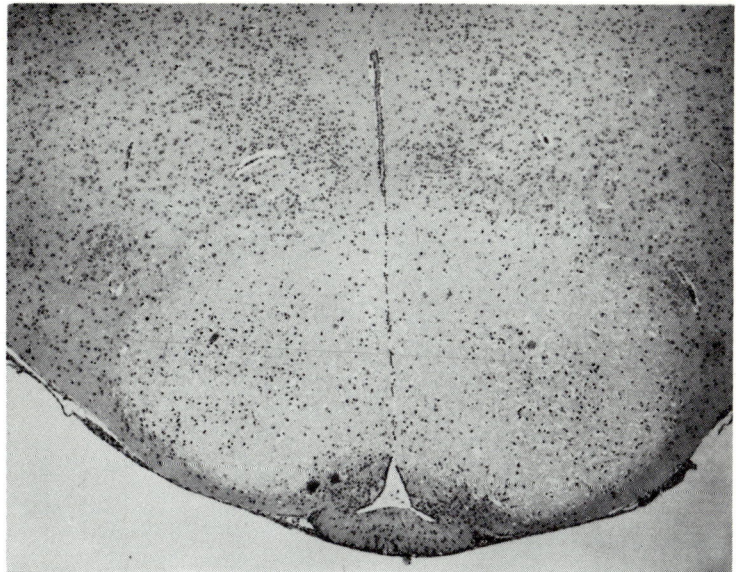

Figure 10.5
Transverse section through the hypothalamus at the level of the median eminence of an alloxan-diabetic mouse given gold thioglucose 1½ hours after insulin injections.

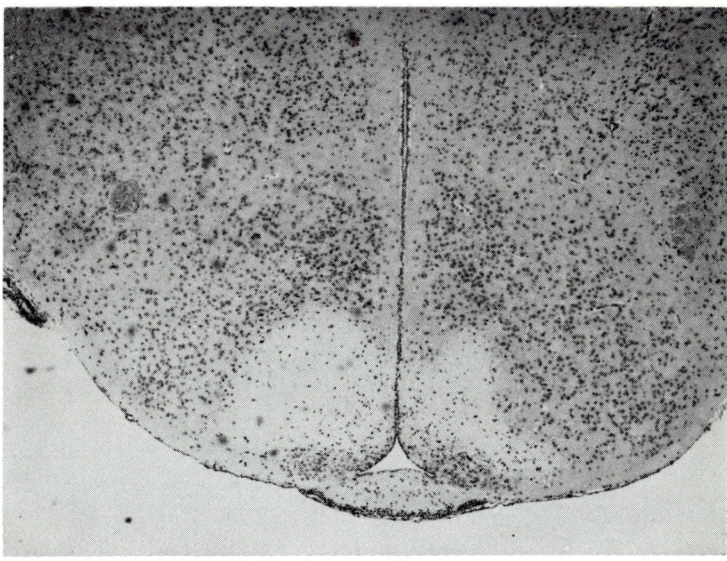

Figure 10.6
Transverse section through the hypothalamus of a mouse treated with anti-insulin serum and gold thioglucose.

tion of insulin to alloxan-diabetic mice caused a return of the sensitivity of the satiety centre to gold thioglucose.

Figure 10.4 shows a transverse section through the hypothalamus at the level of the median eminence. The mouse had been made diabetic with alloxan and then injected with gold thioglucose. No departure from normal structure is seen under the light microscope. Figure 10.5 shows a comparable section through the hypothalamus of a mouse which had been made diabetic by treatment with alloxan and then given insulin. Gold thioglucose was given one and a half hours after insulin injection. A typical area of necrosis is seen 20 hours after administration of gold thioglucose. The lesion appears to be the same as that in a normal animal given gold thioglucose. Figure 10.6 is a section through the hypothalamus of a mouse treated with a single injection of anti-insulin serum and then given gold thioglucose two and a half hours later. It is seen that the area of necrosis is greatly reduced.

We determined the rapidity with which the diabetic effect (the resistance of the satiety centre to gold thioglucose) could be reversed by insulin. The sensitivity of the satiety centre of diabetic mice to gold thioglucose was restored by insulin within five minutes (Debons et al, 1969). This suggested that insulin may be acting directly on the satiety centre. Therefore the effect of an intrahypothalamic injection of insulin on restoration of the sensitivity of the centre to gold thioglucose was investigated in diabetic mice (Debons et al, 1970). Intrahypothalamic injection of insulin restores the sensitivity of the centre (Table 10.1). This amount of insulin when given intravenously also restored the sensitivity. However, when the diabetic mice were injected intravenously with insulin antiserum, the intrahypothalamic administration of insulin was still effective whereas intravenous insulin was without effect. This shows that the intrahypothalamically injected insulin was not acting by way of the circulatory system.

It has been known for some time that the severity of alloxan induced diabetes mellitus in mice can be decreased by administration of glucose shortly before the alloxan (Arteta et al, 1953-4; Bhattacharya, 1954; Carter & Younathan, 1962; Kaneko & Logothetopoulos, 1963; Ratsimamanga et al, 1970). Using this means of modifying the effects of alloxan we found that resistance of the satiety centre to gold thioglucose was decreased in proportion to the decrease in hyperglycaemia, gluconeogenesis and hyperphagia (Debons et al, 1974). Thus a close parallel was seen between alterations in peripheral glucose metabolism and alterations in sensitivity of the satiety centre to gold thioglucose in relation to feeding behaviour. This suggests that factors such as insulin which control

Table 10.1

Gold thioglucose necrosis of the satiety centre in mice: Inhibition in diabetes; Reversal by intrahypothalmic injection of insulin

Animal Type	No. of Animals	Intrahypothalamic Injection	Occurrence of gold thioglucose Necrosis in satiety centre
Normal	10	None	100%
Normal	15	Saline	100%
Diabetic	26	None	12%
Diabetic	19	Insulin, 6 mU	79% *
Diabetic	11	Insulin, 3 mU	63% *
Diabetic	12	Insulin, 1 mU	50% **
Diabetic	13	Inactivated Insulin, 6 mU ***	0%
Diabetic	5	Saline	0%

mU = milliunits
* $P < 0.01$ (comparison was made with diabetic group receiving no treatment)
** $P < 0.05$ (comparison was made with diabetic group receiving no treatment)
*** Insulin was inactivated by exposure to 0.1N NaOH for 3 hr at 37°C then neutralized with HCl

glucose utilization in the periphery are effective in modifying the activity of the satiety centre and, through this, feeding behaviour.

Acknowledgements

We acknowledge the technical assistance of Mrs. Annette From and Mr. H. Pattinian. We are indebted to Mr. R. Cloutier of the Medical Division, Oak Ridge Associated Universities, Tennessee for his cooperation in experiments involving neutron activation for quantitation and localization of gold in the brain.

We are also indebted to Dr. L. Roizin, Chief, Psychiatric Research (Neuropathology), New York Psychiatric Institute, for examination of the ^{3}H-phlorizin autoradiographic preparations and for his helpful criticism and advice.

REFERENCES

ANAND, B.K., CHHINA, G.S., SHARMA, K.N., DUA, S. & SINGH, B.(1964) Activity of single neurons in the hypothalamic feeding centers: effect of glucose. *Am. J. Physiol.*, 207, 1146.

ARTETA, J.L., KONIG, C. & CARBALLIDO, A. (1953-4) The effects of glucose and insulin on the diabetogenic action of alloxan. *J. Endocrinol.*, 10, 342.

BACH, L.M.N., O'BRIEN, C.P. & COOPER, G.P (1964) Some observations concerning the hypothalamic regulation of growth and of food intake. *Progress in Brain Research*, 5, 114.

BHATTACHARYA, G. (1954) On the protection against alloxan diabetes by hexoses. *Science*, 120, 841.

BRECHER, G. & WAXLER, S.H. (1949) Obesity in albino mice due to single injection of gold thioglucose. *Proc. Soc. Exp. Biol. Med.*, 70, 498.

CARTER, W.J. & YOUNATHAN, E.S. (1962) Studies on protection against the diabetogenic effect of alloxan by glucose. *Proc. Soc. Exp. Biol. Med.*, 109, 611.

DEBONS, A.F., KRIMSKY, I. & FROM, A. (1970) A direct action of insulin on the hypothalamic satiety center. *Am. J. Physiol.* 219, 938.

DEBONS, A.F., KRIMSKY, I. & FROM, A. (1973) Modification of alloxan-induced diabetes: correlated changes in hypothalamic satiety center. *Am. J. Physiol.*, 224, 862.

DEBONS, A.F., KRIMSKY, I., FROM, A. & CLOUTIER, R.J. (1969) Rapid effects of insulin on the hypothalamic satiety center. *Am. J. Physiol.*, 217, 1114.

DEBONS, A.F., KRIMSKY, I., FROM, A. & PATTINIAN, H. (1974) Phlorizin inhibition of hypothalamic necrosis induced by gold thioglucose. *Am. J. Physiol.*, 226, 574.

DEBONS, A.F., KRIMSKY, I., LIKUSKI, H.J., FROM, A. & CLOUTIER, R.J. (1968) Gold thioglucose damage to the satiety center: inhibition in diabetes. *Am. J. Physiol.*, 214, 652.

GLICK, Z. & MAYER, J. (1968) Hyperphagia caused by cerebral ventricular infusion of phlorizin. *Nature*, 219, 1374.

KANEKO, M. & LOGOTHETOPOULOS, J. (1963) Sensitivity of beta cells to alloxan after inhibition or stimulation by glucose. *Diabetes*, 12, 433.

LIKUSKI, H.J., DEBONS, A.F. & CLOUTIER, R.J. (1967) Inhibition of gold thioglucose induced hypothalamic obesity by glucose analogues. *Am. J. Physiol.*, 212, 669.

MARSHALL, N.B., BARRNETT, R.J. & MAYER, J. (1955) Hypothalamic lesions in gold thioglucose injected mice. *Proc. Soc. Exp. Biol. Med.*, 90, 240.

MAYER, J. (1960) The Hypothalamic control of gastric hunger contractions as a component of the mechanism of regulation of food intake. *Am. J. Clin. Nutr.*, 8, 547.

MAYER, J. & THOMAS, D.W. (1967) Regulation of food intake and obesity. *Science*, 156, 328.

PASSMORE, R. & DRAPER, M.H. (1964) In *Biochemical Disorders in Human Disease*, p.31 (Ed. Thompson, R.H.S. & King, E.J.), New York: Academic Press.

RATSIMAMANGA, A.R., CHIRVAN-NIA, P. & BIBAL-PROT, P. (1970) Inhibition of the diabetogenic effect of alloxan by the intraperitoneal administration of glucose in the mouse. *Compt. Rend.*, 271, 599.

STEVENSON, J.A.F. (1969) In *The Hypothalamus*, p.524 (Ed. Haymaker, W., Anderson, E. & Nauta, W.J.H.), Springfield, Illinois: Charles C. Thomas.

DISCUSSION

Dr. Curtis-Prior. Dr. Anand has suggested that the brain monitors glucose utilization in order to control short-term intake. Would he like to comment on Harvey's hypothesis that a hypothetical fat soluble substance circulates in the blood and regulates the long-term intake?

Dr. Anand. In terms of long-term regulation we have to think of something which will be in equilibrium with the fat present in the fat depots. In fat animals with hypothalamic lesions, as the fat continues to accumulate in the depots, hyperphagia continues to decrease. When the animals are starved, so decreasing the fat in the fat depots, the hyperphagia returns. In other words, there is some common denominator between the fat present in the depots and the intact feeding centre when the satiety effect has disappeared. Nobody has yet been able to show the link between the two.

Dr. Stock. From my understanding of the literature, it would seem that gold thioglucose is only effective in mice. It does not appear to have any effect in rats or other rodents. Can you explain this in any way?

Dr. Debons. I did not mention that gold thioglucose causes lesions in almost all strains of mice, other than abnormal hereditarily diseased mice. We are using three strains of mice at present; the dose may vary in the different strains. It has been reported in the past that gold thioglucose is very toxic to mice—the dose we use on our CBA and CF-1 mice is toxic to other strains of mice, such as CBL-57. In rats it is possible to obtain lesions but the doses required are toxic and death occurs.

Dr. Horton. In diabetes where there is an insufficiency of insulin there is no uptake of gold thioglucose or glucose and hyperphagia develops. Is insulin necessary to get gold thioglucose into the cells?

Dr. Debons. Yes, with reservations. We have done some studies recently on a diabetic animal in which the diabetes and sensitivity to gold thioglucose can be ameliorated if the pituitary is removed. Also, in another diabetic animal, if the adrenal is abolished the lesion will return. There will also be a diminished blood sugar and gluconeogenesis in these animals.

Dr. Anand. This is a controversial topic: are the cells glucostatic as Dr. Debons has stated, or glucose-sensitive as we think? When studies are carried out with gold thioglucose there is one point which must be remembered; this area of the hypothalamus has a much greater concentration of blood vessels. Thus, the concentration of glucose may be greater here. Glucose will enter every neurone because each one requires glucose for its activity.

I do not think we have yet answered the question whether the glucose concentration is increased in these cells and they are glucostatic, or whether the glucose utilization all over the body—including the neurones—is increased and whether these cells have some mechanism, perhaps enzymatic, or membrane receptors, such that with an increase in normal glucose utilization these cells fire more.

We have taken slices of the satiety centre and of the feeding area from monkeys, which had been fed normally and then starved. *In vitro,* slices from the satiety area in the fed animals took up more glucose than the feeding area, but in starved animals the satiety area picks up less glucose as compared to the feeding area. Thus, glucose does not always concentrate in these neurones. In different states, depending upon the normal utilization of glucose, these cells have some special mechanism such that they are activated more, even when normal utilization of glucose is occurring. They are, therefore glucose-sensitive rather than glucostatic.

Dr. Bray. You used the words 'glucose-sensitive' or 'glucostatic' for your discussion. This implies that local application of glucose ought to modulate feeding behaviour. What experiments are there which show that direct application of glucose to the ventromedial nucleus modulates feeding behaviour? Dr. Debons' study has shown that insulin has an effect, so perhaps he would comment on whether he gets an effect when doses lower than one milliunit are used. This is an enormous quantity of insulin to put on to a ventromedial nucleus. It is sufficient to treat the whole rat who is diabetic. I cannot find data to show that glucose has an effect—in view of that, is it fair to talk about a glucostatic or a glucose-sensitive system?

INSULIN REQUIREMENTS FOR SATIETY CENTRE ACTIVITY 157

Dr. Anand. Electrophoretically, glucose has been applied both to the satiety neurones and the feeding neurones; this work is still being carried out. The firing of the satiety neurones increases tremendously, provided the animal is not already completely bereft of insulin. The normal amount of insulin must be circulating. On the other hand, if glucose is applied electrophoretically to the lateral hypothalamus, the firing of the satiety neurones is inhibited. This is another mechanism whereby neurones receiving external glucose are inhibited rather than increasing their activity. Ordinarily this would not make sense. Glucose can be applied directly to the lateral hypothalamic cells, and it can be shown that their firing rate has been diminished. In the medial cells, the opposite effect occurs.

Dr. Debons. In answer to Dr. Bray's second point, we have gone down to as low as 15 microunits of insulin and have had a return of sensitivity of the hypothalamic ventromedial area to gold thioglucose. The only difficulty is that this is not reproducible and this is why it was not reported. The procedure of applying the material directly to the area is extremely difficult.

Professor Keen. In relation to the gold thioglucose experiments, what is the relationship between the dose of gold thioglucose given to the animal and the concentration of blood sugar? I have in mind the question of the dilution of gold thioglucose by the circulating glucose concentration. If, in the animal given insulin, the blood sugar is 30 mg/100 ml then the amount of gold thioglucose reaching the neurones will presumably be much greater than if the blood sugar is 300 mg/100 ml.

Dr. Debons. That is a good point. We do have some data to show that if intravenous insulin is given within five minutes, when the blood sugar is still quite high, usually between 300 and 400 mg/100 ml, the sensitivity of the centre is restored. Thus, despite the high blood sugar, insulin acts promptly in restoring utilization of glucose to these cells, and gold thioglucose is a glucose analogue.

Professor Adadevoh. I am sure that the mechanisms involved are more complex than they appear. Dr. Anand mentioned that there are differences between the lower and the higher animals, in terms of whether force-feeding can or cannot be carried out. From those experiments in which you force-fed, say, the monkey, do you have any information about the relationship between force-feeding and the glucose and insulin mechanism? This would seem to be relevant in terms of the other mechanisms, such as the level of glucose in blood and the insulin level which can initiate glucose utilization.

Dr. Anand. In animals in which the feeding centre has been destroyed, the cells which respond to glucose utilization are also destroyed. In this case it is necessary to force-feed in order to keep the animal alive. In spite of the fact that in higher primates the hunger feeling is gone, their higher nervous conditioning still leads them to accept food if they are given it. This is the difference between the lower and the higher animals. A rat or a cat will not do this and tube-feeding will be necessary for survival. A monkey, and I believe, even a human being, in whom the lateral area is gone can be made to feed.

Professor Adadevoh. If you are proposing that there is an influence of insulin and glucose, have you measured them in this situation to discover whether they are important or not?

Dr. Anand. We have not measured the arterial/venous glucose differences but, after feeding the animals, the blood sugar reaches normal values.

Dr. York. Would either Dr. Anand or Dr. Debons like to comment on the possible role of free fatty acids and keto acids in the regulation of food intake, and what mechanism exists in ruminants, for example?

Dr. Anand. I cannot answer the question on ruminants. Free fatty acids given intravenously will not produce any immediate effect on the firing rate, either of the satiety neurones or of the feeding neurones. At the same time, it is possible that on a long-term basis they may have some influence which is not apparent from the electrophysiological responses. In terms of these electrophysiological responses, only the changes in glucose utilization seem to be effective. Amino acid mixtures, fatty acids, sodium, potassium, dehydration and hydration are all ineffective.

Dr. Quaade. Is the site of the phlorizin activity the same as that of radioactive gold thioglucose?

Dr. Debons. No. We published some earlier studies with gold thioglucose, which we have made radioactive in a number of ways, taking the brain and putting it into a reactor and activating the cold gold, or by using a commercial glucose with C^{14} attached to the gold. In neither case was the resolution good, although we appeared to see some areas where there was localization, near oligodendrocytes. All gold thioglucose compounds seem to bind in this area as the permeability is high.

Professor Wynn. Would Dr. Debons or Dr. Anand care to speculate on the relevance of their experimental findings to human obesity?

Dr. Debons. Our indications are that there are cells in the ventromedial hypothalamus which are responsive to changes in peripheral metabolism. I think that there is an extremely delicate balance in the periphery affecting the activity of the satiety centre and feeding behaviour. Small changes in adrenal hormones—perhaps also growth hormone, certainly insulin—have their effect on the total output of the satiety centre, which can be measured ultimately in total calorie intake.

Dr. Anand. I think that Dr. Bray provided the best answer to this question. The hypothalamus can only explan one type of obesity, which will be produced in response to hyperphagia. Many factors are involved in human obesity. I have only considered the factor which controls hunger and the feeling of satisfaction, but metabolic, endocrine, genetic, even emotional and social factors play an important role in human obesity.

11. Energy Balance and Obesity

D. S. MILLER

Man cannot escape the laws of thermodynamics but these are often misquoted when applied to the problem of obesity (Durnin & Passmore, 1962; Redfern, 1965). Since fat is the chief energy store of the body it is clear that the obese have at some time or other been in positive energy balance. Equally clear is the need to go into negative energy balance if one wishes to lose fat. However true these statements of the obvious are, in the present state of knowledge they can be shown to be an oversimplification of a rather complex situation (Miller & Mumford, 1966). In fact they are examples of the first law of thermodynamics which states that energy cannot be created or destroyed:

Energy Balance = Energy Intake—Energy Expenditure

The second law in biological terms makes a subtle distinction between the potential energy of food, useful work, and heat. It says that when food is utilized by the body for either physical activity or the laying down of new tissue these processes must inevitably be accompanied by a loss of heat. In thermodynamic terms some energy is degraded. If this were not so, Carnot's engine would have been capable of perpetual motion, and obesity would be far more commonplace than it is.

The examination of these physical laws leads to some important conclusions for those studying the aetiology of obesity.
 1. It is important to account for all the energy turnover in man.
 2. Changes in energy balance should not be confused with changes in body weight. It is important to estimate the energy content of weight gains and losses.
 3. The energy cost of tissue synthesis must be included in the calculations. This is lost as heat.
 4. There are fundamental differences between the energetics of

gaining fat and losing fat. Energy gain per calorie available for gain must be less than unity, whereas energy lost is equal to the calorie deficit.

METHODS

Unfortunately these theoretical considerations do not match the practical methods that we have to study energy balance in man, and it is appropriate to examine these methods critically because they frequently lead to opposed interpretations of the same experimental data. In particular there is controversy about the importance of thermogenesis in man, and many theories concerning the mechanisms involved in the maintenance of energy homoeostasis over long periods of time, both in the thin and the obese. These difficulties will probably not be resolved until better methods are available. The precision required is of a different order from that of most clinical measurements. For example, an error of plus five per cent in the estimation of energy intake and minus five per cent in the estimation of expenditure of a man with a turnover of 3000 kcals/day would lead to an error of 300 kcals/day in the estimation of balance. Over a period of a year this error would amount to 110,000 kcals or approximately equal to 12 kg of fat or 13 kg of body weight. Over four years this would be 72 kg of body weight, equivalent to the weight of the subject. Remember too that daily energy balance calculated from the difference between intake and expenditure is a small difference between two large numbers, and that all the errors of the large numbers are also applied to the small balance. But are our errors as small as ± 5 per cent?

It is usual to assess scientific methods in terms of statistical reproducibility. The standard deviation of a series of measurements tells of the method, and the standard error of the certainty of the mean value. But accuracy is much more elusive. If a large series of measurements is available the standard error will be very small even if all the results are biased from the true value. What is more, there is evidence that in all balance studies there is a positive bias because for technical reasons there is a tendency to overestimate intakes and underestimate expenditure.

Another problem with energy balance in obesity is the peripatetic nature of man's everyday life. Methods have been devised that might meet the above criteria, but they are only suitable for captive subjects in the laboratory. If physiologists are to make contributions to the general field of human obesity they have to study the condition in its natural habitat. We are still largely ignorant of the influence of stress on either intake or expenditure, to say nothing of love, anger, fear, excitement, or of the three addictive drugs commonly taken in the western world—caffeine, alcohol and nicotine. But there is enough information to recognize that these factors cannot be ignored.

ENERGY INTAKE

The most precise method for determining energy intake is to take a duplicate sample of all the food eaten by each subject and to determine energy intake by bomb calorimetry. In practice this is rarely done, and most investigators rely on weighing the food as eaten and then calculating energy intake from food tables. Comparison between the two methods shows reasonable agreement (±2 per cent) if the raw ingredients of the meals are weighed but poorer agreement if prepared foods are included (±7 per cent). Unfortunately most clinical investigators estimate food intake by recall where weights have to be estimated, but the number of subjects is often large and the calculated standard error of the groups small, giving a false sense of precision. This technique is not appropriate to the obese because of the suspicion that this group will underestimate the amount of food consumed. Most government estimates of food consumption are based on the consumption of social groups, such as households, geographical areas or even whole countries. These give no indication of the distribution of food within the group and yield what I have called a meaningless mean (Miller, 1970). Nevertheless such data do provide valid comparisons between groups and show that the affluent countries consume about 3000 kcals per head of population compared with 2000 kcals in the underdeveloped world. Similarly it can be shown that the rich in Britain eat about 20 per cent more than the poor. This is an apparent paradox because whereas there is more obesity in the western world it is more common amongst our poor.

ENERGY EXPENDITURE

Direct calorimetry was popular at the beginning of this century but because of the high cost of the apparatus and the need to encase subjects in a confined space, the method was soon abandoned for indirect calorimetry. However the method has much to commend it in terms of accuracy and there are moves to reintroduce the technique by building larger calorimeters (Durnin *et al*, 1973). It is essentially the method of reference and could be used for proving the indirect methods which rely mainly on measuring oxygen consumption. The energy expenditure per litre of oxygen consumed depends upon the nature of the metabolic mixture burnt. This can be estimated from a knowledge of the respiratory quotient, since fats are richer in carbon than are carbohydrates. However in practice Weir (1949) has shown that it is only necessary to measure the volume of expired air and its oxygen content, and many types of apparatus have been designed to do this. None of them are really socially acceptable and tend to interfere with everyday life. Also it is impossible to persuade even army cadets to wear them for twenty-four hours, although it is the total daily energy expenditure that is important. This problem has been avoided by using a diary card whereby the subject records his activities during the day and the time spent is multiplied by an appropriate minute-energy-cost, but with much loss of accuracy. More recently an instrument for measuring heart rate has become available which is much more socially acceptable, and if there were a correlation between heart rate and energy expenditure it would provide an ideal instrument. Unfortunately there is some doubt about this correlation, but improved models which differentiate between heart rate whilst the subject is supine and erect are more promising (de Looy, 1973). It is doubtful if present techniques are capable of measuring the energy expenditure in man during his everyday life to an accuracy of greater than ±10 per cent. Moreover, there are very few measurements on the obese.

ENERGY BALANCE

If energy expenditure is difficult to measure, a possible alternative would be to measure energy balance directly. This requires an estimate of body energy content before and after a period of time. The energy-containing components of the body are fat, protein and glycogen. In the obese individual fat is the largest component both in energy density and in absolute wieght. There are many indirect methods for estimating body fat but these have been essentially based on an analysis of seven cadavers. On the assumption that this small sample is representative, fat may be determined from measurements of body density, body water, or body protein. Such estimates do not always agree, and the errors involved are probably large. More recently convenient methods have been suggested for the estimation of body fat from skinfold thickness, but these are based on the methods listed above and thus include the errors inherent in them.

The situation is however not as bad as indicated because it is possible to design experiments to reduce the importance of these technical errors. For example, if the fat content of a subject ±20 per cent is known before and after a period of a year, it can be shown that daily energy balance may be estimated to within ±5 per cent of energy turnover. It may well be that improved methods for indirect carcass analysis will provide a solution to our present difficulties.

FACTORS INFLUENCING ENERGY TURNOVER

Bearing in mind the shortcomings of these techniques, it is not surprising that there is some controversy as to why it is that some people become fat and the exact aetiology of their obesity. Some factors, however, do seem clear because of their simplicity.

Determinants of food intake

Whereas many investigators almost axiomatically attribute overweight to overeating, the evidence in man is very poor indeed. Davidson & Passmore (1963) have warned against the assumption that all obese people are big eaters and many surveys (Johnson et al, 1956; McCarthy, 1966; Stefanik et al, 1959; Swanson et al, 1955) have shown that the obese do not generally eat more than lean individuals. In fact the obese often eat less. Of course it must be pointed out that the measurements referred to were made after they became obese, and it may be that they consumed more during their dynamic phase of obesity. However, it must be said that psychiatrists would better be directed to helping the obese to restrict their diet rather than trying to cure gluttony. Seen in this way dietitians try to persuade their obese patients to deny their fundamental instinct which is to eat a normal amount of food. It is not surprising therefore that follow-up studies yield data which are very disappointing.

However, if it is to be assumed that the obese ate more than they expended during the dynamic phase of obesity it is pertinent to ask how relevant hypothalamic control is in man. In experimental animals it is generally believed that the regulation of energy balance is achieved by a control of food intake. But the evidence in man is non-existent. Edholm (1973) in numerous studies of a wide range of subjects insists that there is no obvious relationship between energy expenditure and food intake in individuals. Certainly there is none from day to day. Also the range of food intakes of individuals of the same sex, age and occupation is known to vary twofold (Widdowson, 1947). In man the hypothalamic control of food intake appears to be weak and can be over-ridden by good food, good company and the good rewards given by experimental scientists. Marathon overfeeding experiments by Sims *et al* (1973) show that some individuals can be persuaded to eat 10,000 kcals/day for 200 days without any biological control mechanism intervening to stop them. Another important difference between man and the rat is the monotony of the latter's diet. With rising income man has switched from relatively bulky diets to high energy density foods containing fat and sugar, enabling those in the developed world easily to consume diets containing 3000 kcals/day, whereas man in the developing countries would have to consume 2 kg of food to achieve his meagre 2000 kcals/day. Bulk is therefore no longer a factor in our diet. However, if the control of food intake is poor in man, it can be reinforced by the administration of drugs. In experiments with fenfluramine in our laboratories, subjects reduced their energy intake by 25 per cent over a seven week period without being aware of it or knowing that they were taking an anorectic agent.

Determinants of energy expenditure

It is customary to consider energy expenditure as being made up of a number of factors, the most important of which is the basal metabolic rate (BMR). Thus the total cost of any given activity is equal to the BMR plus the work done plus the heat production due to the inefficiency of that work. It is thus assumed that BMR is a constant part of all energy expenditure and for most of us in the affluent society it may be calculated to amount to considerably more than half of the total. But it should be realized that BMR is defined as the oxygen consumed under very precise experimental conditions which only occur once a day. The value will certainly be lower during sleep and is indeterminate during the waking day. Even so, the accepted range of normal BMR is ±10 per cent, which can account for some of the differences between similar individuals consuming widely differing food intakes. Also one must be careful to examine the dimensions of expressed values of BMR. It is customary to express these as kcals per square metre of body surface, whereas food intakes are expressed per day. A short middle-aged obese woman may have a normal BMR expressed per surface area. But the same data expressed as kcals per day would be low in comparison with a tall young lean male. Nor should it be forgotten that BMR falls with starvation (Apfelbaum, *et al*, 1971; Keys *et al*, 1950) and an obese patient may reduce his or her BMR when following dietary advice. However there remains the problem that some individuals apparently consume less than their measured BMR and yet maintain weight.

Such individuals probably depress their oxygen consumption during the night as do hibernating animals.

The energy expended in BMR is associated with the useful work of vital functions. However, since the potential energy of the working system is unaltered, all the energy appears as heat. Man exists in a flux of degrading energy transformations which are necessary for life. He differs from machines which can be switched off when not in use, but like a machine, when he is performing physical work only a relatively small proportion of the fuel is usefully available and there are further losses of heat. Such considerations apply whether the work is physical as in exercise or synthetic as in the formation of new tissue, even adipose tissue. The efficiency of these processes has been studied extensively in animals (Blaxter, 1971), but the relevance of this work to obesity has been challenged (Miller, 1974). Experimental animals, especially farm animals, have been genetically selected, a factor which reduces individual variation; whereas the obese are a group of individuals within the human population clearly different from the mean. There is some evidence, albeit insufficient, to suggest that the obese are more efficient in both synthesis of fat and performing physical work. Such a facility is valuable in pigs or bullocks and an advantage in man when subjected to chronic starvation, but a severe disadvantage in an affluent society.

Thermogenesis

In recent years interest has revived in the phenomenon of thermogenesis, that is to say heat production unassociated with BMR or physical work. There are three well defined phenomena:
1. *Cold induced or non-shivering thermogenesis* where heat is produced for thermoregulation. The phenomenon is rare but biochemically interesting because it has lead to the study of metabolic processes that do not yield ATP. Biochemists had hitherto been primarily concerned with explaining how food energy may be transformed into muscular work; now they are interested in futile cycles and energy leaks.
2. *Dietary-induced thermogenesis* where heat production rises in association with the consumption of food. The old terms specific dynamic action (SDA) and *luxuskonsumption* are now so confused and controversial that they should be dropped. The phenomenon is however well established and is important in human energetics and may explain some of the differences between the lean and the obese.
3. *Drug-induced thermogenesis.*

Thermogenesis induced by diet was first described by Rubner who demonstrated that dogs fed a meal energetically equivalent to their BMR remained in negative energy balance as a result of an increased heat production. He was of the view that dietary protein had a greater effect than fat or carbohydrate but the present view is that the phenomenon depends more on the nutrient balance of the diet. Thermogenesis also depends upon the size of the meal. More recently Fabry (1969) has shown that the heat production associated with a given caloric intake depends upon the distribution of meals within the day, nibblers producing more heat than gorgers. This work is relevant to the design of slimming regimens, and there is evidence that it is better to spread 1000 kcal diet over the whole day then to eat it in one meal (Kudlicka et al, 1966). Dietary-induced thermogenesis may also be potentiated by physical activity (Miller et al, 1967), an effect that suggests that dieters should be advised to exercise after meals and to eat earlier in the day in order to take advantage of the potentiating effect of normal activities.

Dietary-induced thermogenesis may also provide a mechanism to explain how the lean achieve energy homoeostasis. As described earlier, an error of 10 per cent in balancing energy intake with expenditure would lead to a doubling of body weight every four years. Since at least some individuals can maintain weight without trying there must be a precise homoeostatic mechanism. In animals this regulation may be achieved primarily by control of food intake, but the evidence in man is equivocal. If food intake is not controlled, energy expenditure must be. Increased expenditure as a result of increased intake in man is now well established (Apfelbaum et al, 1973; Kasper et al, 1973; Miller & Mumford, 1967; Miller et al, 1967; Sims et al, 1973) but because of the errors inherent in the techniques available it is still controversial whether the phenomenon is enough to provide a control for regulation of energy homoeostasis. Volunteers who double their food intake either do not gain weight or gain very slowly in comparison with the extra load. These experiments have shown that this cannot be explained by changes in the digestibility of the food or in spontaneous activity. There are some changes in carcass composition as well as increased heat production and the two could be related inasmuch as the energy cost of synthesizing fat is significant. But there are limits to the process of gaining fat and losing water in order to maintain weight, and the length of some of the experiments is such as to indicate a lowered overall efficiency of energy utilization. It has been suggested that fat stores are monitored by the surface area of adipocytes which in turn would control the entry of hormones into the cells which in turn would control the metabolic rate of adipose tissue (Shapiro, 1973). The theory is intellectually elegant and could provide an explanation for the regulation of energy balance in man but lacks experimental proof.

These overfeeding experiments have mainly been conducted on lean individuals and it is pertinent to ask whether the obese would behave differently and if so, why. Bray (1972) showed that previously reduced obese subjects when overfed regain weight very rapidly compared with the lean, but also when compared with untreated obese. This suggests that the obese have a homoeostatic mechanism which is simply set too high. In looking at differences between the lean and the obese therefore it is important to establish whether obese subjects are in a dynamic or static phase of obesity. This is not always easy, and may explain why the literature is contradictory on whether the obese have impaired dietary-induced thermogenesis. Rony (1940) reviewing the subject cites six other authors who claim that it is low in the obese, and three who claim it is normal. In our own work, obese subjects in general show a low response but we cannot demonstrate this in all individuals. Perhaps this indicates that there are at least two forms of obesity. However, Sims *et al* (1973) have established that the energy cost of maintenance between hospitalized obese and overfed lean subjects differs by a factor of two, clearly indicating a metabolic difference. But unequivocal evidence to prove that the obese have a causal metabolic defect depends upon an accurate assessment of their daily energy turnover as they go about their everyday life as distinct from laboratory measurements. This is still lacking.

PHARMACOLOGICAL AGENTS

It is not the purpose of this chapter to review pharmacological agents used in the treatment of obesity, but there are clearly two possible types to consider, namely anorectic and thermogenic compounds. It is perhaps important to point out that some drugs taken as part of the diet have marked anorectic and thermogenic properties. Thus smoking acts as an appetite suppressant, alcohol is a peripheral vasodilator that potentiates thermogenesis (Stock, *et al*, 1973) and caffeine is specifically thermogenic (Miller *et al*, 1974). These substances refute the argument that pharmacological interference with energy metabolism is likely to be hazardous. It is my view that thermogenic drugs will be extensively used in the future, if only because they will enable the obese to lose weight without enduring the severe discipline of dietary restriction and consequent loss of one aspect of the *'dolce vita'*. Such compounds may be used as tools in establishing the aetiology of obesity.

REFERENCES

APFELBAUM, M., BOTSARRON, J. & LACATIS, D. (1971). Effect of Calorie Restriction and Excessive Calorie Intake or Energy Expenditure. *Am. J. Clin, Nutr.*, 24 1405.

APFELBAUM, M. BOTSARRON, J. & LACATIS, D. (1973) Adaptation of Energy Expenditure to the Level of Intake in Man. *Energy Balance in Man. Paris: Masson*, p. 71.

BLAXTER, K. (1971) Methods of Measuring the Energy Metabolism of Animals and Interpretation of Results Obtained. *Fed. Proc.*, 30, 1436.

BRAY, G.A. (1972) Lipogenesis in Human Adopose Tissue: Some Effects of Nibbling and Gorging. *J. Clin. Invest.*, 51, 537.

DAVIDSON, S. & PASSMORE R. (1963) *Human Nutrition and Dietetics* London: E. & S. Livingstone.

DE LOOY, A. (1973) Socially Acceptable Measurement of Energy Expenditure in Man. *Ph.D. Thesis, London.*

DURNIN, J.V.G.A., EDHOLM, O.G., MILLER, D.S. & WATERLOW, J.C. (1973) How Much Food Does Man Require? *Nature, Lond.*, 242, 418.

DURNIN, J.V.G.A. & PASSMORE, R. (1962) Effect of Nightly Food Supplements on Food Intake in Man (letter). *Lancet*, 2, 884.

EDHOLM, O.G. (1973) Energy Expenditure and Food Intake. *Energy Balance in Man. Paris: Masson*, p. 51.

FABRY, P. (1969) Feeding Patterns and Nutritional Adaptations (book). *London: Butterworth.*

JOHNSON, M.L., BURKE, B.S. & MAYER, J. (1956) Relative Importance of Inactivity and Overeating in the Energy Balance of Obese High School Girls. *Am. J. Clin. Nutr.*, 4, 37.

KASPER, H., THIEL, H. & EHL, M. (1973) Response of Body Weight to a Low Carbohydrate, High Fat Diet in Normal and Obese Subjects. *Am. J. Clin. Nutr.* 26, 197.

KEYS, A., BROZEK, J., HERSHEL, A., MICKELSON, O. & TAYLOR, H.L. (1950) The Biology of Human Starvation. *University of Minnesota Press.*

KUDLICKA, V., FABRY, P., DOBERSKY, P. & KUDLICKOVA, V. (1966) 'Nibbling' and 'Meal-Eating' in the Treatment of Obesity. *Proc. Vllth Internat. Congr. Nutrition, Hamburg*, 2, 264.

McCARTHY, M.C. (1966) Dietary and Activity Patterns of Obese Women in Trinidad. *J. Am. Diet. Ass.*, 48, 33.

MILLER, D.S. (1970) Evaluation of Diets in Relation to Nutritional Status. *Proc. Nutr. Soc.*, 29, 191.

MILLER, D.S. (1974) Overfeeding in Man. *Fogarty Internat. Center Conf. on Obesity* (in press).

MILLER, D.S. & MUMFORD, P. (1966) Obesity: Physical Activity and Nutrition. *Proc. Nutr. Soc.*, 25, 100.

MILLER, D.S. & MUMFORD, P. (1967) Gluttony. 1. An Experimental Study of Overeating Low or High Protein Diets. *Am. J. Clin. Nutr.*, 20, 1212.

MILLER, D.S., MUMFORD, P.M. & STOCK, M.J. (1967) Gluttony. 2. Thermogenesis in Overeating in Man. *Am. J. Clin. Nutr.*, 20, 1223.

MILLER, D.S., STOCK, M.J. & STUART, J.A. (1974) The Effects of Caffeine and Carnitine on the Oxygen Consumption of Fed and Fasted Subjects. *Proc. Nutr. Soc.*, 33, 28A.

REDFEARN, E.R. (1965) Energy and Life. An Inaugural Lecture. *Leicester University Press.*

RONY, H.R. (1940) Obesity and Leanness. *Philadelphia: Lea and Febiger.*

SHAPIRO, B. (1973) Regulation of Adipose Tissue Size. *Energy Balance in Man. Paris: Masson,* p. 247.

SIMS, E.A.H., DANFORTH, E.Jr., HORTON, E.S., BRAY, G.A., GLENNON, J.A. & SALANS, L.B. (1973) Endocrine and Metabolic Effects of Experimental Obesity in Man. *Recent Progr. Hormone Res.*, 29, 457.

STEFANIK, P.A., HEALD, F.P.Jr. & MAYER, J. (1959). Calorie Intake in Relation to Energy Output of Obese and Non-Obese Adolescent Boys. *Am. J. Clin. Nutr.*, 7, 55.

STOCK, A.L., STOCK, M.J. & STUART, J.A. (1973) The Effect of Alcohol (ethanol) on the Oxygen Consumption of Fed and Fasting Subjects. *Proc. Nutr. Soc.*, 32, 40A.

SWANSON, P., ROBERTS, H. WILLIS, E., PESEK, I. & MAIRS, P. (1955) *Weight Control. Iowa: Iowa College Press,* 80.

WEIR, J.B. de V., (1949) New Methods for Calculating Metabolic Rate with Special Reference to Protein Metabolism. *J. Physiol. Lond.*, 109, 1.

WIDDOWSON, E.M. (1947) A Study of Individual Children's Diets. *Spec. Rep. Ser. Med. Res. Coun,* 257.

12. The Effects of Exercise in Human Obesity

P. BJÖRNTORP

The hyperinsulinaemia frequently seen in human obesity is an important abnormality because of its presumed association with diabetes mellitus and hyperlipidaemia. It seems possible that if hyperinsulinaemia could be prevented, then the risk for metabolic complications might be diminished.

Like several other groups we became interested in the cause of the elevated plasma insulin levels in spontaneously obese man. The interesting findings of Rabinowitz & Zierler (1962) suggesting that in obesity muscle is insulin insensitive, focused interest on muscle metabolism. Hultman (1967) also demonstrated that muscle is an important assimilator of glucose, particularly after exercise. Furthermore, studies by Holloszy (1967) had shown that physical training may cause adaptation of muscle metabolism. These observations demonstrated the potential for adaptations of glucose metabolism in muscle. The quantitative aspects of these metabolic changes must be of considerable importance to the organism when one considers that muscle mass constitutes the main part of the cellular mass of the body. The adaptation of insulin insensitive muscle in obesity to physical training might have an effect on the total peripheral insulin sensitivity, and on the hyperinsulinaemia of that condition; we therefore studied hyperinsulinaemic obese subjects after physical training.

PHYSICAL TRAINING

Obese man

Severely obese subjects were selected, primarily those who had been obese since childhood and who had an increased body cell mass and hyperplastic adipose tissue. These patients were instructed not to restrict their diet, but to eat freely during the period of physical

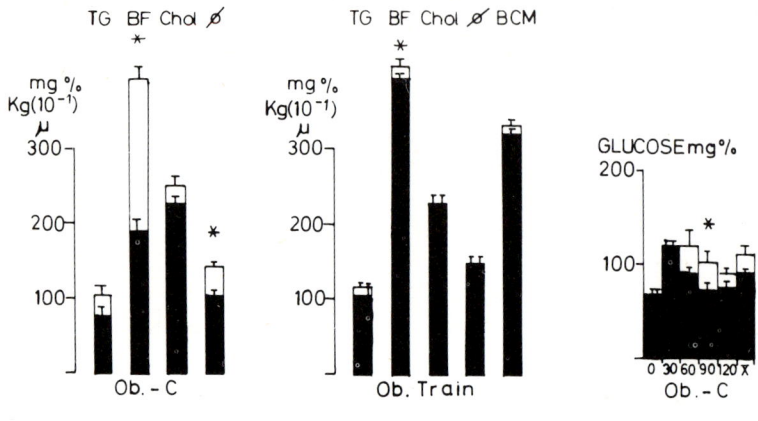
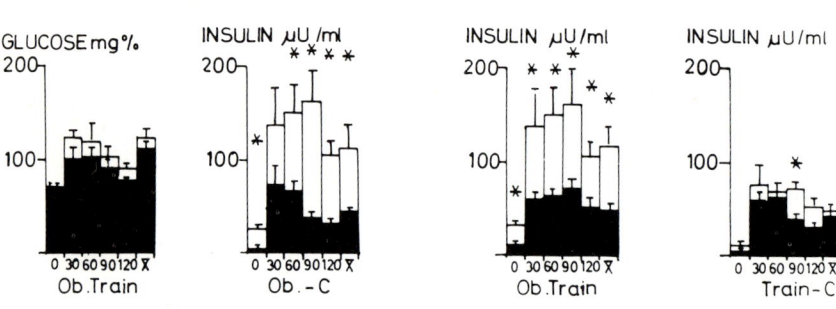

Abbreviations:
TG: Plasma triglycerides
BF: Body fat
Chol: Plasma cholesterol
ϕ: Fat cell diameter
BCM: Body cell mass
Ob.C: Comparisons between obese subjects (white bars) and controls (black bars)
Ob.train: Comparisons between obese subjects before (white bars) and after (black bars) physical training.
Train-C: Comparisons between obese subjects after physical training (white bars) and controls (black bars). x = $p < 0.05$.
Figures under glucose and insulin bars denote times after ingestion of 100g glucose by mouth. x is average of all values.
For reference to original literature, see text.

Figure 12.1
Comparison between metabolic parameters and body composition in severely obese subjects and control women before and after physical training.

training. These instructions were motivated by the suspicion that addition of a dietary regime to the physical training programme would probably decrease effective training. After the programme of training on free diet was finished, a combined programme of continued training plus diet would presumably have a better effect on body weight. The training was mainly obtained on the bicycle ergometer and by similar exercise.

In the initial study (Björntorp et al, 1970a) the training period of eight weeks caused an increase of aerobic power and muscular strength. Figure 12.1 shows the body composition and metabolic data before and after training in comparison with non-obese, non-training women (Björntorp, 1971a). Before training the obese subjects had a higher body fat content and enlarged fat cells when compared to controls. Glucose tolerance tests showed an increased glucose concentration only at 90 minutes. Insulin values were however considerably elevated. Physical training caused no decrease in body fat. On the contrary, a small increase was seen. There was no change in glucose tolerance. Insulin concentrations were now considerably lower and showed only slightly different values from those of the non-obese controls. These results show that it is possible to decrease plasma insulin in obese hyperinsulinaemic subjects without decreasing body fat.

The next subjects to be studied were obese and had a lower glucose tolerance and less marked hyperinsulinaemia (Björntorp et al, 1973a). None were frankly diabetic. The training was not so intensive in this group due to their higher age and less cooperation. The effects on plasma insulin were less marked but were demonstrable on fasting values and on the insulin values during an intravenous glucose tolerance test. They were not found during the oral test. The fact that the effect was found only during the intravenous test seems to indicate that the effect of physical training on insulin secretion is not mediated via enteric insulinogenic hormones.

In a third and similar study (Björntorp et al, 1973b) the training schedule was strictly standardized and maintained three times weekly for as long as six months. The maximum work loads during these training sessions were individualized according to each subject's maximal working capacity, and kept so that the pulse was 10-15 beats per minute below this level. Aerobic power increased in all these subjects both after three and six months. Plasma insulin decreased both on fasting and after the oral glucose tolerance test. In these subjects glucose tolerance was improved after six months, but on average body fat did not decrease (Fig. 12.7).

One problem with these studies is that difficulty arises in separating acute effects of the last training session from the long-term adaptation of metabolism after physical training. An acute work load of two-thirds of maximal working capacity, performed by obese subjects on the bicycle ergometer during one hour, lowers plasma insulin concentration. Such work comes close to complete exhaustion and almost empties the muscle glycogen stores (Hultman, 1967). The insulinogenic index, as a crude index of insulin sensitivity at the periphery, decreases for a few days after such work (Fahlen et al, 1972). In chronically trained obese subjects using lower work loads this acute effect did not seem to be present four and seven days after the last exercise as the insulin curves were similar and both below that before training (Björntorp et al, 1973b). The effect of physical training on plasma insulin is therefore at least partly an adaptation lasting for longer than a few days.

Physical training exerts a lowering effect on plasma insulin in obesity. The effect on glucose tolerance is less striking and the decrease in insulin seems best detectable on the intravenous test indicating that the effect is to be found at the periphery.

These studies have provided interesting findings, first the diminution of hyperinsulinaemia and second the absence of weight loss in the training obese subjects. Some aspects of these findings will be discussed.

METABOLISM OF THE NON-OBESE

In order to be able to evaluate the results obtained from training obese patients, the effects in non-obese subjects must be known. Surprisingly little seems to be understood about the effects of physical training on metabolism in non-obese subjects, in contrast to the well-known effects on circulation and respiration. Studies have mainly concentrated on the effects on plasma lipids (Holloszy et al, 1964). It is well-known that exercise has acute effects on the insulin requirement of juvenile diabetics; this was described during the first years of use of insulin (Lawrence, 1926).

Usually the effects of physical training are followed in young subjects simply because it is easier to train young people. From the metabolic point of view this is an unfortunate selection because it has been shown that several of the alterations in metabolism following ageing seem similar to those which accompany a sedentary life. Metabolic changes caused by physical training are therefore easier to detect in older subjects. Therefore we studied a group of well-trained, middle-aged men and compared them with sedentary controls (Björntorp et al, 1972a). These physically active men have

THE EFFECTS OF EXERCISE IN HUMAN OBESITY 175

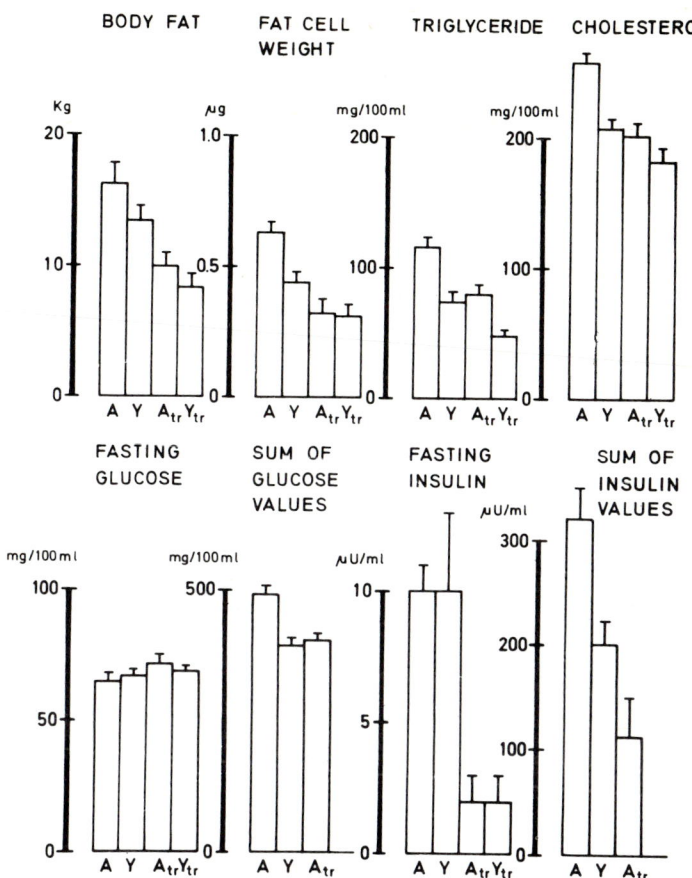

Sum of glucose or of insulin values refer to the sum of these values after a 100g oral glucose tolerance test.

For reference to original literature, see text.

Figure 12.2
Comparison between metabolic parameters and body composition in middle-aged, randomly selected, mainly sedentary men (A), young, sedentary men (Y) and middle-aged (A_{tr}) and young (Y_{tr}) physically well-trained men.

been training regularly all their lives and are still active competitors in cross-country running or skiing. They train for at least an hour three times weekly and they frequently compete.

Figure 12.2 compares the metabolic data of these middle-aged, well-trained men with sedentary controls of the same age, selected at random from the same city. The values for young men are included for comparison. The later were sedentary medical students and well-trained men from a football team (Björntorp et al, 1972b). Body fat was lower in both well-trained groups but there was no difference between the young and middle-aged well-trained men. This lower body fat was associated with a difference in fat cell size. Plasma lipids were lower in the trained groups, young trained men having lower triglycerides than the middle-aged trained men. Glucose tolerance was similar in young sedentary men and middle-aged trained men. These data were not available for young trained men. Fasting insulin was low in both trained groups. The insulin values during a glucose tolerance test were lower in middle-aged trained men than in young or middle-aged sedentary men. The well-trained men had low insulin/glucose ratios indicating a high peripheral insulin sensitivity.

The variables examined seem to be dependent on ageing because all values were higher in the middle-aged than in the young sedentary men, with the exception of fasting blood glucose and insulin. All these variables are lowered by physical training. Physical training thus seems to be associated with a rejuvenation of carbohydrate and lipid metabolism in non-obese subjects, and the age-dependence disappears, middle-aged trained men having values similar to those of young trained men.

It is obvious that the well-trained groups studied in the previous comparison are highly selected, and that the results might be caused by effects other than those of physical training. Studies during training on patients who have suffered myocardial infarction suggest that these results are indeed the effects of physical training (Björntorp et al 1972c).

Men who had had a myocardial infarction before the age of 55 were physically trained for nine months. They constituted the total population of surviving infarction patients at the age and sex in question during a limited period of time in Gothenburg. Every second patient was studied as a control and did not undergo a training programme. These patients were given no recommendations to change their diet, except in a few cases where obvious dietary peculiarities were at hand. They followed a training programme identical to that of the third obesity study (III) described previously. Some of them were slightly obese. The group showed a decrease in body fat during the training period (Fig. 12.7). Plasma insulin decreased and so did plasma triglyceride, while glucose tolerance showed only minor improvements and plasma cholesterol remained unchanged.

Comparisons between the effects of physical training in obese and non-obese subjects have been performed utilizing only the results of the myocardial infarction group because the intensity and duration of training of the athletic groups are not comparable with those of the obese patients. In non-obese or slightly obese subjects body fat, plasma insulin and triglycerides decreased, and there was a slight improvement of glucose tolerance. In severely obese subjects plasma insulin decreased and, after prolonged training (obese training study III), glucose tolerance was also improved. However, body fat did not decrease. Plasma triglyceride showed no clear decrease either but this may be because the effect would be found after a comparably light training programme only when plasma triglycerides are initially elevated as in the myocardial infarction patients. The main difference of the effect of training between severely obese and non-obese or slightly obese subjects seems to be the lack of any decrease of body fat in the severely obese patients.

ADIPOSE TISSUE AND HYPERINSULINAEMIA IN OBESITY

In the search for an explanation of hyperinsulinaemia in obesity the findings after physical training of severely obese subjects can be studied. One might first ask whether or not adipose tissue is involved here.

The observation that during weight decrease the hyperinsulinaemia of obesity decreases in parallel with body fat seems to indicate that adipose tissue mass and hyperinsulinaemia are associated in some way. Recent studies indicate that adipose tissue fat cell size rather than the number of fat cells is the factor associated with plasma insulin (Fig. 12.3). This has been demonstrated both in randomly selected middle-aged men (Björntorp et al, 1970b; Stern et al, 1972) and in men who have survived a myocardial infarction (Berchtold et al, 1972). In women fat cells need to be enlarged before this association is found. The relationship is not found in randomly selected middle-aged women (Björntorp et al, 1971a). Obese or hypertriglyceridaemic men and women show the same significant correlation, however, and both of these groups have enlarged fat cells (Björntorp et al, 1971b; Björntorp & Sjöström, 1971). It should be noted, however, that the association in obesity is demonstrated only under strictly standardized conditions without dietary restriction and without exercise (Sjöström & Björntorp, 1973). Brook & Lloyd (1973) have recently found a significant correlation between fat cell size and plasma insulin in obese children.

The association between fat cell size and plasma insulin is not very strong, and it can be disturbed by a number of factors (Fig. 12.3). Diabetes mellitus causes the correlation to disappear (Björntorp et al,

	Fat cell size v.s. Fasting insulin	
Middle-aged men	0.51***	(n:49)
Post-MI men	0.42**	(n:23)
Hypertriglyc. men+women	0.42**	(n:40)
Obesity men+women	0.42**	(n:26)
Obesity restricted diet	n.s.	(n:16)
Obesity after training	n.s.	(n:30)
Middle-aged women	n.s.	(n:23)
Maturity onset D.M.	n.s.	(n:24)

MI: Myocardial infarction.
DM: Diabetes mellitus.
For reference to original literature, see text.

Figure 12.3
Correlations between adipose tissue fat cell size and fasting plasma insulin concentration in different groups.

1972d) probably because insulin secretion is abnormal in this situation. Obese subjects who are dieting do not show the correlation (Sjöström & Björntorp, 1973). This may be due to the importance and relationship of carbohydrate intake and plasma insulin concentration in obese subjects (Grey & Kipnis, 1971). Physical training also effectively removes the association between adipose tissue mass or fat cell size and plasma insulin as described above.

The correlation between fat cell size and plasma insulin might be interpreted as a causal relationship. Enlarged fat cells might theoretically be responsible for an increased insulin secretion. Several explanations are possible, including mechanisms whereby fat cells affect glucose uptake and insulin sensitivity of tissues other than adipose tissue. At present it seems equally possible that a causal association might be the reverse, namely that plasma insulin regulates fat cell size by several known mechanisms, which cause an accumulation of adipose cell triglyceride.

THE INFLUENCE OF EXERCISE ON ADIPOSE TISSUE METABOLISM

Even if the role of adipose tissue is only minor in creating hyperinsulinaemia it is still of interest to see what effects exercise and physical training have on fat cell metabolism. Are the effects only secondary to the lowered plasma insulin concentration or are there other adaptive phenomena? I propose to discuss this problem on the basis of preliminary and as yet incomplete studies performed in our laboratory.

Rats subjected to repeated forced swim exercises decreased in body weight and total body fat. Epididymal fat pads were diminished because of a decrease in the size of the fat cells rather than in fat cell number. Muscle aerobic capacity increased while fasting plasma insulin decreased. One swim had no effect. With repeated swimming there was evidence of a physical training effect on muscle and plasma and in adipose tissue morphology. In the fat cells of the trained rats basal glucose incorporation into triglycerides decreased while the response to insulin (1000 μU) was elevated. The fat cell size dependence of triglyceride labelling in adipose tissue disappeared both after training and after one swim (Kral et al, 1974).

The fact that fat cell size was diminished by physical training complicates conclusions about adipocyte metabolism because variation in fat cell size is associated with variation in fat cell metabolism. This was suggested by the finding that in obese non-diabetic subjects with enlarged fat cells glucose incorporation into carbon dioxide and triglyceride is increased (Björntorp, 1966). Definite conclusions are not possible in such experiments because circulating substrates and hormones in the adipose tissue donor interfere with fat cell metabolism and such host differences may well obscure any differences in metabolism caused by the size of the fat cells.

This problem was studied by an examination of fat cells of different size from the same tissue. Therefore a simple method was devised for this purpose, utilizing the smaller density of larger fat cells to separate them by flotation from smaller fat cells (Björntorp & Karlsson, 1970). With this method it was possible to show that in the basal state both triglyceride synthesis and breakdown was increased in larger fat cells rather than in smaller ones (Björntorp & Sjöström, 1972). Uptake of exogenous fatty acids is also increased in larger fat cells, probably due to an increase of lipoprotein lipase activity (Björntorp et al, 1974).

Similar exercise studies in man, focused on adipose tissue metabolism, are currently being performed. In obese subjects we have so far only the results after one bout of work performed on the bicycle ergometer at two-thirds of maximal working capacity for one hour (Fahlen et al, 1972 and unpublished results). As in controls treated in the same way, glucose tolerance was decreased four hours afterwards and plasma insulin values were higher. These changes are perhaps remnants of the stress of hard, prolonged work in untrained individuals. After one day, however, glucose tolerance returned to its original value and plasma insulin was diminished. Adipose tissue

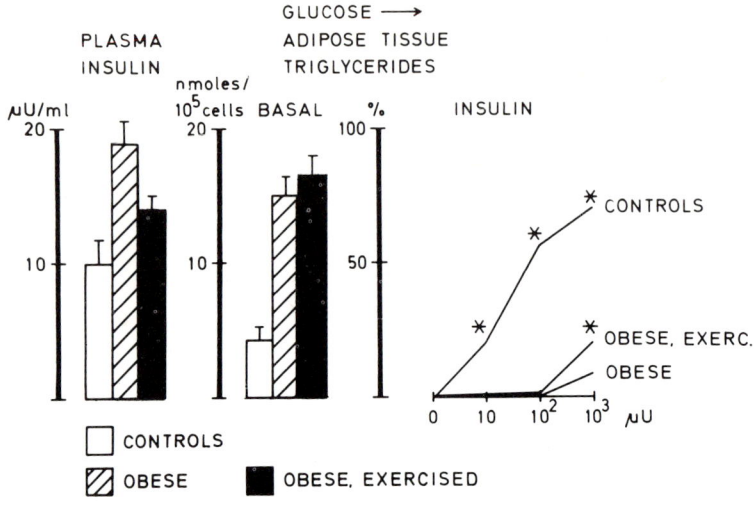

Figure 12.4
Fasting plasma insulin concentration and incorporation of $1-^{14}C$ glucose into adipose tissue triglycerides in the basal and insulin stimulated state in non-obese controls and in obese subjects before and 24 hours after bicycle ergometer exercise of 1 hour duration and at 2/3rd maximal working capacity. Insulin addition *in vitro* in μU. Increases indicated as percentage of basal value.

triglyceride synthesis from glucose was increased in comparison with controls but did not change after work. The response to insulin in the controls was not found in obese subjects who were totally unresponsive to insulin. After work there was a response (Fig. 12.4). The fat cell size dependence of glucose metabolism disappeared. These results are summarized in Figure 12.5.

The changes in fat cell metabolism after work might be due to a decreased availability of glucose. To test this possibility dietary carbohydrate was varied and fat cell metabolism examined (Smith *et al*, 1973). A diet containing 75 per cent of calories as carbohydrate was accompanied by lower blood glucose and plasma insulin, confirming an increased peripheral insulin sensitivity after carbohydrate feeding, as suggested by Brunzell *et al* (1971). Basal and insulin stimulated incorporation of labelled glucose into fat cells was increased. A low carbohydrate diet caused the dependence of fat cell metabolism on fat cell size to disappear.

These results are summarized in Figure 12.6. The blood glucose and plasma insulin values in the carbohydrate fed and in the exercised rats might, in the light of other results, be interpreted as an increased peripheral insulin sensitivity. Such an increased insulin

THE EFFECTS OF EXERCISE IN HUMAN OBESITY

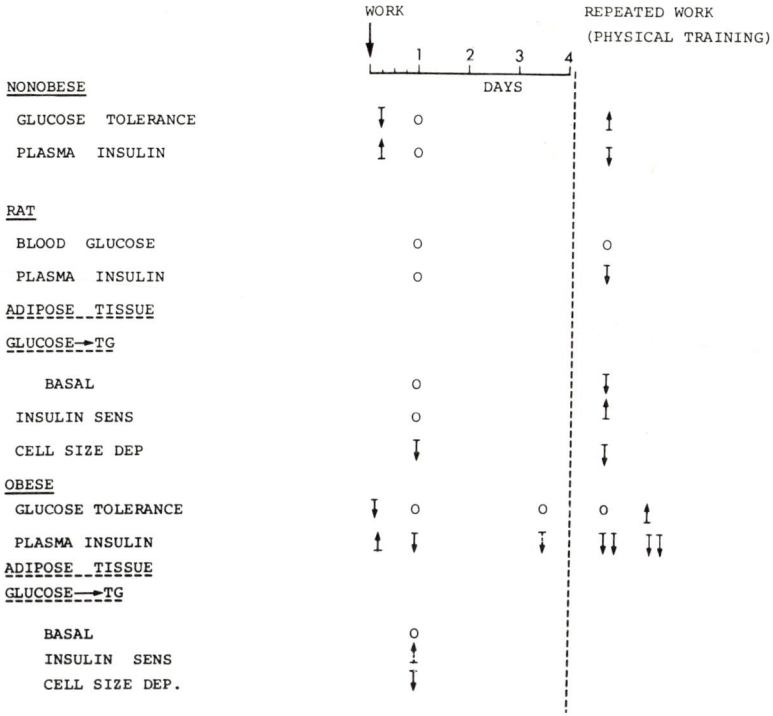

Figure 12.5
Summary of information on the effects of exercise (one or repeated work sessions) on glucose tolerance, plasma insulin and adipose tissue glucose metabolism and insulin sensitivity. Cell size dependence: the dependence of incorporation of $1-{}^{14}C$ glucose into fat cell triglyceride on the size of the fat cells.
TG = triglyceride

sensitivity was actually seen in adipose tissue. Physical inactivity and fat feeding yield opposite results.

The results of the studies on the basal glucose metabolism in adipose tissue, and on the cell size dependence on activity, are less readily interpreted. It has been shown that the fat cell surface area is best correlated with glucose metabolism, indicating that a factor close to the cell membrane is rate-limiting for metabolism under certain conditions (Björntorp & Sjöström, 1972; Jacobsson & Smith, 1972; Zinder et al, 1967). Such cell membrane factors might be associated with glucose transport and insulin receptors on the cell surface (Cuatrecasas, 1973). Carbohydrate feeding was shown to be associated with a dependence of metabolism on fat cell surface, indicating that increased availability of glucose to adipose tissue is making the fat cell membrane factor rate-limiting for metabolism. An increased basal glucose metabolism also seems to be associated with this situation. This interpretation infers that physical inactivity would also be a condition where there is an increased availability of glucose for the adipose cells while physical activity and fat feeding would be conditions resulting in less glucose being available. Hypothetically the condition after physical activity would be characterized by a high peripheral insulin sensitivity with little glucose metabolism in adipose tissue. The reverse would be the case during physical inactivity, namely a decreased peripheral insulin sensitivity and an increased adipose glucose uptake. A diet high in carbohydrate causes an increased peripheral insulin sensitivity and an increased

	GLUCOSE TOLERANCE	PLASMA INSULIN	INSULIN SENS.	ADIPOSE TISSUE GLUCOSE → TG BASAL	CELL SIZE DEP.
CARBOHYDRATE DIET	↑	↓	↑	↑	↑
PHYSICAL ACTIVITY	↑	↓	↑	↓	↓
PHYSICAL INACTIVITY	↓	↑	↓	↑	↑
FAT DIET	↓	↕	↓	↓	↓

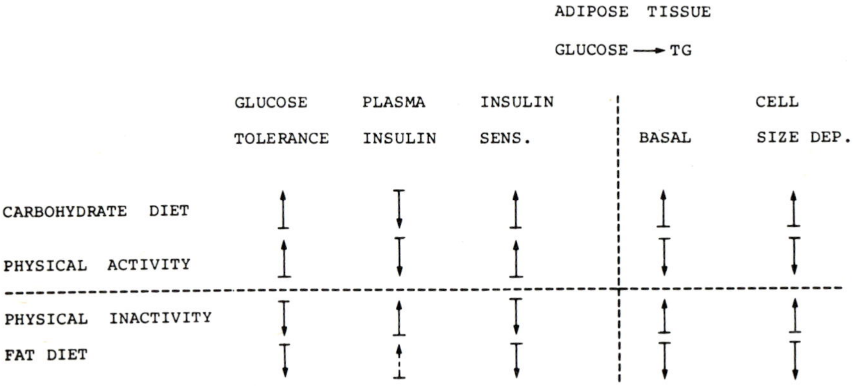

Figure 12.6
Summary of information on the effects of exercise and carbohydrate feeding on plasma and adipose tissue metabolic variables.
Abbreviations as in Fig. 5.
TG = triglyceride

glucose metabolism in adipose tissue while fat feeding reverses the situation.

Failure to lose body fat in the obese during training

Another striking feature of the studies involving training severely obese subjects is that body fat seems to decrease abnormally slowly.

The results of the body fat measurements in the trained obese subjects and in control groups are seen in Figure 12.7. In the first and second training study the obese subjects showed no measurable decrease in body fat after training. This was studied more closely in the third training study. The training period was extended over half a year and the programme was rigidly standardized so that an evaluation of the amount of work performed by the training subjects could

THE EFFECTS OF EXERCISE IN HUMAN OBESITY 183

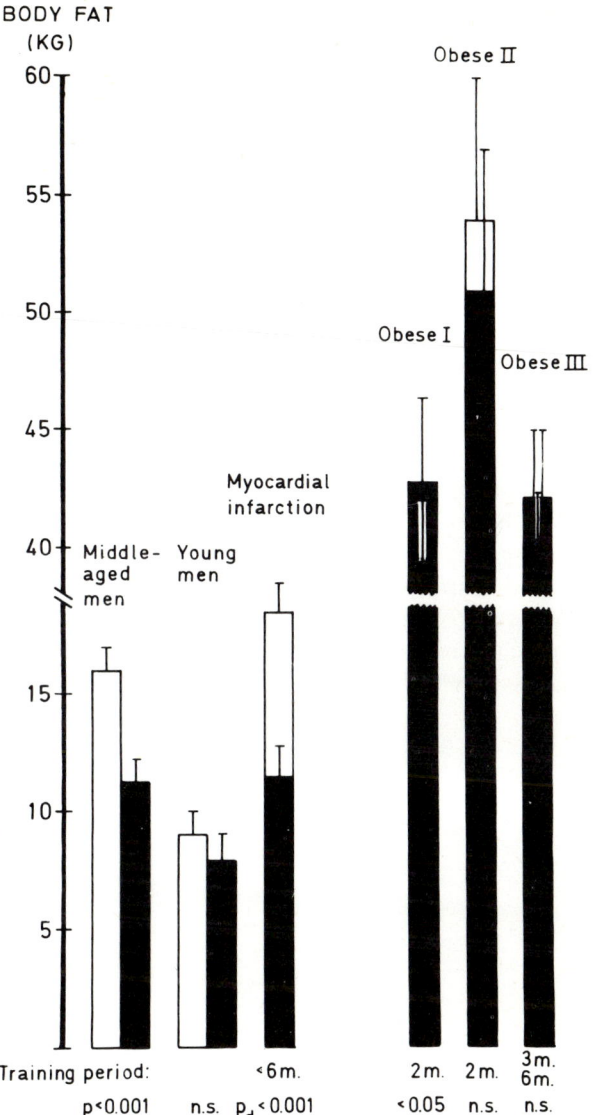

m: months.
For reference to original literature, see text.

Figure 12.7
Body fat values in various groups of subjects who were physically untrained (white bars) or trained (black bars).

be made. This also enabled a comparison to be made with other groups.

The detailed results of this third study are shown in Figure 12.8. There was no decrease in average body fat although in some subjects there appeared to be some slight decrease in body fat towards the end of the experiment (HF, TH and possibly GP). This weight decrease is, however, clearly smaller than that obtained in similarly trained non-obese individuals. In patients with myocardial infarction exactly the same training programme was followed for six months. Both this group and the obese group worked on the same relative work load for the same period of time three times a week, but this meant that in absolute terms the patients with infarctions actually worked less because they had less maximal working capacity. The myocardial infarction patients decreased their body fat by an average of 7 kg, or almost 40 per cent of their original body fat (Fig. 12.7). Similar results have been experienced previously not only from athletes (Pařízková, 1963), but also from studies with middle-aged moderately obese men in training programmes of comparable intensity to that applied in this study of obese subjects (Oscai & Williams, 1968). The obese groups consisted mainly of women, while all the non-obese subjects referred to were men. Physical training causes a

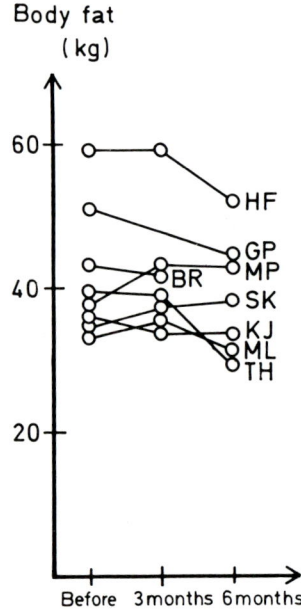

Figure 12.8
Body fat changes in seven obese men subjected to physical training.

decrease in weight in female athletes (Parizkova, 1963; Wilmore, 1973) but it is not clear whether non-obese women suffer a decrease in body fat when they undergo moderate training. Physically trained female rats apparently do not lose body fat (Holloszy, 1973).

In total, seven men have taken part in the three studies of physical training in obesity. These men did not show a significant decrease of body fat. The loss of weight ranged from 0.5 to 0.9 kg., TH clearly decreased his body fat between three and six months, although others (e.g. SK and KJ) did not do so (Fig. 12.8).

It would seem possible that severely obese subjects reduced body fat abnormally slowly or not at all when subjected to physical training on an *ad libitum* diet. It should be emphasized that in all studies patients have been selected to be severely obese, they have usually been obese since childhood and have an increased body cell mass and hypercellular adipose tissue (hyperplastic obesity) (Björntorp & Sjöström, 1971; Hirsch & Knittle, 1970).

Non-obese subjects usually decrease their body fat during physical training. This means that they encounter a negative caloric balance during the training period in spite of the fact that food intake might be increased particularly in training athletes. They have, however, an appetite regulation which is set to decrease adipose tissue mass during training. It seems an attractive possibility that appetite regulation is in some way deranged in hyperplastic obese subjects, and therefore they do not decrease weight during physical training on *ad libitum* diet. Alternatively, regulation of caloric expenditure might be insufficient. The difficulties encountered in treating such patients by ordinary dietary regime supports this suggestion (Björntorp *et al*, 1971e).

Data reported by Brook and his co-workers (1972) suggest that the first years of life are of particular importance in the development of adipose tissue hyperplasia. Knittle & Hirsch (1968) have shown that adipose tissue hypercellularity can be induced by increased caloric intake in the rat during a limited period early in life. It is possible that some of the obese patients who seem to have abnormal appetite regulation have had this abnormality from early in life. It should be emphasized that other mechanisms may lead to the development of hypercellular adipose tissue. For instance genetic factors may well be a primary event; abnormal appetite regulation and the resultant hypercellular state may follow.

SUMMARY

Severely obese patients were subjected to physical training without restriction of food intake. Plasma insulin concentration was decreased but glucose tolerance and body fat did not change. These results are compatible with an increased peripheral insulin sensitivity after physical training.

In order to evaluate these findings similar studies were performed in non-obese groups. Results from comparisons of body composition and lipid and carbohydrate metabolic variables in sedentary and well-trained young and middle-aged men suggested that physical training causes a juvenation of several of these variables. The main difference between the results of physical training in severely obese and non-obese subjects seems to be the lack of decrease in body fat in the former. Whether a normalization of plasma insulin occurs in obesity is not yet possible to state.

These findings offer a means for evaluating different explanations of hyperinsulinaemia in obesity. Positive correlations between fat cell size and plasma insulin have been found repeatedly, but these significant correlations are disturbed by several factors, including physical training in obesity, indicating that the hyperinsulinaemia of obesity is not caused by the adipose tissue fat cell enlargement.

Physical training produces changes in adipose tissue metabolism. These are at least partly due to a diminution of fat cell size which by itself causes metabolic differences as has been demonstrated by separation of different size fat cells from the same tissue. Comparisons between the metabolic situation after exercise and after variation in the carbohydrate content of the diet showed that exercise and carbohydrate both produce an increased insulin sensitivity.

The slow decrease in fat during physical training on *ad libitum* diet might be characteristic for the hyperplastic juvenile onset obesity syndrome studied. It might be considered that these patients have abnormal regulation of appetite or caloric expenditure offering a possible pathogenetic mechanism for their hypercellular obesity.

REFERENCES

BERCHTOLD, P., BJÖRNTORP, P., GUSTAFSON, A., LINDHOLM, B. TIBBLIN, G. & WILHELMSEN, L. (1972) Glucose tolerance, plasma insulin and lipids in relation to adipose tissue cellularity in men after myocardial infarction. *Acta Med. Scand.*, **191**, 35.

BJÖRNTORP, P. (1966) Studies on adipose tissue from obese patients with or without diabetes mellitus. II. Basal and insulin-stimulated glucose metabolism. *Acta Med. Scand.*, **179**, 229.

BJÖRNTORP, P., BENGTSSON, G., BLOHM, A., JOHNSSON, L. SJÖSTRÖM, L., TIBBLIN, E., TIBBLIN, G. & WILHELMSEN, L. (1971a) Adipose tissue fat cell size and number in relation to metabolism in randomly selected middle-aged men and women. *Metabolism*, 20, 927.

BJÖRNTORP, P., BERCHTOLD, G., GRIMBY, B., LINDHOLM, B. SANNE, H., TIBBLIN, G. & WILHELMSEN, L. (1972c) Effects of physical training on glucose tolerance, plasma insulin and lipids and on body composition in men after myocardial infarction. *Acta Med. Scand.*, 192, 439.

BJÖRNTORP, P., DE JOUNGE, K., KROTKIEWSKI, M., SULLIVAN, L. & SJÖSTRÖM, L. (1973b) Physical training in human obesity. III. Effects of long-term physical training on body composition. *Metabolism.* 22, 1467.

BJÖRNTORP, P., DE JOUNG, K., SJÖSTRÖM, L. & SULLIVAN, L. (1970a) The effect of physical training on insulin production in obesity. *Metabolism*, 19, 631.

BJÖRNTORP, P., DE JOUNGE, K., SJÖSTRÖM, L. & SULLIVAN, L. (1973a) Physical training in human obesity. II. Effects on plasma insulin in glucose intolerant subjects without marked hyperinsulinemia. *Scand. J. Clin. Lab. Invest.*, 32, 41.

BJÖRNTORP, P., ENZI, G., PERSSON, B., SPONBERGS, P. & SMITH, U, (1974) Lipoprotein lipase activity uptake of exogenous triglyceride in fat cells of different size. Submitted for publication.

BJÖRNTORP, P., FAHLÉN, M., GRIMBY, G., GUSTAFSON, A., HOLM, J., RENSTRÖM, P. & SCHERSTEN, T. (1972a) Carbohydrate and lipid metabolism in middle-aged, physically well-trained men. *Metabolism*, 21, 1037.

BJÖRNTORP, P., GRIMBY, G., SANNE, H., SJÖSTRÖM, L., TIBBLIN, G. & WILHELMSEN, L. (1972b) Adipose tissue fat cell size in relation to metabolism in weight-stabile, physically active men. *Horm. Metab. Res.*, 4, 182.

BJÖRNTORP, P., GUSTAFSON, A. & PERSSON, B. (1971b) Adipose tissue fat cell size and number in relation to metabolism in endogenous hypertriglyceridemia. *Acta Med. Scand.*, 190, 363.

BJÖRNTORP, P., GUSTAFSON, A. & TIBBLIN, G. (1970b) Relationships between adipose tissue cellularity and carbohydrate and lipid metabolism in a randomly selected population. In *Atherosclerosis—Proceedings of the 2nd International Symposium*, p. 374, Ed. Jones, R.J. Berlin: Springer-Verlag.

BJÖRNTORP, P., JONSSON, A. & BERCHTOLD, P. (1972d) Adipose tissue celularity in maturity onset diabetes mellitus. *Acta Med. Scand.*, 191, 129.

BJÖRNTORP, P. & KARLSSON, M. (1970) Triglyceride synthesis in human subcutaneous adipose tissue cells of different size. *Europ. J. Clin. Invest.*, 1, 112.

BJÖRNTORP, P. & SJÖSTRÖM, L. (1971) Number and size of adipose tissue fat cells in relation to metabolism in human obesity. *Metabolism*, 20, 703.

BJÖRNTORP, P. & SJÖSTRÖM, L. (1972) The composition and metabolism in vitro of adipose tissue fat cells of different sizes. *Europ. J. Clin. Invest.*, 2, 78.

BJÖRNTORP, P., SJÖSTRÖM, L, BERCHTOLD, P., JONSSON, A. FAHLEN, M., KRAL, J., SULLIVAN, L., KROTKIEWSKI, M., LARSSON, B., VRANA, J., SOMLO-SZÜCS, Z. & ENZI, G. (1971c) Diagnose und Behandlung der Adipositas. *Schwiez Rundschau. Med.* (Praxis), 60, 698.

BROOK, C.G.D. & LLOYD, J.K. (1973) Adipose cell size and glucose tolerance in obese children and effects of diet. *Arch. Dis. Childh.*, 48, 301.

BROOK, C.G.D., LLOYD, J.K. & WOLF, O.H. (1972) Relation between age of onset of obesity and size and number of adipose cells. *Brit. Med. J.*, 2, 25.

BRUNZELL, J.D., LERNER, R.L., HAZZARD, W.R., PORTE, D.Jr., & BIER-

MAN, E.L. (1971) Improved glucose tolerance with high carbohydrate feeding in mild diabetes. *New Eng. J. Med.*, 284, 521.
CUATRECASAS, P. (1973) Insulin receptor of liver and fat cell membranes. *Fed. Proc.*, 32, 1838.
GREY, N. & KIPNIS, D.M. (1971) Effect of diet composition on the hyperinsulinemia of obesity. *New Eng. J. Med.*, 285, 827.
FAHLEN, M., STENBERG, J. & BJÖRNTORP, P. (1972) Insulin secretion in obesity after exercise. *Diabetol.*, 8, 141.
HIRSCH, J. & KNITTLE, J.L. (1970) Cellularity of obese and non-obese human adipose tissue. *Fed Proc.*, 29, 1516.
HOLLOSZY, J.O. (1971) Biochemical adaptations in muscle. Effects of exercise on mitochondrial oxygen uptake and respiratory enzyme activity in skeletal muscle. *J. Biol. Chem.*, 242, 2278.
HOLLOSZY, J.O. (1974) The effects of endurance exercise on body composition. In the regulation of the adipose tissue mass. (Eds Vague, J. & Boyer, J.) *Excerpta Medica.* p. 254.
HOLLOSZY, J.P., SKINNER, J.S., TORO, C. & CURETON, T.K. (1964) Effects of a six month programme of endurance exercise on the serum lipids of middle-aged men. *Amer. J. Cardiol.*, 14, 753.
HULTMAN, E. (1967) Studies on muscle metabolism of glycogen and active phosphate in man with special reference to exercise and diet. *Scand. J. Clin. Lab. Invest.*, 19, suppl. 94.
JACOBSSON, B. & SMITH, U. (1972) Effect of cell size on lipolysis and antilipolytic action of insulin in human fat cells. *J. Lipid. Res.*, 13, 651.
KNITTLE, J.L. & HIRSCH, J. (1968) Effect of early nutrition on the development of rat epididymal fat pads; Cellularity and metabolism. *J. Clin. Invest.*, 47, 2091.
KRAL, J.G., JACOBSSON, B., SMITH, U. & BJÖRNTORP, P. (1974) The effects of physical exercise on fat cell metabolism in the rat. *Acta Physiol. Scand.*, in press.
LAWRENCE, R.D. (1926) The effect of exercise on insulin action in diabetes. *Brit. Med. J.*, 1, 648.
OSCAI, L.B. & WILLIAMS, B.T. (1968) Effect of exercise on overweight middle-aged males. *J. Amer. Ger. Soc.*, 16, 794.
PARIZKOVA, J. (1963) Impact of age, diet and exercise on man's body composition. *Ann. N.Y. Acad. Sci.*, 110, 661.
RABINOWITZ, D. & ZIERLER, K.L. (1962) Forearm metabolism in obesity and its response to intraarterial insulin. Characterization of insulin resistance and evidence for adaptive hyperinsulinism. *J. Clin. Invest.*, 41, 2173.
SJÖSTRÖM, L. & BJÖRNTORP, P. (1974) Body composition and adipose tissue cellularity in human obesity. *Acta Med. Scand.*, In press.
SMITH, U., KRAL, J. & BJÖRNTORP, P. (1973) Influence of dietary fat and carbohydrate on the metabolism of adipocytes of different size in the rat. *Biochim. Biophys. Acta.*, 337, 278.
STERN, M., OLEFSKY, J., FARQUHAR, J. & REAVEN, G. (1972) Relationship between fat cell size and insulin resistance in vivo. *Clin. Res.*, 20, 557 (abstract)
WILMORE, J.H. (1974) Physical exercise and body composition. In *The regulation of the adipose tissue mass* (Eds Vague, J. & Boyer, J.) *Excerpta Medica.* p. 265.

ZINDER, O., ARAD, R. & SHAPIRO, B. (1967) Effect of cell size on the metabolism of isolated fat cells. *Israel J. Med. Sci.*, 3, 787.

DISCUSSION

Professor Wynn. Surely we should look at body fat. Mr. Miller described data derived from Dr. Bray's study which refer to changes in body weight. Fifty to sixty per cent of the body is water, thus, the extremely large changes in weight could be predominantly due to changes in water balance. If obese people lose weight, and are then re-fed, they have a tremendous disturbance of water balance and very large gains in weight over a period of 14 days.

Mr. Miller. I do not dispute this. What is interesting about Dr. Bray's data is that there was a difference between the two groups. It is not that those obese who have previously been put on a reduction diet, gain weight rapidly, but that the other obese, who had not been reduced, did *not* gain weight so spectacularly. This is not conclusive but it is evidence that there might be a homoeostatic control mechanism which is set too high.

Dr. Horton. We have just completed some rather short-term over-feeding studies in two individuals who were previously obese and who had lost weight. Their results were compared with those of normal weight individuals. The study lasted only six weeks, and we found that the weight gain in both groups of individuals was equivalent for the excess number of calories. In other words, we did not pick up any difference in efficiency of weight gain over that short period.

With regard to Dr. Björntorp's elegant studies on the effects of physical conditioning, I am interested in the possible effects of the composition of the diet, as it interacts with physical conditioning. I have recently had the opportunity to study four members of our national cross-country team who are in training. Their fasting insulin levels are very low. Intravenous glucose tolerance tests showed that two individuals had K values less than one and very low insulin responses. The other two individuals had K values of 1.4 and 1.5, and had considerably higher insulin responses to intravenous glucose. On questioning it was found that the two individuals with low K values take diets very low in carbohydrates, whereas the two with higher insulin responses and higher K values ate higher carbohydrate diets. Do you have any data on the dietary habits of your cross-country runners and skiers?

Dr. Björntorp. I have the impression that their diets are not low in carbohydrates. In fact, some of them seem to have more carbohydrate than would be expected of people of their age. I think it is the general experience that athletes, at least when competing, eat more carbohydrate.

Professor Yudkin. I would like to make the plea that when we talk about carbohydrate a distinction should be made as to the kind of carbohydrate. For example, when we feed sucrose rather than starch, there is an impaired glucose tolerance, and a rise in insulin, accompanied by a fall in insulin sensitivity. It matters, therefore, what sort of carbohydrate is being used.

Professor Keen. Would Dr. Björntorp speculate a little on the mechanisms of the change in insulin sensitivity or in glucose tolerance in these individuals? How rapidly does it occur; in which tissues of the body is insulin sensitivity increased; how does it agree, for example, with current thoughts about insulin receptor sites on adipose cell surfaces?

Dr. Björntorp. These are interesting questions. We have been studying this problem for several years and have never reached the answers to these particular questions, which are the key ones. We wanted to define the problem as clearly as possible before doing such experiments as glucose uptake in liver and muscle, and I would guess that something is happening in the liver, or in muscle, with regard to insulin sensitivity.

Dr. Galton. It has been shown that exercise and anoxia can accelerate glucose transport into muscle cells, heart and adipose tissue. This may be due to a metabolite accumulating in exercise, or a reduction in the phosphorylation potential, or an alteration in the ATP-ADP ratio. Do you think that these metabolic factors could account for the insulin-sparing effect of exercise which you noticed?

Dr. Björntorp. Certainly it could account for the acute effect, but perhaps not the chronic effects.

Dr. Salans. I find it surprising that exercise has no effect on the basal state of glucose metabolism by the adipose tissue. From what is known about the effects of exercise and anoxia on basal glucose metabolism, I would have thought that there would aslo have been an alteration in the basal state.

I should like to make a general plea that when we are trying to assess the influence of any factor on the metabolic variables in plasma which have been discussed today. Whether it be exercise or dietary changes, we are extremely careful in the interpretation of the data derived from acute measurements of plasma glucose and insulin, or triglyceride, in response to an oral glucose challenge, and in relating or extending this to happenings throughout the day as the individual lives his life, exercises or does not exercise, and eats his meals.

I refer to the observation that although a diet high in carbohydrate may improve the tolerance to glucose and lower the levels of insulin, if the levels of insulin and glucose in the plasma are measured in response to the meals taken over a period of 24 hours, the opposite is seen. Do you have any data which relates exercise to this observation?

Dr. Björntorp. No, we have glucose tolerance in the postabsorptive state only. As to the first question, the decrease in basic glucose transformation through triglyceride might be present earlier than we have measured it, i.e. before one day.

Dr. Durnin. Mr. Miller is absolutely correct in saying that part of our problem in this whole field is due to technological difficulties, in that we are unable at present to measure the energy intake and expenditure sufficiently accurately.

Secondly, I should like Dr. Björntorp to say, not that he is comparing obese subjects to non-obese, but what sort of obese subjects they are, what are the levels of obesity and how long have they had this?

Mr. Miller. We must distinguish between measurements in the very carefully controlled conditions of our laboratories on the one hand and the rather poor studies of everyday life on the other. These do not always agree. This is the nature of our difficulties. Clearly, it is possible, and more straightforward, to measure thermic responses to food or to drugs, or differences for the energy cost of maintenance, under laboratory conditions. However, the difficulties start when it comes to investigating the influence of walking about a big city and engaging in life. Until better techniques are available, I do not see how this question can be answered.

Dr. Björntorp. Of course, it is important that we remember that the subjects we have studied are severely obese, have had juvenile onset obesity and have many fat cells. Moderately obese subjects probably do not follow the same pattern. In fact, some of the myocardial infarction patients we studied were only slightly obese, and their weight fell. Thus, the phenomena are probably related to a limited group only.

13. The Human Adipocyte and Its Disorders

D. J. GALTON

The occurrence of enzymatic defects in various cell types associated with abnormal cell function is now well-established. Most of the defects described so far occur on an inherited basis and constitute the rare group of 'inborn errors of metabolism'. Examples of such disorders in erythrocytes, hepatocytes and melanocytes are already well-known, and lead to diseases such as haemolytic anaemia, glycogen storage disease and albinism. However, recent studies of human adipocytes have extended this concept and revealed that in addition to inherited abnormalities of enzymes there is a group of acquired disorders of enzyme action giving rise to 'errors of metabolic regulation' (Galton, 1971). In these conditions the enzyme is present but not subjected to regulation by environmental factors such as hormones, inhibitor or activator metabolites. This leads to an abnormal over-use or under-use of metabolic pathways, or a reversed direction of metabolic pathways, which may be one of the initial events of the disease process and may give rise to the secondary complications of the disease. Good examples of acquired errors of metabolic regulation are the abnormal lipolytic state of adult diabetes and the failure of citrate to regulate the activity of phosphofructokinase in lipoma adipocytes. In this chapter I therefore wish to review both types of metabolic disorder, inborn errors and acquired errors of metabolic regulation which occur in the human adipocyte.

The major function of the adipocyte is to act as a fuel cell where circulating fuels such as glucose and lipoprotein-fatty acids are taken up by the cell and synthesized into triglycerides for storage. Under fasting condition, triglycerides are broken down to fatty acids and glycerol for release into the blood stream. The disorders of the adipose cell therefore fall naturally into three categories:

(a) failure to store glucose and fatty acids

(b) excessive storage of triglycerides
(c) excessive release of fatty acids

Both inherited and acquired metabolic defects occur on each of these metabolic segments and will be described.

FAILURE OF STORAGE

FAMILIAL HYPERTRIGLYCERIDAEMIA
(Type I Hyperlipaemia)

This is a good example of a storage defect in adipose tissue (Havel & Gordon, 1960). There is a failure of adipose and other tissues to clear circulating chylomicra from the blood stream and store the fatty acids in neutral lipid. It is a rare inborn error of metabolism inherited as an autosomal recessive (Brown & Greten, 1973).

The disease is probably due to a defect in the enzyme lipoprotein lipase. This enzyme is located close to the capillary endothelium of heart, muscle and adipose tissue; and is responsible for the hydrolysis of chylomicron-triglycerides to free fatty acids. The fatty acids then traverse the capillary wall and are taken up for oxidation by peripheral tissues or for storage in adipose tissue. Failure to remove chylomicra leads to excessive accumulation of triglycerides in the blood and to the clinical features of bouts of severe abdominal pain, eruptive xanthomata and moderate hepatosplenomegaly, and these are often present in early infancy. The evidence that this disease is in fact due to a defect in lipoprotein lipase derives from two sources. First, in normal subjects, lipoprotein lipase is released from capillary sites into the blood stream on injection of heparin intravenously. However, patients with Type I hyperlipaemia show very low levels of triglyceride-lipase activity after injection of heparin. On the other hand, lipolytic activities against diglycerides, monoglycerides and phospholipids appear to be normal. Secondly, acetone-ether extracts of adipose tissue of patients with this disease contain very low activities of lipoprotein lipase compared to normal subjects (Harlan *et al*, 1967). The data are therefore compatible with the suggestion that a defect in lipoprotein lipase is the causative factor of this rare condition.

ADULT DIABETES

Failure to remove glucose from the blood stream results in hyperglycaemia and although in juvenile-onset diabetes this is due to a deficiency of insulin, in adult diabetes changes occur in peripheral tissue which increase the body's requirements for insulin. These metabolic changes are of a reversible nature, they can be induced by environmental factors such as obesity, pregnancy, over-secretion of growth hormone or cortisol and fall into the category of errors of metabolic regulation. They have been intensively studied in the human adipocyte because the tissue is readily accessible, but similar changes may occur at other sites, such as muscle and heart, which are responsible for clearing blood glucose. The nature of these metabolic changes in the adipocyte of adult diabetics are of great interest. It has been shown that the conversion of glucose into neutral lipid by adipose tissue is defective and that this may be due to either a transport defect or a defect in intracellular phosphorylation of glucose (Galton et al, 1971).

The evidence for a transport defect comes from 'cross-over plots' of glycolytic intermediates in adipose tissue. During a glucose tolerance test (Page & Galton, 1974), glycolytic intermediates (glucose-6-phosphate, fructose-6-phosphate, fructose 1:6 diphosphate, glycerol phosphate) are measured in adipose tissue at zero-time and at 1 h after an oral glucose load in obese diabetic and non-diabetic patients, and the 1 h values are expressed as a percentage of the initial values (Fig. 13.1). It is observed that the values for glucose and glucose-6-phosphate (between which a transport step

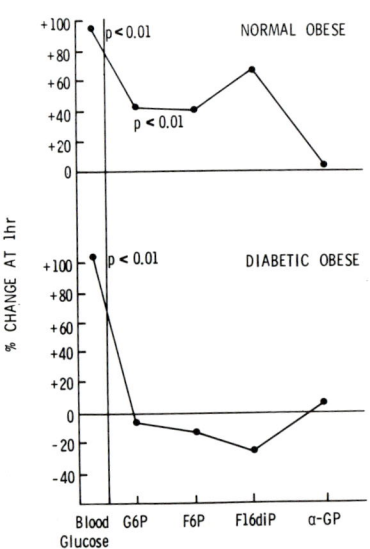

Figure 13.1

A cross-over plot for glycolytic intermediates in human adipose tissue measured at zero time and 1 h after an oral glucose load (100 g). Each point represents a mean of four determinations on 10 obese and nine diabetic patients G6P = glucose-6-phosphate; F6P = fructose-6-phosphate; Fl6diP = fructose diphosphate; αGP = glycerol phosphate (Page & Galton, 1974).

intervenes) both rise in the non-diabetic obese patients; but that in the obese diabetic the blood glucose values rise and the intra-cellular glucose-6-phosphate levels fall below initial values (i.e. there is a 'cross-over' of the baseline values). This suggests that there is a defect in entry of glucose into the adipocyte of adult diabetics. The defect in glucose transport into the diabetic adipocyte may be secondary to a defect in intracellular phosphorylation. Phosphofructokinase is probably one of the rate-determining enzymes in glycolysis and phosphorylates fructose-6-phosphate to fructose 1:6 diphosphate. The activity of this enzyme is impaired in adult diabetes (Galton & Wilson, 1971) and is inversely related to the degree of hyper-glycaemia (Fig. 13.2). A consequence of this may be a build-up in intracellular levels of glucose-6-phosphate proximal to the block. Glucose-6-phosphate is a non-competitive inhibitor of hexokinase

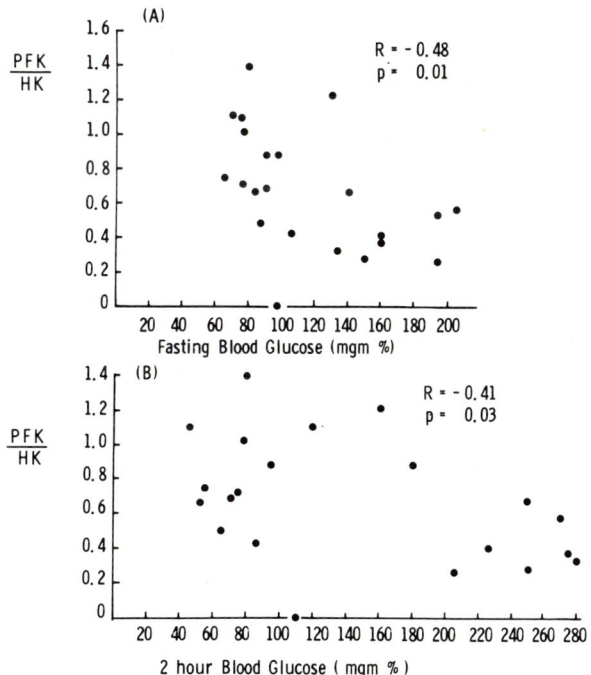

Figure 13.2
The activity of phosphofructokinase (PFK) related to hexokinase (HK) in extracts of adipose tissue from obese diabetic and non-diabetic patients. Points represent individual patients with biopsies at zero time or two hours during a glucose tolerance test (50 g).

with Inhibitor Constants for ATP of 0.17 mM and for glucose of 0.16 mM; and values of glucose-6-phosphate found in obese diabetic patients compared to obese non-diabetics after an overnight fast were 7.09 ± 2.16 (10) nmoles/g net weight, versus 5.78 ± 0.83 (11) nmoles/g (Page & Galton, 1974). The accumulation of glucose-6-phosphate in the diabetic was not observed when the results were expressed on the basis of cell number or triglyceride content but if the difference is real it may lead to feedback inhibition of hexokinase. This may then account for the failure to observe an increase in intracellular levels of glucose-6-phosphate in the diabetic adipocyte following a glucose load because hexokinase is in an inhibited state. If similar changes were to occur in other insulin-sensitive tissues, such as muscle or heart, this defect in glucose metabolism could contribute considerably to the hyperglycaemia found in adult diabetics.

There are other disorders of adipose tissue which lead to a failure of uptake of fatty acids and glucose. In the rare disorder of lipoatrophic diabetes, there is a generalized atrophy of the adipose organ with the development of diabetes, hyperlipaemia and fatty infiltration of the liver which can lead to cirrhosis. However, the factors underlying this lipoatrophy are poorly understood, although the consequences may be a failure to store blood glucose and fatty acids (Schwartz et al, 1960).

EXCESSIVE STORAGE

TRIGLYCERIDE STORAGE DISEASE

A kindred has been recently described (Galton et al, 1974) in which three close members (mother, sister and daughter) appear to have a defect in the mobilization of glycerol from adipose tissue following stimulation with isoprenaline (Fig. 13.3). The defect is not located at the β-receptor or adenyl cyclase, because isoprenaline stimulates the levels of cyclic-AMP in tissue from the mother and daughter. However, there appears to be a failure of cyclic-AMP to activate the triglyceride-lipase and the defect may lie at the level of protein kinase responsible for phosphorylation of the inactive triglyceride-lipase. The evidence for this is that protein kinases extracted from adipose tissue of the mother respond poorly to cyclic-AMP with regard to phosphorylation of histones, whereas protein kinases from control tissue of obese patients are more active (Fig. 13.4). This assay probably measures several protein kinases in the cell (phosphorylase and nuclear kinases) as well as the lipase kinase. A defect in the pathway between triglyceride and glycerol was excluded by finding normal amounts of mono- and di-glycerides on thin layer chromatography in adipose tissue of the mother.

Triglyceride storage disease may be somewhat analogous to glycogen storage disease; and it is of relevance that the reactions controlling the activity of the phosphorylase are similar to those regulating triglyceride-lipase in adipose tissue. They both involve β-receptors, adenyl cyclase, phosphodiesterase and protein kinases (and probably phosphatases). Of the nine types of glycogen storage disease, Types *VIII* and *IX* are due to defects in the activation of phosphorylase by protein kinases in the liver. It is quite possible that a similar group of defects occur on the pathways of triglyceride mobilization and now that attention has been drawn to this, other variants may perhaps come to light (Galton *et al,* 1974).

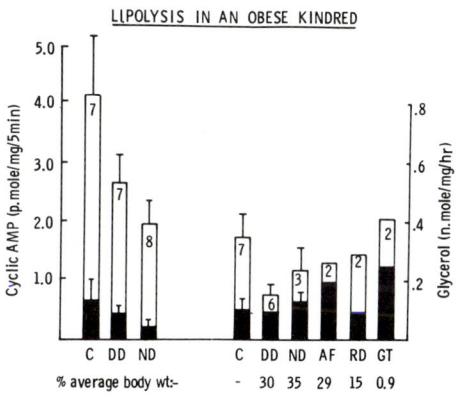

Figure 13.3

Lipolysis in an obese kindred. Release of glycerol and levels of cyclic-AMP were measured in biopsies from adipose tissue from obese controls and from the kindred in the absence (filled columns) and presence (open columns) of isoprenaline (10^{-5} M). Results are means of the number of observations with the SEM marked by bars. Methods are as described by Gilbert *et al,* 1974.

Key: C = controls;   DD = propositus;
      ND = daughter;   AF = sister;
      RD = brother;   GT = twin sister (non-identical) of propositus

Significance of difference calculated by Students t test: glycerol increment in DD versus controls, $p < 0.05$; mean glycerol increment in obese kindred versus controls, $p < 0.01$; glycerol release of obese kindred versus controls, $p < 0.05$; glycerol release from DD, basal versus isoprenaline, p = NS (Not Significant).

THE LIPOMA ADIPOCYTE

Lipomata are benign tumours of adipose tissue which accumulate neutral lipid at slightly greater rates and undergo slightly faster rates of growth than surrounding tissue. Several factors could contribute to this increased deposition of lipid; these include increased rates of lipogenesis from glucose or decreased mobilization of triglycerides. However, maximal rates of lipolysis stimulated by isoprenaline and rates of lipogenesis from glucose or palmitate are similar to those of normal tissue. A more subtle defect occurs in these tumour cells. Although maximal rates of conversion of glucose to glyceride-glycerol are normal, this pathway is insensitive to inhibition by citrate (Atkinson et al, 1973; Galton & Wilson, 1970). Citrate is an allosteric inhibitor of phosphofructokinase in many tissues, including normal adipose tissue, but in lipoma cells the enzyme appears to respond poorly to citrate (Fig. 13.5). There is also evidence that cyclic-AMP is a poor stimulator of the tumour enzyme compared to normal phosphofructokinase (Galton & Wilson, 1970). This may be due to a structural defect (either conformational or an amino-acid substitution) of the ensyme in the region of regulatory sites for citrate and cyclic-AMP, but not affecting the catalytic binding site for fructose-6-phosphate.

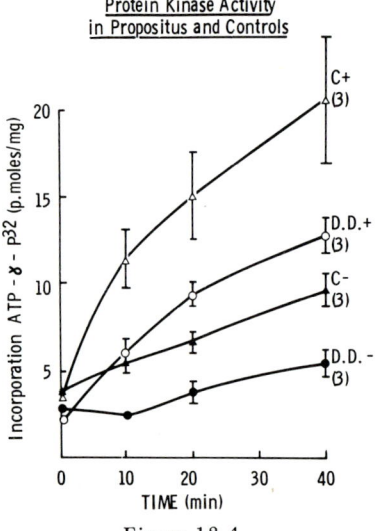

Figure 13.4

The activity of protein kinase in extracts of adipose tissue from the propositus (DD) of Figure 13.3 and obese controls, in the presence (open symbols $\circ, \triangle$) and absence (filled symbols, $\bullet, \blacktriangle$) of cyclic-AMP (5×20^{-7} M). Points are means of 32P incorporated into histones ± SEM using the methods of Corbin and Krebs (1969).

These changes may render the enzyme less sensitive to environmental controls; one consequence may be that although maximal rates of synthesis of glyceride-glycerol are unaltered, the pathway is always operating under conditions of maximal stimulation and may not be able to modulate with environmental changes in levels of citrate or cyclic-AMP. This represents a possible example of an acquired error of metabolic regulation of a key enzyme in glycolysis and may be linked to the increased deposition of glyceride-glycerol found in these tumours. It is also of interest to speculate on the relationship of such enzyme defects and the development of neoplasia. Lipomata represent 'minimal-deviation' tumours of adipose tissue since they are biochemically and morphologically very similar to adipose tissue. Abnormalities in such tumours may therefore be closely related to the development of neoplasia. If, for example, loss of negative feedback control occurs as a general phenomenon with tumour enzymes on other metabolic pathways such as those involved in the control of cell division, increased rates of mitosis may result.

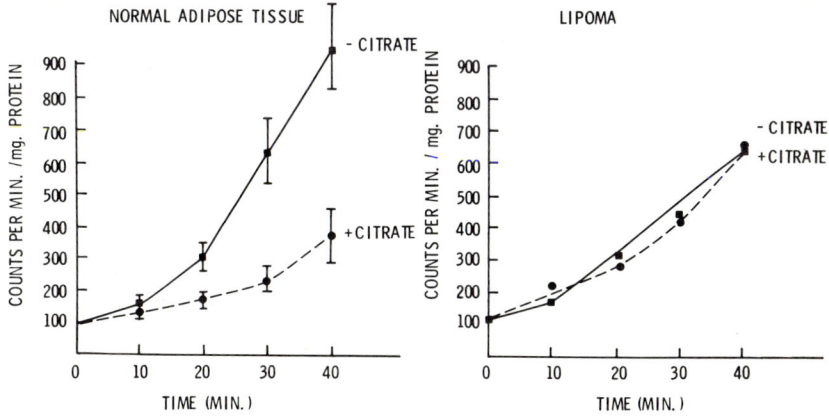

Figure 13.5
The effect of citrate on the conversion of glucose-6-phosphate to glyceride-glycerol in extracts of lipoma and normal adipose tissue. Points are means of 7 lipomata and 6 control tissues incubated in the presence and absence of citrate (10 mM). Methods are as described in Galton & Wilson (1970).

EXCESSIVE RELEASE

DIABETES MELLITUS

In diabetes there is excessive release of fatty acids from adipose tissue which produces an elevation of plasma levels. With insulin-dependent diabetics, this is probably due to a failure of the antilipolytic action of insulin on adipose tissue, since the abnormal levels of fatty acids are corrected by replacement with insulin. Insulin can exert an antilipolytic effect in two ways. One is by stimulating glucose metabolism and, therefore, the re-esterification of fatty acids to neutral lipid in adipose tissue. However, insulin can exert an antilipolytic effect on adipose tissue *in vitro* in the absence of external glucose. This is termed the direct antilipolytic action of insulin and is possibly mediated by a decline in intracellular levels of cyclic-AMP. Insulin can be shown to lower levels of cyclic-AMP in adipocytes which have been previously stimulated with catecholamines, but not to affect basal levels. The effect of insulin on levels of cyclic-AMP, although rather small, is accompanied by inhibition of glycerol output from the tissue and may therefore be a physiologically significant effect. It is not yet established how insulin acts on cyclic-AMP; it may be by direct inhibition of the enzyme adenyl cyclase responsible for conversion of ATP to cyclic-AMP, or by

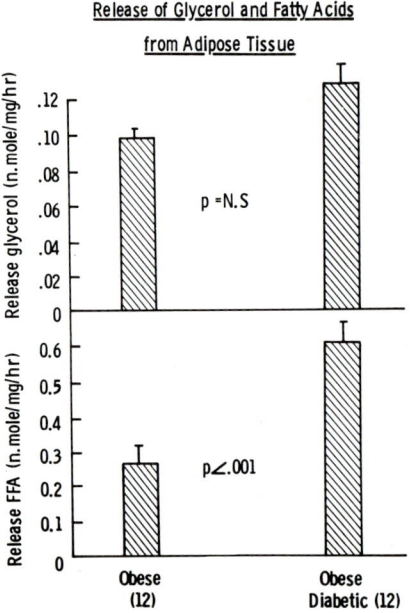

Figure 13.6
The release of glycerol and fatty acids from adipose tissue of obese diabetic and non-diabetic patients. Samples of adipose tissue (200 mg) were incubated in 0.5 ml of bicarbonate buffer and the appearance of glycerol and fatty acids in the medium was measured according to previously described methods (Gilbert et al, 1974). Results are means with SEM enclosed within bars.

stimulation of the phosphodiesterase which converts cyclic-AMP to 5/AMP.

In adult, or insulin-independent, diabetes, there is also an elevation of plasma fatty acids and an augmented release of fatty acids from adipose tissue (Fig. 13.6). This occurs under conditions of raised concentrations of glucose and insulin, which would be expected to exert a marked antilipolytic action. The fact that antilypolysis does not occur has led to two proposals. First, there are lipolytic hormones, such as growth hormone or cortisol, circulating in the blood stream to account for the increased lipolytic state; but these hormone levels have never been convincingly shown to be abnormal. Moreover the lipolytic sequence in adipose tissue of obese diabetics appears to be capable of full stimulation by catecholamines as judged by rises in cyclic-AMP and release of glycerol, so that the lipolytic sequence appears not to be grossly altered in adult diabetes. However, during an oral glucose tolerance test there is usually a precipitate

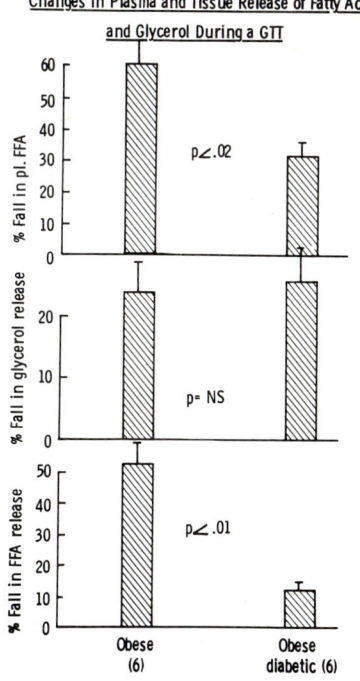

Figure 13.7
The changes in plasma and tissue release of fatty acids and glycerol during a glucose tolerance test in obese and diabetic patients. Methods are as described by Gilbert et al, (1974). Results are means with SEM enclosed within bars.

reduction in the concentrations of plasma fatty acids (Hales & Randle, 1963) and a decline in release of fatty acids of about 50 per cent from adipose tissue of obese patients. In the obese diabetic, however, this fall in plasma fatty acids and decrease in release of tissue fatty acids occurs to a much lesser extent (Fig. 13.7). This may suggest that in the adult diabetic there is perhaps a defect in the termination of the lipolytic state following a period of stimulation. The metabolic abnormality leading to this failure to terminate lipolysis in the adult diabetic has as yet to be clarified, but may well be responsible for the raised plasma concentrations of fatty acids.

CONCLUSION

The human adipocyte is one of the more recent cells to come under careful investigation in clinical medicine. Like the study of the erythrocyte before it, the study of the adipocyte is yielding new concepts for the investigation of diseases. Because of its integrated structure with nucleus, hormone-receptor site and full complement of metabolic pathways, the cell provides a valuable model for the study of errors in metabolic regulation. Study of the adipocyte has led to the probable identification of a new group of inborn errors of metabolism, the triglyceride storage diseases. Finally, the adipocyte is a focal point in the metabolism of body lipids and is likely to be intimately involved in the development of some types of hyperlipaemia. Diabetes, obesity and the hyperlipaemias are amongst the commonest of present-day diseases, and the role of the adipocyte requires further exploration in these disorders.

REFERENCES

ATKINSON, J.N.C., GALTON, D.J. & GILBERT, C. (1973) Regulatory defect of glycolysis in human lipoma. *Brit. Med. J.*, 1, 101.

BROWN, W.V. & GRETEN, H. (1973) Type I hyperlipoproteinaemia. *Clinics in Endocrinol. and Metab.*, 2, 73.

CORBIN, J.D. & KREBS, E.G. (1969) A cyclic AMP stimulated protein kinase in adipose tissue. *Biochem. Biophys. Res. Commun.*, 36, 649.

GALTON, D.J. (1971) In *The Human Adipose Cell:* a model for errors in metabolic regulation, London: Butterworth.

GALTON, D.J., GILBERT, C., RECKLESS, J.P.D. & KAYE, J. (1974) Triglyceride storage disease: a group of inborn errors of triglyceride metabolism. *Quart. J. Med.* 43, 63.

GALTON, D.J. & WILSON, J.P.D. (1970) Lipogenesis in homogenates of human adipose tissue. *Clin. Sci.*, 38, 649.

GALTON, D.J. & WILSON, J.P.D. (1971) The effect of starvation and diabetes on glycolytic enzymes in human adipose tissue. *Glin. Sci.*, 41, 545.

GALTON, D.J., WILSON, J.P.D. & KISSEBAH, A.H. (1971) The effect of adult diabetes on glucose utilization and esterification of palmitate by human adipose tissue. *Europ. J. Clin. Invest.*, 1, 399.

GILBERT, C., GALTON, D.J. & KAYE, J. (1973) Triglyceride storage disease: a disorder of lipolysis in adipose tissue in two patients. *Brit. Med. J.*, 1, 25.

GILBERT, C., KAYE, J. & GALTON, D.J. (1974) The effect of a glucose load on plasma fatty acids and lipolysis in adipose tissue of obese diabetic and non-diabetic patients. *Diabetologia*, 10, 135.

HALES, C.N. & RANDLE, P.J. (1963) Effects of low-carbohydrate diet and diabetes mellitus on plasma concentrations of glucose, non-esterified fatty acids and insulin during oral glucose tolerance tests. *Lancet*, 1, 790.

HARLAN, W.R., WINESETT, P.S. & WASSERMAN, A.J. (1967) Tissue lipoprotein lipase in normal individuals and in individuals with exogenous hypertriglyceridaemia and the relationship of this enzyme to assimilation of fat. *J. Clin. Invest.*, 40, 239.

HAVEL, R.J. & GORDON, Jr.R.S. (1960) Idiopathic hyperlipaemia: metabolic studies in an affected family. *J. Clin. Invest.*, 39, 1777.

PAGE, A. & GALTON, D.J. (1974) In preparation.

SCHWARTZ, R., SCHAFER, I. & RENOLD, A.E. (1960) Lipoatrophy, disturbed carbohydrate metabolism and accelerated growth. *Am. J. Med.*, 28, 973.

14. Hormones and the Adipocyte: Factors Influencing the Metabolic Effects of Insulin and Adrenaline

L.B. SALANS, S.W. CUSHMAN, E.S. HORTON, E. DANFORTH, Jr. and E.A.H. SIMS

In man, adipose tissue is the major energy storage organ of the body. Storage and mobilization of energy in the specialized cells of this tissue, the adipocytes, is an active metabolic process involving lipogenic and lipolytic activities. As with most metabolic processes of the body, these functions are regulated by a variety of hormones. Lipogenic activity consists of the *de novo* synthesis of fatty acids from glucose and the esterification of these fatty acids, and of others derived from lipoprotein and chylomicrons, with glycerophosphate to form triglycerides. This energy storage activity is stimulated by increased substrate availability and, more specifically, by insulin. Lipolytic activity comprises the breakdown of stored triglyceride by a specific lipase and the subsequent release of energy from the cell of fatty acids and glycerol. This activity is stimulated by a variety of hormones including adrenaline, adreno-corticotrophic hormone (ACTH), glucagon and growth hormone. Fatty acids may also be re-esterified with glycerophosphate and re-stored as triglyceride, a process which is enhanced by insulin and glucose and inhibited by the lipolytic hormones.

Integration of these activities occurs at several levels. At the cell membrane, hormones bind to specific receptors, triggering a sequence of events which culminate in the various metabolic activities of the cell. Insulin and the lipolytic hormones appear to act antagonistically towards the activity of the membrane bound ensyme, adenyl cyclase (Butcher, 1970); at the same time insulin and the lipolytic hormones appear to alter the concentration of specific cyclic nucleotide second messengers: cyclic guanosine monophosphate (cGMP) is altered by insulin (Illiano *et al*, 1973) and cyclic adenosine monophosphate (cAMP) by the lipolytic hormones (Butcher, 1970). Intracellularly, the availability of glycerophosphate for esterification relative to the rate of fatty acid liberation from triglyceride by lipolysis appears to determine whether energy is released from the cell as fatty acid or stored as triglyceride.

The balance between the energy storage and energy mobilization function of the adipose cell, and therefore the size of the adipose tissue mass, depends upon the state of energy supply in relation to energy need. In obesity energy intake is excessive relative to energy expenditure; thus, triglyceride storage in the adipose tissue is increased and the adipose depot is enlarged.

In obesity, expansion of the adipose depot is accompanied by alterations in the metabolic character of this tissue. Studies in our laboratory indicate that the metabolic function of the adipose tissue and its control by hormones is influenced by a variety of factors including the cellular character of the tissue, the nature of the diet and the state of growth of the organism at the time tissue is obtained

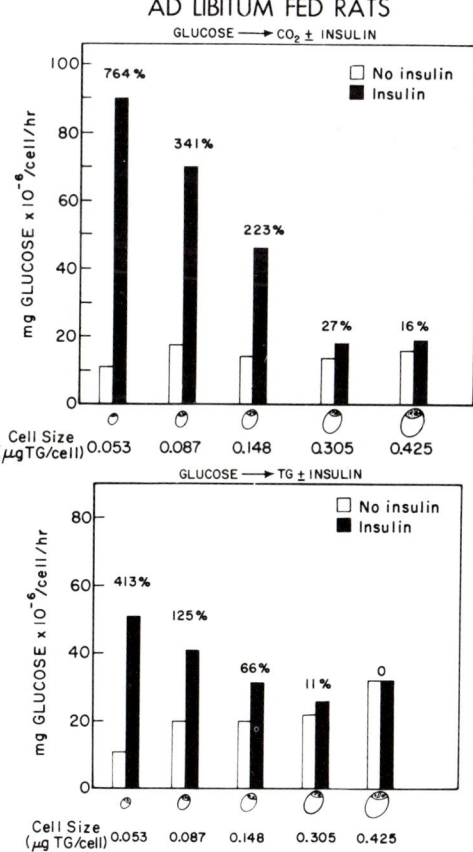

Figure 14.1

for study (Salans *et al*, 1972; Salans & Dougherty, 1971; Salans *et al*, 1968).

Thus, when adipose tissue is obtained from animals ingesting diets of similar carbohydrate, fat and protein composition, and during similar growth states, increasing adipose cell size is associated with unchanging rates of glucose oxidation and increasing rates of glucose-1-^{14}C incorporation into triglyceride-glycerol in the absence of insulin. There is a decreased stimulation of these two parameters of glucose metabolism by insulin (Fig. 14.1) (Salans & Dougherty, 1971). Similar relationships have been observed when adipose tissue from obese and non-obese patients have been compared and in human adipose cells of different size (Salans *et al*, 1972; Salans *et al*, 1968; Smith, 1971). These alterations of fat cell metabolism associated with cellular enlargement can not only be reversed through weight loss and reduction in cell size in obese patients (Fig. 14.2a) Salans *et al*, 1968) but can also be induced through weight gain and

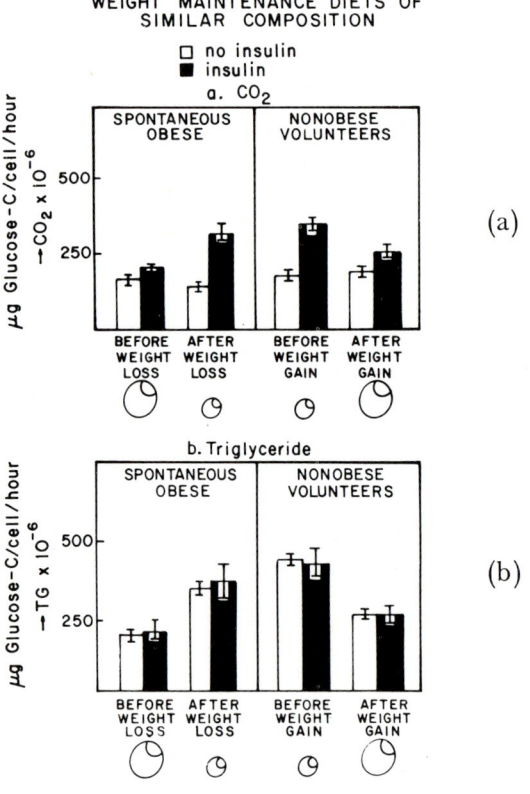

Figure 14.2

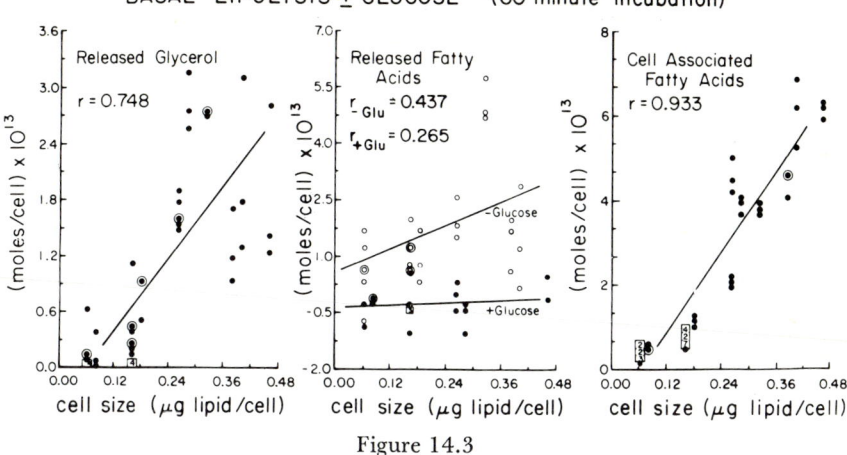

Figure 14.3

increase in cell size in non-obese subjects (Fig. 14.2b) (Salans et al, 1972).

Figure 14.3 indicates that the basal rate of lipolysis by rat adipocytes, as reflected by glycerol release, increases with increasing cell size and is accompanied by increasing fatty acid release in the absence but not in the presence of glucose (Cushman & Salans, 1973a). This figure also illustrates the association between increasing adipose cell size, increased basal lipolytic activity and an elevation of cell associated nonesterified fatty acid (CAFA) levels. Figure 14.4

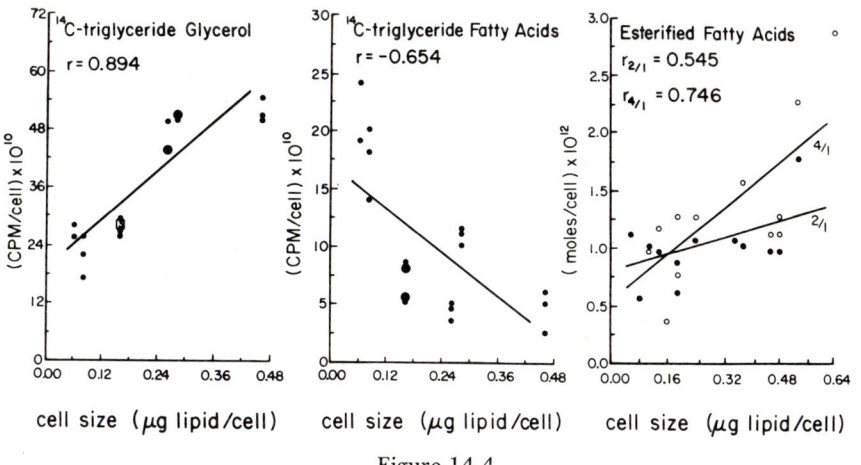

Figure 14.4

shows that the enhanced rate of basal lipolysis associated with increasing cell size is accompanies by a marked decrease in the rate of *de novo* fatty acid synthesis from glucose. However, the capacity for re-esterification, as measured by the incorporation of glucose carbon into triglyceride-glycerol increases with increasing cell size. Esterification of exogeneous fatty acids by enlarged cells may be equal to or slightly greater than that observed in smaller cells, when exposed to excessive levels of preformed fatty acids.

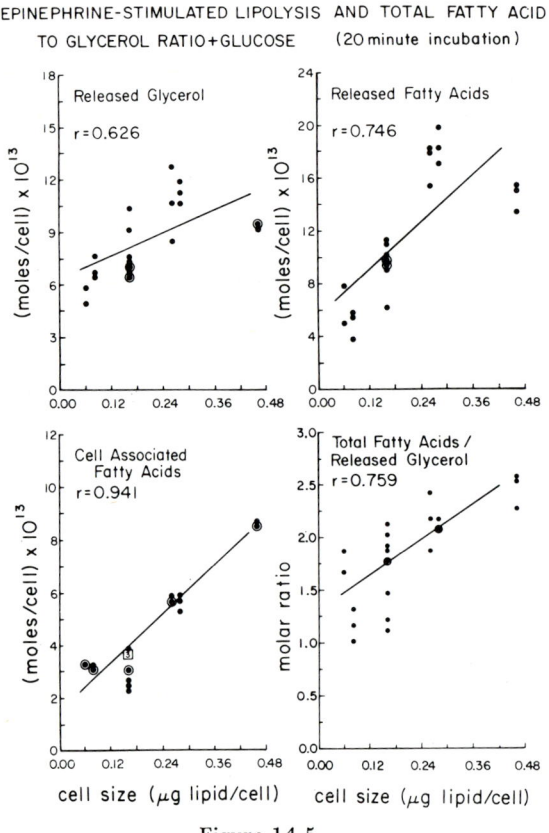

Figure 14.5

In the presence of adrenaline, lipolysis or glycerol release increases only slightly with increasing adipose cell size (Fig. 14.5), but is accompanied by a marked increase in fatty acid release and elevation of CAFA levels. However, as indicated by the increasing ratio of total fatty acids measured, i.e. the sum of released fatty acids and CAFA per unit of glycerol release, esterification in the large cell decreases. Enlargement of the adipose cell, under conditions of similar nutri-

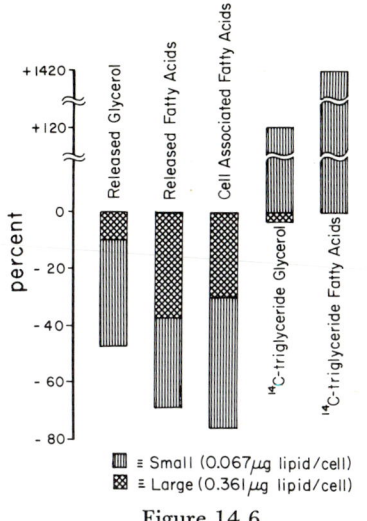

Figure 14.6

tional intake and growth, is therefore accompanied by increasing adrenaline stimulated lipolytic activity, increasing net triglyceride mobilization and increasing intracellular fatty acid levels.

Figure 14.6 illustrates the decreasing antilipolytic and lipogenic effects of insulin with increasing rat adipose cell size. The inhibition of adrenaline stimulated glycerol and fatty acid release, the reduction of adrenaline elevated CAFA levels and the stimulation of triglyceride-glycerol and fatty acid synthesis by insulin is diminished in the large adipose cells. Thus, the association between cellular enlargement and increased basal and adrenaline stimulated triglyceride-turnover is paralleled by a decreasing insulin response. Increases in CAFA levels accompany all of these cell size related alterations.

This evidence for a relationship between the size and the *in vitro* metabolism of adipose cells has been derived from studies in patients and animals having widely different cell size, but in whom the state of nutrition and growth was similar. Recent studies in our laboratory however indicate that these cell size associated functions can be altered considerably by the state of nutrition and growth of the organism (Salans & Dougherty, 1971).

Thus, basal glucose metabolism and the response to insulin by large adipose cells obtained from obese individuals who maintain their weight while ingesting high carbohydrate diets may be equal to or even greater than that of smaller cells from non-obese subjects

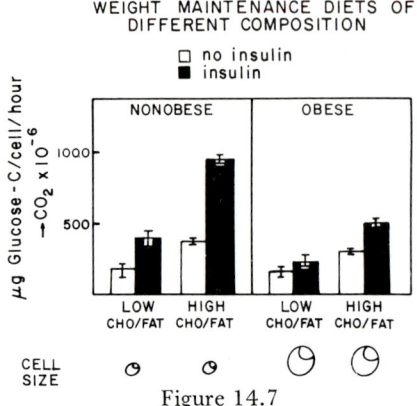

Figure 14.7

during ingestion of isocaloric low carbohydrate diets (Fig. 14.7). Dietary control, therefore, is a critical factor in comparisons of the metabolic character of the adipose tissue between and within individuals.

Furthermore, Figure 14.8 indicates that when adipose tissue is studied during active weight gain, basal glucose metabolism and the insulin response of large cells from obese patients who are actively gaining weight may be greater than that observed in smaller cells obtained from non-obese subjects at constant body weight and obese

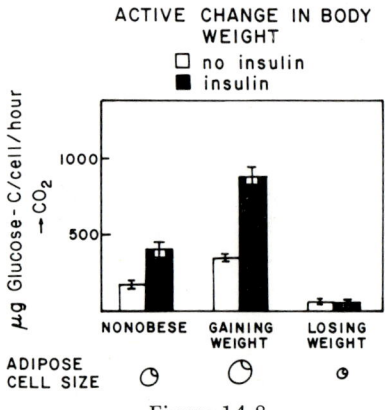

Figure 14.8

patients actively losing weight. Similar observations have been made in the rat (Salans & Dougherty, 1971). Thus, it is important to distinguish between the enlarging and the enlarged adipose cell; that is between the state of becoming obese from that of being obese.

Since these alterations in the metabolic character of the adipose tissue are not only reversed by weight loss in obese patients but can also be induced by weight gain in non-obese subjects, the altered *in vitro* metabolism of adipose tissue in obesity may represent adaptive rather than primary changes in adipose cell function. The reduced effect of insulin coupled with the increased rate of lipolysis suggests that the enlarging adipose cell progressively loses its capacity for net triglyeride storage. Whether these adaptive responses are mediated through the increased concentration of nonesterified fatty acid within the enlarged cell (Cushman & Salans, 1973b), through altered hormonal binding to the cell (Kahn *et al*, 1973) or through some other factor, is not known. Since these adaptive changes can be overcome either by high carbohydrate or high caloric intake, the delivery of excessive lipogenic substrate may be responsible for the maintenance of the increased storage of triglyceride in the adipose tissue of obese individuals. The source and nature of this lipogenic substrate remains to be more fully examined.

The function of the adipose tissue is triglyceride storage and mobilization; these metabolic activities are regulated principally by insulin and adrenaline. The lipogenic and lipolytic functions of adipose tissue and their hormonal control are influenced by the cellular character of the tissue and by the nutritional and growth state of the organism.

When studied under conditions of similar dietary intake and growth, increasing adipose cell size is associated with a diminished stimulation of glucose metabolism by insulin, an enhanced rate of basal and adrenaline-stimulated lipolysis and a relative decrease in esterification, a reduced rate of *de novo* fatty acid synthesis from glucose and an elevation of cell associated—probably intracellular—nonesterified fatty acids. These cell size associated metabolic alterations can not only be reversed by weight loss and reduction of cell size in the obese, but also be induced through weight gain and adipose cellular enlargement in non-obese subjects.

Following ingestion of a high carbohydrate diet, or during active weight gain, basal glucose metabolism and the insulin response of adipocytes are enhanced; thus, even large fat cells from the obese can be at least as responsive to insulin as are smaller cells from the non-obese. Furthermore, in the presence of high concentrations of free fatty acids, the capacity of the enlarged adipocyte for esterification of exogenous fatty acids may be equal to or even greater than that observed in smaller cells. Thus, the alterations in function observed in the enlarged adipocyte represent secondary rather than primary changes in obesity.

Such alterations result in a progressive reduction in the capacity of the adipose cell for net triglyceride storage. These adaptive changes can, however, be overcome by the continued delivery of excess lipogenic substrate.

REFERENCES

BUTCHER, R.W. (1970) The role of cyclic AMP in the actions of some lipolytic and antilipolytic agents. In *Adipose Tissue, Regulation and Metabolic Functions*, p.5, Ed. Jeanrenaud, B. & Hepp, D. New York: Academic Press.

CUSHMAN, S.W. & SALANS, L.B. (1973a) Lipolysis and triglyceride turnover in rat adipose cells: effects of cell size. *Fed. Proc.*, 32, 940.

CUSHMAN, S.W. & SALANS, L.B. (1973b) Cell associated fatty acids: a role in the mediation of cell size effects on adipose cell function. *Clin. Res.*, 21, 620.

ILLIANO, G. TELL, G., SIEGEL, M. & CUATRECASAS, P. (1973) Guanosine 3':5'-cyclic monophosphate and the action of insulin and acetylcholine. *Proc. Soc. Nat. Acad. Sci.*, 70, 2443.

JOHNSON, P.R. & HIRSCH, J. (1972) Cellularity of adipose depots in six strains of genetically obese mice. *J. Lipid Res.*, 13, 2.

KAHN, C.R., SOLL, A., NEVILLE, D.M. & ROTH, J. (1973) Severe deficiency in insulin receptors: a common denominator in the insulin resistance of obesity. *Clin. Res.*, 21, 628.

RODBELL, M. (1965) Modulation of lipolysis in adipose tissue by fatty acid concentration in fat cell. *Ann. N.Y. Acad. Sci.*, 110, 302.

SALANS, L.B., DANFORTH, E.Jr., HORTON, E.S. & SIMS, E.A.H. (1972) Dissociation of the effects of adiposity and diet on glucose, insulin and adipose tissue metabolism in human obesity. *J. Clin. Invest.*, 51, 84a.

SALANS, L.B. & DOUGHERTY, J.W. (1971) The effect of insulin upon glucose metabolism by adipose cells of different size. Influence of cell lipid and protein content, age and nutritional state. *J. Clin. Invest.*, 50, 1399.

SALANS, L.B., KNITTLE, J.L. & HIRSCH, J. (1968) The role of adipose cell size and adipose tissue insulin sensitivity in the carbohydrate intolerance of human obesity. *J. Clin. Invest.*, 47, 153.

SMITH, U. (1971) Effect of cell size on lipid synthesis by human adipose tissue *in vitro*. *J. Lipid Res.*, 12, 65.

DISCUSSION

Dr. Elkeles. Dr. Salans, do you have any explanation of the failure of insulin to stimulate the incorporation of glucose into glyceride/glycerol in human adipose tissue?

Dr. Salans. I wish that I had. This problem has to be approached on the basis of knowledge about the way in which insulin affects the cell. This could be at any one of several levels. For example, it could be that binding to the specific receptor is distorted in some way due to the enlarging adipose cell. There are some data suggesting that insulin binding in enlarged adipose cells is impaired compared to the binding of insulin to smaller adipocytes.

As I have shown, there are many other steps in which insulin can influence the metabolic function of the adipose cell; failure could be in any one of the subsequent steps which occur after insulin binds to a specific receptor. On the basis of the data available now, my own preference would be that the defect, the adaptive change in the enlarging cell, probably occurs after the binding of insulin to its receptor site. This is because we see different changes in the metabolism of the adipose cell, depending on which pathway is investigated.

Dr. Stock. It worried me that there was no incorporation of 14C glucose into lipid in the samples of adipose tissue in the presence of insulin. Yet it is well-known that if the subjects are re-fed first, then there is incorporation, with insulin stimulation. I should like to know what the difference is in the adipose tissue of subjects who have been re-fed.

Dr. Salans. I do not think that I can answer that; it worries us too. All I can say at present is very non-specific because our studies with re-feeding are really normal meal ingestion, and the results are too preliminary to make proper comments. Smith and coworkers have demonstrated an impairment in the ability of insulin to stimulate glucose carbon incorporation into glyceride/glycerol. I do not know why we are unable to demonstrate this effect in our studies.

Dr. Björntorp. In connection with this subject of incorporation into glyceride/glycerol, Smith is able to obtain an insulin effect on human adipose tissue. His techniques are somewhat different from yours; he utilizes slightly larger adipose tissue slices, and the glucose concentration is probably important too. He uses an adipose tissue culture medium, which be considers to be more sensitive for this purpose. Could Dr. Salans speculate about the physiological significance of the cell-associated fatty acids?

Dr. Salans. The one abnormality present in the adipose tissue of obese patients which does not seem to be present in that of non-obese patients, and which seems to fluctuate with changes in diet, is the level of intracellular fatty acid. There is abundant evidence to suggest that this can have a profound effect on the metabolic character of the adipose tissue. There is no evidence to suggest that it may interfere with insulin binding, but there is no reason why it could not. Thus, it may be that the changes which are observed are related in some way to the level of intracellular fatty acid.

Professor Keen. Dr. Salans has spent some time showing us that big adipose cells do not respond to insulin, except under one specific circumstance which is when they are becoming larger, that is, when the individual, or the animal, is in a state of active weight gain. Could that perhaps be re-interpreted as meaning that during the stage of active weight gain the empty adipocytes are being recruited, and that he is looking at the effect of two populations of cells; the stable, adipose cell and a newly-stimulated cell which is, in fact, insulin responsive?

Dr. Salans. This is a most perceptive and important question. We are considering here the age of the cell, or its active growth. I do not know how to study specifically the age of the cell in a given population of cells or the stage of its growth. That we might be looking at two populations makes sense to me.

Professor Keen. Could it be done radioautographically to see which cells enhance glucose uptake?

Dr. Salans. That is possible but I do not know whether it is a feasible process. However, there may be factors in addition to your suggestion. We have shown also that the enlarged adipose cell can respond actively to the effect of insulin, in fact it may be more responsive than the small cell, under conditions of high carbohydrate feeding.

Dr. Galton, in your studies carried out in adipose tissue with lipoma, have you demonstrated any difference in lipoma or other normal tissues at different sites? That is, if a patient has a lipoma in his subcutaneous abdominal fat, and another has a lipoma in the triceps fat, is there any difference in the abnormalities, either quantitatively, or qualitatively.

Dr. Galton. My results were from 21 consecutive lipomas removed from subcutaneous sites. We have not looked at lipomas from other sites.

Dr. Salans. It is important to be very careful about describing in terms of one isolated area the morphological or metabolic character of the tissue as a whole. There is sufficient data to suggest that the variability from site to site is great enough for us not to be able to interpret either *in vivo* or *in vitro* studies in these terms.

Dr. Stock. Could I put an alternative explanation for Dr. Galton's family with the triglyceride storage? The diminished release of glycerol could be due to the presence of glycerol kinase in the adipose tissue of these people. It need not necessarily be a defect in adipolysis, but enhanced re-esterification with glycerol kinase in the tissue. Have you considered this possibility?

Dr. Galton. I have not measured glycerol kinase. It could be due to increased glycerol re-utilization.

Dr. Quaade. Have you extended your lipoma research to the lipodystrophies?

Dr. Galton. We had the opportunity to look at lipodystrophic tissue and adjacent tissue; but it is difficult to make a comparison. Lipodystrophic tissue is very fibrous. We looked basically at lipogenesis and lipolysis. We have not succeeded in demonstrating any convincing differences.

Dr. Durnin. I presume it would be possible to make a calculation of the difference in efficiency of the energy production in the tissues which you are investigating. If such a calculation were made, how much difference would it make in relation to the practical situation of the energy turnover, or expenditure, for obese and none-obese people? It seems to me that it would come to an extremely small quantity finally.

Dr. Salans. We have not done that. I am not sure that we have measured enough of the metabolic functions of the adipose cell to enable us to make any meaningful measure. My guess is that, although the amount of change seen in isolated pieces of adipose tissue is small, when this is added up over billions of adipose cells, particularly in the case of hypercellular obesity, this may well amount to a significant figure. It would be most interesting to have a look at this.

Dr. Durnin. I think it would be possible to work out the relative efficiency of, say, ATP production, and it might be possible to say that the difference between the obese and the non-obese cells might account for, say, five or 10 per cent overall difference. Theoretically anyway, this could be related to total quantities of energy for the whole organism. This would give a clearer picture of whether this is something which is important.

Dr. Björntorp. It is difficult to calculate the ATP losses per cycle of glycerol releases and re-esterification because many assumptions have to be made. We have calculated the metabolic activity at different fat cell sites. If the adipose tissue is decreased there could be a significant difference in caloric expenditure.

Dr. Ashwell. Dr. Salans has shown that there can be a very large difference in cell size in different subcutaneous sites. Has he investigated the metabolic parameters and compared the results with the amount of fat in these particular subcutaneous sites, and are there any correlations?

Dr. Salans. We have observed that there are differences between subcutaneous and deep sites of adipose tissue and we have studied metabolic characteristics too. We have not yet reached the stage at which we have analysed this adequately, but there are differences in the metabolism of the adipose tissue from the same individual between sites. In general, these follow cell size, but not completely. The effects of diet which I have described, the interaction of diet and cell size, are even clearer when we study the influence of cell size on metabolism of the adipose tissue.

In other words, diet influences the metabolic capacity of the adipose tissue at different sites of the body, and the degree of that influence is dependent, in part, upon the size of the cell which is being examined.

Dr. Bray. One perplexing problem to me is the effects of high carbohydrate feeding. When subjects are put on a high carbohydrate diet, as compared to a low one, as Dr. Salans' group did for their measurements of cell function, plasma insulin levels are raised. At the same time the adipose cells and muscle are made more sensitive to insulin *in vitro*. I cannot understand why these subjects do not become hyperglycaemic or do not have lower blood sugars than the people on the high fat diet who have lower insulin, and less sensitivity of their tissues.

Dr. Salans. All the studies which I presented are ones done in the fasting state. In our hands, the switch from a low to a high carbohydrate diet is not associated, in the fasting state, with a change in the level of insulin and glucose in the direction you describe. We do not see much difference between patients on a high or low carbohydrate diet in the fasting state. Moreover, in response to an acute oral glucose challenge, there is an improvement in the glucose utilization, in plasma insulin and plasma glucose levels, rather than an increase in the insulin and glucose levels. Only in response to the meals over a 24 hour period do we see what you describe. Nevertheless, it does not answer the question of why, in that limited time period, these people do not become hyperglycaemic. What prevents this happening? I suspect some adaptation of the liver is involved. This is the primary site for controlling the blood glucose in the first place. I cannot be more specific than that.

Professor Keen. Dr. Galton, do your patients have raised lipid levels when fasting? Can they lipolyse under conditions of food deprivation and, secondly, have you taken the big step of giving them adrenaline to see what happens in terms of fatty acid mobilization *in vivo*?

Dr. Galton. First, I have data on the propositus gained by fasting for 14 days. There was a rise in fatty acids from day zero up to day 14. There is a corresponding drop in weight. Thus, under fasting conditions, they can lipolyse. We think that activation of lipolysis by fasting is different from activation of lipolysis by isoprenaline.

With regard to the second question, I did not mention that they also have a hyperlipidaemia, and the propositus has ischaemic heart disease, so we have neither exercised her nor added adrenaline. Of course, the crucial action to take is to give *in vivo* hormonal stimulus, rather than *in vitro*.

15. Peripheral Metabolism of Carbohydrate in Obesity and Diabetes

MARGARET J. WHICHELOW

Measurements of the arterial or venous blood concentrations of substrate, in the fasting or resting state or in response to stimuli, give indications of total changes in the body but cannot reveal what is happening in individual tissues.

The glucose tolerance test is widely used for the detection and diagnosis of diabetes mellitus. The diagnosis is based on the capillary or venous blood sugar concentrations at various time intervals after glucose loading. However although a number of individuals may have the same concentrations it does not mean that glucose disposal into the various tissues is similar, and therefore that if subjected to stress or additional stimuli their glucose tolerance curves would then be the same. Information about the pattern of glucose disposal in the body can be valuable, since it is important to know not only who has diabetes but also who is likely to develop diabetes.

In view of the large number of people who currently wish or are advised to lose weight, the effects of a low calorie diet, with or without the aid of appetite suppressant drugs, on the patterns of glucose disposal have been studied, as have those due to oral antidiabetic agents in diabetes. The effect of exercise in non-diabetics and diabetics has also been examined since lack of exercise frequently leads to a gain in weight and excess exercise to hypoglycaemia in diabetics.

The forearm technique has been used to study a representative example of one tissue namely the peripheral tissues which consist mainly of skeletal muscle. This Chapter is mainly concerned with glucose and its peripheral disposal in obesity and diabetes during oral glucose tolerance tests and following the local intra-arterial injection of insulin.

METHODS

The forearm preparation, described in detail elsewhere by Butterfield

& Holling (1959) has been used, with minor modifications, in informed volunteer lean and obese non-diabetic and diabetic subjects. Briefly, fine polythene catheters are inserted under local anaesthetic into the brachial artery and into a suitable vein in the antecubital fossa, which is carefully chosen as draining the deep muscle compartment of the forearm. The catheters, kept patent by the slow infusion of saline, facilitate repeated blood sampling over a period of hours. Blood flow is measured with a water filled venous occlusion plethysmograph, and the hand circulation is excluded for one minute before and during all sampling procedures by inflating a cuff at the wrist to 200 mm Hg. Simultaneous arterial and venous blood samples are collected over one minute periods with concommitant blood flow measurements.

Tissue glucose uptake is calculated from the product of the blood flow and the arterio-venous glucose difference. The cell glucose uptake is derived from the tissue glucose uptake and the changes in the venous glucose concentration since the venous and extracellular glucose concentrations equilibrate rapidly (Butterfield et al, 1963).

During glucose tolerance tests glucose uptake measurements are made three to five times in the fasting state and then at 15 minute intervals for two hours following the oral administration of 50 g glucose. In the studies where insulin is injected into the brachial artery, glucose uptake is measured at intervals in the fasting state, and then at 10 minute intervals for one hour following a two minute injection of 0.1 unit ^{131}I insulin (Butterfield et al, 1962).

The tests are all carried out after an overnight fast, and in the case of the diabetics all antidiabetic therapy is withdrawn for 16 hours prior to the test.

RESULTS AND DISCUSSION

GLUCOSE UPTAKE IN THE FASTING STATE

In all subjects, lean or obese, diabetic or non-diabetic, the arterio-venous difference is small, usually 1 to 3 mg/100 ml, and the glucose uptake is low and similar, so that meaningful comparisons between individuals or groups cannot be made (Whichelow & Butterfield, 1971). However, after glucose loading or an intra-arterial insulin injection peripheral glucose uptake rises and differences between groups become apparent.

GLUCOSE UPTAKE IN LEAN AND OBESE SUBJECTS

In lean non-diabetic men and women the arterial blood sugar concentration rises more rapidly than the venous concentration. This results in a widening arterio-venous glucose difference, and since the blood flow usually remains steady, an increase in glucose uptake. This reaches a peak between 30 and 75 minutes, and then returns to the fasting level by 120 minutes. Thus the mean glucose uptake after glucose is considerably higher than before—up to 1.5 mg/100 ml/min. In contrast the increase in glucose uptake after glucose administration in grossly obese subjects and even the mildly obese is much less (Butterfield *et al*, 1965; Whichelow & Butterfield, 1971). This is a very consistent finding and there is in fact a close inverse correlation between the mean cell glucose uptake and the skinfold thickness, as a measure of obesity (Fig. 15.1) (Whichelow & Butterfield, 1971). Calculations have shown that, despite the fact that skinfold thickness is measured at different sites in men (sub-scapular) and women (mid-triceps), the relationship between skinfold thickness and glucose uptake is the same; these have thus been grouped together in Figure 15.1.

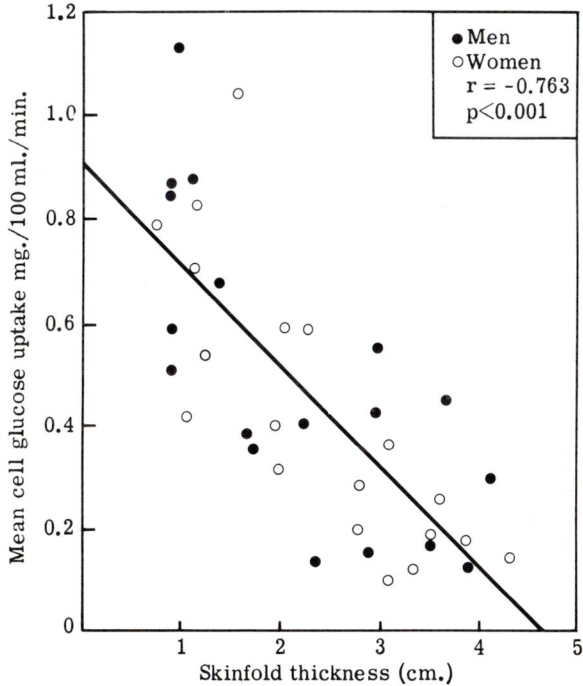

Figure 15.1
Relationship between glucose uptake and skinfold thickness during a 50 g oral glucose tolerance test in non-diabetic subjects. (Reproduced by permission of the Editor of the Quarterly Journal of Medicine).

The rise in blood sugar is accompanied by a rise in the arterial and venous plasma insulin concentrations and with a widening arterio-venous difference there is an increase in peripheral insulin uptake which tends to be greater in obese subjects (Asmal *et al,* 1971).

Thus it is apparent that with increasing obesity the muscles become less and less metabolically active with respect to glucose and less sensitive to insulin. Calculations based on the estimated muscle mass (30 kg) of the average man, show that in a lean subject 40 g or more of the 50 g glucose load enters the muscles during the test, whereas in a grossly obese subject only 5 to 10 g do so. The fate of

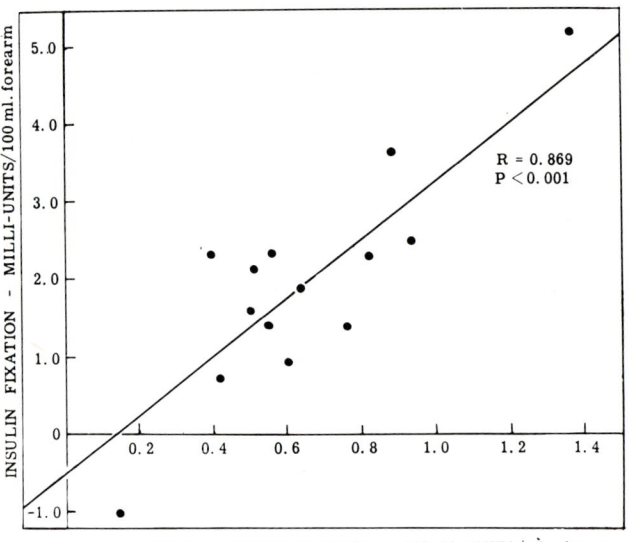

Figure 15.2
Relationship between peripheral insulin fixation and plasma insulin concentration achieved by the intra-arterial injection of 0.1 unit insulin in non-diabetic subjects. (Reproduced by permission of the Editor of Clinical Science).

the rest of the glucose is not known with certainty but the liver, a large metabolically active organ with a large blood flow, seems the most likely site for its disposal.

Malaisse (1968) has found in animals that most of the glucose load in a glucose tolerance test enters the liver during the first hour. This does not necessarily contradict the present findings since in lean subjects it may be that glucose first enters the liver and then is released to find its way to the peripheral tissues, whereas in obese subjects it enters the liver but does not subsequently leave it. This would fit in well with the observation that although peripheral glucose uptake is so different in obese and lean subjects their glucose tolerance curves are so similar. Thus in the non-diabetic the liver appears responsible for maintaining glucose homoeostasis.

The low peripheral glucose uptake in obesity is due to peripheral insulin resistance, since plasma insulin concentrations during glucose tolerance tests are normal or even higher than normal and insulin uptake also high (Asmal *et al*, 1971). Furthermore Rabinowitz & Zierler (1962) have shown that the peripheral tissues of obese subjects are less sensitive to intra-arterially injected insulin than those of lean subjects, in terms of glucose uptake.

In studies where ^{131}I insulin was injected intra-arterially, it has been found that insulin uptake by the peripheral tissues correlates closely with the concentration of insulin achieved in the blood (Fig. 15.2) and that there is also a close correlation between insulin uptake and the mean glucose uptake after the insulin injection (Butterfield *et al*, 1963).

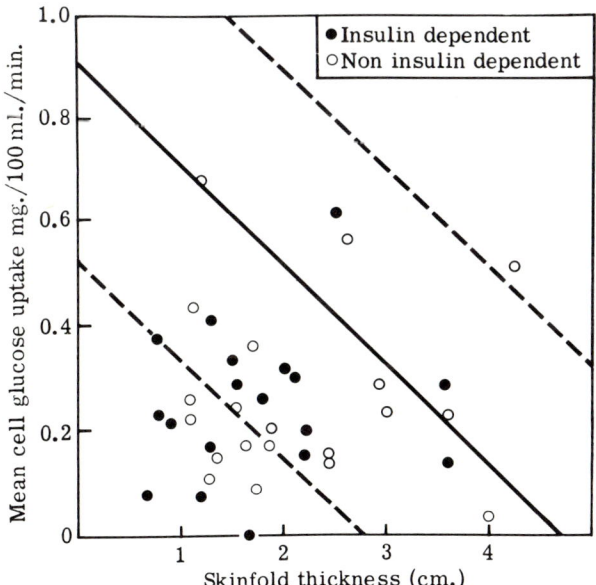

Figure 15.3
Relationship between glucose uptake and skinfold thickness during a 50 g oral glucose tolerance test in diabetic subjects with the regression line (solid) and 95% confidence limits (dotted line) for non-diabetics. (Reproduced by permission of the Editor of the Quarterly Journal of Medicine).

GLUCOSE UPTAKE IN DIABETES

The response of peripheral glucose uptake to hyperglycaemia produced by an oral glucose load in diabetics is variable. In insulin-dependent subjects who have been deprived of their insulin, only a small increase in glucose uptake occurs and in general the rise above the fasting level in the non-insulin dependent case is less than that observed for non-diabetics of similar skinfold thickness (Fig. 15.3). There is no relationship between glucose uptake and skinfold thickness in what are termed 'true diabetics'—i.e. those with a two hour blood sugar above 200 mg/100 ml (Butterfield, 1968). Thus the mechanism which controls the level of peripheral glucose uptake in relation to obesity in non-diabetics fails to operate in diabetics. Furthermore, in diabetics the liver cannot apparently compensate for the low peripheral glucose uptake by assimilating the glucose load in order to maintain glucose homoeostasis.

Undoubtedly in many diabetics the low glucose uptake is due at least in part to low circulating insulin levels due to islet cell failure.

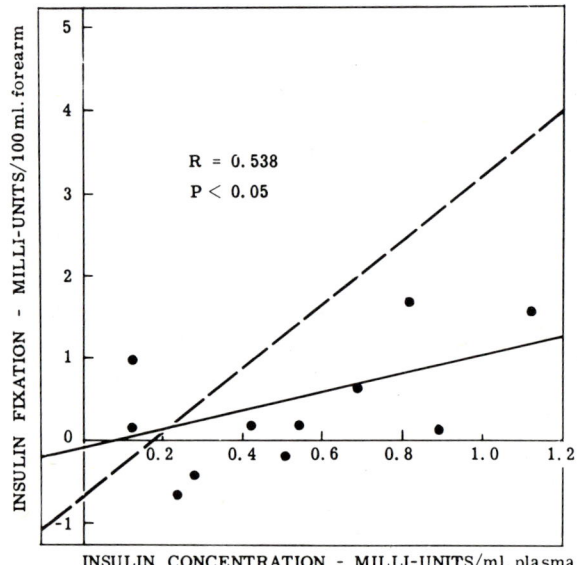

Figure 15.4
Relationship between peripheral insulin fixation and plasma insulin concentration achieved by the intra-arterial injection of 0.1 unit insulin in diabetics (solid line). Dotted line shows the regression line for non-diabetics. (Reproduced by permission of the Editor of Clinical Science).

However, in addition, the intra-arterial injection of ^{131}I insulin in diabetics results in a much smaller fixation of insulin for any one concentration achieved than occurs in non-diabetics (Fig. 15.4) (Butterfield *et al*, 1963). The relationship between insulin uptake and glucose uptake is, however, unaffected. Therefore insulin resistance in diabetes is due to a failure of insulin to leave the circulation and reach the muscle. This is in contrast to the insulin resistance of obesity. In some diabetics the liver appears to remain remarkably sensitive to insulin at any rate at high blood sugar levels (Butterfield & Whichelow, 1965), but the absolute lack of insulin during a glucose tolerance test probably impairs hepatic glucose uptake, and in some cases the liver may also become insulin resistant.

It is therefore possible to see why obese subjects tend to become diabetic. In these obese persons where insulin secreting capacity is barely adequate a low peripheral glucose uptake will throw an intolerable burden on the hepatic tissues and the blood sugar level will rise.

EFFECT OF WEIGHT REDUCTION IN OBESITY

If the low glucose uptake found in obesity is genetically determined and irreversible, then however much weight is lost the muscles of previously obese subjects will still be acting in an 'obese' fashion. If this is not the case then weight reduction should result in a marked increase in peripheral glucose uptake.

Three obese women were studied before and after weight loss (range 6.75 to 11.25 kg) produced by low calorie diet. Before weight loss glucose uptake was low, in accordance with their large skinfold thickness, but afterwards was increased considerably, in accordance with their new, smaller skinfold thickness (Fig. 15.5). These results show that the block to glucose uptake in obesity is reversible, and suggests that obesity leads to peripheral insulin resistance, rather than peripheral insulin resistance leading to obesity (Butterfield & Whichelow, 1968).

Studies have also been made on overweight subjects before and after treatment with fenfluramine. In those subjects who lost weight, all of whom had admitted eating less, there was an increase in peripheral glucose uptake and a decrease in skinfold thickness so that the same relationship between the two factors was maintained (Fig. 15.5) (Whichelow & Butterfield, 1970). The evidence from studies of peripheral glucose uptake suggests that fenfluramine does not affect glucose uptake directly, but since it is an effective appetite suppressant, the weight loss following the reduction in calorie intake results in increased glucose uptake.

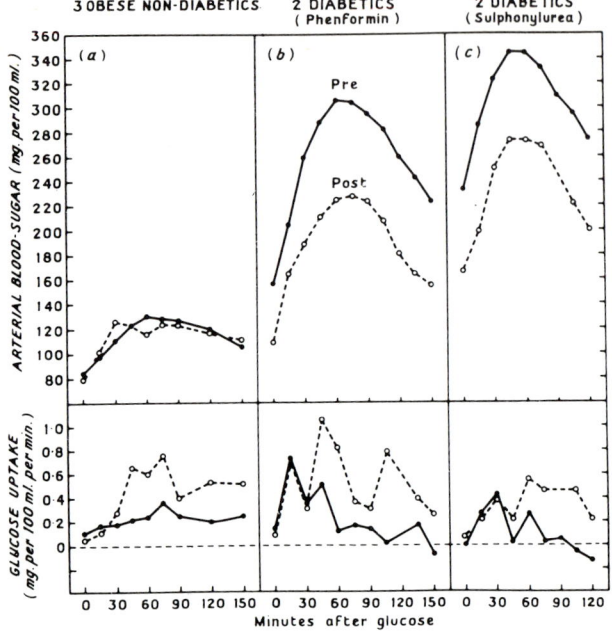

Figure 15.5
Effect of weight reduction by diet in non-diabetics (a), and successful anti-diabetic therapy with phenformin (b) and sulphonylureas (c) on the glucose tolerance curve and peripheral glucose uptaken in diabetics. (Reproduced by permission of the Editor of the Lancet).

EFFECT OF EXERCISE

The effect of light exercise on peripheral glucose uptake during a glucose tolerance test has been examined by adapting the forearm technique so that both arms can be studied simultaneously, one at rest and the other squeezing a rubber bulb once every 10 seconds throughout the test. The usual forearm preparation is set up in both arms except that only one artery is catheterized (Whichelow *et al*, 1968).

In all non-diabetic subjects following glucose administration glucose uptake is increased to a much greater extent (on average threefold) in the exercising arm than the resting arm. This is not just due to the increased blood flow in the exercising limb since the arterio-venous glucose difference is also greater on that side (Table 15.1). This effect of exercise appears to be dependent on the presence of circulating insulin since glucose uptake is also found to be higher in the exercising arm of non-insulin dependent diabetics and in an insulin dependent diabetic given a dose of insulin half an

Table 15.1

Effect of Exercise during Glucose Tolerance Test

Subjects	Resting		Exercising	
	Glucose Uptake mg/100ml/min	Blood Flow ml/min	Glucose Uptake mg/100ml/min	Blood Flow ml/min
Non-diabetics (7)	0.347	5.0	0.954	9.7
Mild diabetic	0.107	3.6	1.031	11.0
Insulin-dependent diabetic	0.480	11.0	0.496	15.4
Insulin-dependent diabetic given insulin	0.190	4.9	0.576	9.4

from Whichelow *et al* (1968)

(Reproduced by permission of the Editor of Metabolism)

hour prior to the test, but not in one deprived of insulin (Table 15.1) (Whichelow *et al*, 1968).

The mechanism of the action of exercise has been examined by injecting insulin intra-arterially in the resting and exercising state (Garratt *et al*, 1972). During exercise the peripheral tissues take up a greater amount of insulin in proportion to the concentration achieved, thereby increasing glucose uptake (Fig. 15.6). The relationship between insulin uptake and glucose uptake is unaffected. Exercise then, increases peripheral insulin sensitivity.

The role of the liver in exercise may also be important. In lean non-diabetics the muscles take up most of the glucose load during the two hours of a glucose tolerance test. In a subject performing ordinary light exercise involving many muscle groups, such as walking, peripheral glucose uptake must be very high and would account, during a glucose tolerance test, for much more glucose than the 50 g ingested. The excess glucose would have to be supplied by the liver. Light exercise will not result in the total combustion of all this glucose, so that it is probably metabolized to lactate which is released and taken up by the liver. The liver probably reconverts the lactate to glucose which is in turn released.

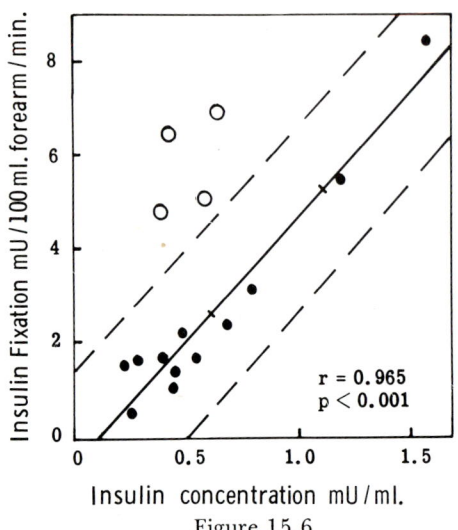

Figure 15.6

Effect of exercise (open circles) on the relationship between insulin fixation and the plasma insulin concentration achieved by the intra-arterial injection of insulin in non-diabetics. (Reproduced by permission of the Editor of Metabolism).

Insulin dependent diabetics not infrequently suffer hypoglycaemia when taking exercise, if they have not increased their carbohydrate intake. It seems probable, therefore, that in these subjects, when peripheral glucose uptake increases during exercise, the liver does not compensate by releasing sufficient glucose to maintain the blood sugar level.

EFFECT OF ORAL ANTIDIABETIC AGENTS

In diabetes the fasting blood sugar is lowered and often the shape of the glucose tolerance curve improved by successful treatment with a sulphonylurea or biguanide. Four newly diagnosed adult onset diabetics were studied before and after successful therapy, one with chlorpropamide, one with tolbutamide and two with phenformin. In all cases glucose uptake was low prior to treatment, considerably lower than would be expected for non-diabetics of similar skinfold thickness. After treatment glucose uptake was markedly increased (Fig. 15.5) (Butterfield & Whichelow, 1968). The reduction in blood sugar is then due, in part at least, to increased peripheral glucose assimilation, although it is not possible from these studies to determine whether hepatic glucose metabolism is also altered.

The sulphonylureas are known to increase insulin secretion from the β-cells, so that higher circulating insulin levels probably play a part in affecting an increasing in glucose uptake in treated cases. Phenformin however has been shown to increase peripheral insulin sensitivity (Whichelow & Butterfield, 1969) thereby increasing glucose uptake, but it does not increase insulin secretion. In view of this and reports by Stowers & Bewsher (1969) that phenformin aided weight reduction in obesity, the effect of biguanide therapy in three obese non-diabetic subjects was studied. However none of them lost weight or showed any changes in glucose uptake or blood sugar concentrations (Butterfield & Whichelow, 1968) again suggesting that the blocks to glucose uptake in diabetes and obesity are different.

REFERENCES

ASMAL, A.C., COX, B.D., BUTTERFIELD, W.J.H., KARAMANOS, B. & WHICHELOW, M.J. (1971) The peripheral uptake of glucose and endogenous insulin. *Postgrad. Med. J.* (suppl), 407.
BUTTERFIELD, W.J.H. (1968) In *Priorities in Medicine*, p.38. London:
BUTTERFIELD, W.J.H. GARRATT, C.J. & WHICHELOW, M.J. (1962) Peripheral hormone action: a method for the study of the action of insulin in the forearm tissues. *Guy's Hosp. Rep.*, 111, 130.
BUTTERFIELD, W.J.H. GARRATT, C.J. & WHICHELOW, M.J. (1963) Peripheral hormone action: studies on the clearance and effect of (^{131}I) iodoinsulin in the peripheral tissues of normal, acromegalic and diabetic subjects. *Clin. Sci.*, 24, 331.
BUTTERFIELD, W.J.H., HANLEY, T. & WHICHELOW, M.J. (1965) Peripheral metabolism of glucose and free fatty acids during oral glucose tolerance tests. *Metabolism*, 14, 851.
BUTTERFIELD, W.J.H. & HOLLING, H.H. (1959) Peripheral glucose metabolism in fasting control subjects and diabetic patients. *Clin. Sci.*, 18, 147.
BUTTERFIELD, W.J.H. & WHICHELOW, M.J. (1965) Peripheral glucose metabolism in control subjects and diabetic patients during glucose, glucose-insulin and insulin sensitivity tests. *Diabetologia*, 1, 43.
BUTTERFIELD, W.J.H. & WHICHELOW, M.J. (1968) Effect of diet, sulphonylureas and phenformin on peripheral glucose uptake in diabetes and obesity. *Lancet*, 2, 785.
GARRATT, C.J., BUTTERFIELD, W.J.H., ABRAMS, M.E., STERKY, G. & WHICHELOW, M.J. (1972) Effect of exercise on peripheral uptake of ^{131}I-iodo insulin and glucose in non-diabetics. *Metabolism*, 21, 36.
MALAISSE, W.J. (1968) Personal communication.
RABINOWITZ, D. & ZIERLER, K.L. (1962) Forearm metabolism in obesity and its response to intra-arterial insulin. Characterization of insulin resistance and evidence for adaptive hyperinsulinism. *J. Clin. Invest.*, 41, 2173.
STOWERS, J.M. & BEWSHER, P.D. (1969) Studies on the mechanism of weight reduction by phenformin. *Postgrad. Med. J.* (suppl), 13.
WHICHELOW, M.J. & BUTTERFIELD, W.J.H. (1969) *In vivo* studies in man on the hypoglycaemic action of phenformin. *Postgrad. Med. J.* (suppl), 24.
WHICHELOW, M.J. & BUTTERFIELD, W.J.H. (1970) In *Amphetamines and*

Related Compounds, p. 614. Ed. Costa and Garrattini. New York: Raven Press.

WHICHELOW, M.J. & BUTTERFIELD, W.J.H. (1971) Peripheral glucose uptake during the oral glucose tolerance test in normal and obese subjects and borderline and frank diabetics. *Quart. J. Med.*, **40**, 261.

WHICHELOW, M.J., BUTTERFIELD, W.J.H., ABRAMS, M.E., STERKY, G. & GARRATT, C.J. (1968) The effect of mild exercise on glucose uptake in human forearm tissues in the fasting state and after oral glucose administration. *Metabolism*, **17**, 84.

16. Endocrine and Metabolic Alterations Associated with Over-feeding and Obesity in Man

E.S. HORTON, E. DANFORTH, Jr., E.A.H. SIMS and L.B. SALANS

Numerous endocrine and metabolic alterations have been observed in human obesity but it is not yet clear which, if any, of the deviations from normal might be primary abnormalities operating to promote or perpetuate the obese state and which are secondary changes occurring in association with factors such as enlargement of the adipocyte, the increased intake of calories, the composition of the diet, the level of physical activity or other conditions found in association with obesity.

For the past several years we have been conducting studies to determine which of the abnormalities found in spontaneous obesity might be induced in lean volunteers who have no family history of obesity or diabetes mellitus and who gain 20–25 per cent above their normal weight by consuming a balanced, high caloric diet (Sims et al, 1968, 1973). While a detailed review of these early studies is beyond the scope of this chapter, the major findings in a total of 19 subjects who completed the original programme are summarized in Table 16.1 and compared with the changes which have been observed in spontaneous obesity. It can be seen that with few exceptions, lean individuals develop endocrine and metabolic changes in a direction similar to those observed in spontaneous obesity when they overeat and increase their adipose tissue mass. It should be emphasized however that these changes are primarily directional and that with few exceptions actual values remained within the conventionally accepted limits of normal.

Only three major differences were observed between the findings

---

[1] This paper was also presented as part of the Fogarty International Center Conference on Preventative Medicine on occasion of the Conference on Obesity, National Institutes of Health, Bethesda, Maryland, October 1-3, 1973.

[2] Supported in part by U.S.P.H.S. grants 5 RO1 AM 13307 (Dr. Horton), 5 RO1 AM 10254 (Dr. Sims), AM 13321 (Dr. Salans) and RR-109 (General Clinical Research Center)

Table 16.1

Endocrine and metabolic changes in spontaneous and experimental obesity, the latter induced by increased intake of all elements of the diet (19 subjects)

	Spontaneous Obesity	Experimental Obesity
Adipose Tissue		
Cell size	↑	↑
Cell number	↑	Unchanged
Caloric Balance		
Calories required to maintain obese state	1300 kcal/M²	2700 kcal/M²
Return to starting weight	rapid	rapid
Spontaneous physical activity	↓	↓
Appetite late in the day	↑	↑
Fasting Concentrations in Blood		
Cholesterol	↑	↑
Triglycerides	↑	↑
Free fatty acids	↑	Unchanged or ↓
Amino acids	↑	↑
Glucose	N or ↑	↑
Insulin	↑	↑
Glucagon	N	
Growth hormone	N or ↓	Unchanged or ↓
Glucose Tolerance		
Oral	↓	↓
Intravenous	↓	↓
Insulin Release		
To oral glucose	↑	↑
To I.V. glucose	↑	↑
To I.V. arginine	↑	↑
Evidence of Insulin Resistance		
Insulin:glucose ratio	↑	↑
Adipose tissue metabolism		
— sensitivity to insulin *in vitro*	↓	↓
— sensitivity to insulin *in vivo*	↓	↓
Forearm muscle metabolism		
— insulin-stimulated glucose uptake	↓	↓
— insulin inhibition of release of amino acid		↓

(Cont'd)

Table 16.1 Contd.

Hormones possibly affecting insulin resistance		
Glucocorticoids		
Plasma cortisol	N or ↓	Unchanged
Cortisol production rate	↑	↑
Urinary 17-hydroxycorticoids	↑ *	↑ *
Growth Hormone		
Response to glucose	↓	↓
Response to arginine	↓	↓
Nocturnal rises		↓
Glucagon		
Fasting plasma concentration	N	
Response to glucose	N	
Response to amino acids		
Arginine	↑	
Alanine	↓	
Beef meal	N	

* Normal/kg body weight

in experimental obesity and the spontaneously obese state. First, all subjects studied to date have increased their adipose tissue mass by increasing only adipose cell size without any change in the total cell number. This is in contrast to the findings by Hirsch & Knittle (1970) of a significant increase in adipose cell number in spontaneous obesity of early age onset.

Second, in subjects who gained weight by increasing all elements of the diet there was a marked increase in the daily caloric requirement to maintain the obese state. Spontaneously obese individuals maintain a constant weight on a daily intake of as little as 1300 kcal/M^2 (Bray, 1970), whereas the subjects with experimental obesity required approximately 2700 kcal/M^2 to maintain their gained weight, an increase of 50 per cent above the 1800 kcal/M^2 they required for maintenance of their usual lean weight. The mechanism responsible for the apparent caloric inefficiency which develops during overfeeding of a mixed diet has not yet been fully defined and is currently under investigation by us in collaboration with the U.S. Army Research Institute of Environmental Medicine (Goldman et al, 1974).

Finally, the subjects with experimental obesity showed a decrease of free fatty acid, in contrast to the increased plasma concentrations frequently found in spontaneous obesity. This has subsequently been explained on the basis of the composition of the diet, the suppression of plasma free fatty acids being associated with a high carbohydrate intake rather than with the development of obesity (Sims et *al*, 1973). In all other respects, the changes observed in experimental obesity parallel those found in spontaneous obesity.

HYPERINSULINAEMIA AND INSULIN RESISTANCE

Perhaps the most striking endocrine alteration in obesity is the combination of hyperinsulinaemia and the presence of peripheral insulin resistance. An understanding of this phenomenon is of particular importance because of its apparent relationship to the development of decreased glucose tolerance and diabetes mellitus which is frequently associated with obesity.

The finding of increased plasma insulin concentrations in obese subjects, both in the fasting state and following glucose stimulation, was first observed by Karam *et al* (1963) and has subsequently been well documented in many laboratories. In addition, a general increased responsiveness of the β-cells has been demonstrated by many investigators using a wide variety of stimuli including amino acids, insulin secretogogues and pharmacological agents (Rabinowitz, 1970).

Perley & Kipnis (1967) have demonstrated that the hyperinsulinaemia is related primarily to obesity and not to co-existant diabetes mellitus in which the abnormal glucose tolerance is associated with a relative deficiency of insulin secretion. The presence of decreased sensitivity of peripheral tissues to insulin action has been demonstrated in both adipose tissue and muscle using *in vitro* and *in vivo* techniques (Rabinowitz & Zierler, 1962; Salans *et al*, 1968).

However the aetiology of hyperinsulinaemia and insulin resistance in obesity is still unknown. Does the hyperinsulinaemia develop first as the result of chronic stimulation of the β-cell by excessive intake of specific elements in the diet with peripheral insulin resistance developing as a secondary phenomenon, or is the development of insulin resistance the primary change with increased insulin secretion occurring in a compensatory manner? Whichever the sequence, the net result is a combination of high plasma insulin concentrations, increased insulin:glucose ratios and frequently diminished glucose tolerance. Several hormones which might be implicated in the development of impaired glucose tolerance and insulin resistance have been studied, but to date none can be incriminated as a primary factor.

Growth Hormone

In obesity, the secretion of growth hormone in response to a wide variety of stimuli is decreased. This includes suppression of the rise in growth hormone which normally occurs four to six hours after an oral glucose challenge and decreased growth hormone responses following stimulation by insulin induced hypoglycaemia, infusion of L-arginine, muscular exercise or prolonged fasting (Sims & Horton, 1968).

Cortisol

Although both the production rate and urinary excretion of cortisol and its metabolites are increased in obesity this is proportional to the increased body mass and plasma concentrations are generally within the normal range or decreased (Sims *et al,* 1971). No specific role for cortisol in the pathogenesis or perpetuation of the obese state has yet been elucidated. Since plasma concentrations are normal, it is difficult to accept the hypothesis that cortisol may be a significant factor in the production of peripheral insulin resistance in obesity.

Glucagon

Despite early reports that glucagon concentrations may be increased in obesity (Paulsen & Lawrence, 1968) the bulk of evidence now points to normal fasting glucagon concentrations, normal suppression following glucose administration and variable responses to stimulation by amino acid infusions. Wise *et al* (1973) have found a diminished glucagon response to infusion of L-alanine in obese subjects whereas Kalkhoff *et al* (1973) have found the response to arginine infusion to be increased. Thus, on the basis of the information presently available, neither growth hormone, cortisol nor glucagon appear to be important in the development of insulin resistance and hyperinsulinaemia in obesity.

Physical training

It is now clear that factors other than the size of the adipose tissue mass influence the degree of hyperinsulinaemia in obesity and must be carefully controlled in studies of this problem. Björntorp & coworkers (1970) have shown that physical training influences plasma insulin concentrations in obesity and their work has been reviewed in this book (page 171). Despite an insulin lowering effect of physical conditioning in obese subjects plasma insulin concentrations remain higher than in comparably trained lean individuals.

Diet

One obvious question is whether or not the intake of a high carbohydrate diet results in chronic stimulation of the β-cells leading to hyperinsulinaemia and development of peripheral insulin resistance as a secondary phenomenon. Both the hyperinsulinaemia and peripheral insulin resistance are reversed by weight reduction (Kalkhoff *et al,* 1971). In addition plasma insulin concentrations in the obese are influenced by the composition of the diet without any change in the total intake of calories. Grey & Kipnis (1971) found a 50 per cent decrease in basal insulin concentrations in obese subjects fed iso-caloric low carbohydrate diets for three weeks despite only a slight decrease in the fasting blood glucose concentration. Insulin concentrations increased when the subjects were changed to iso-caloric high carbohydrate diets.

We have done similar experiments in lean volunteers in whom the effect of varying the carbohydrate content of the diet on plasma insulin and glucose inter-relationships was studied (Danforth, 1971). Subjects were studied first on an isocaloric diet containing 40 per cent of calories as carbohydrate, 40 per cent as fat and 20 per cent as protein; then following a second diet phase of two weeks duration in which carbohydrate was decreased to 10 per cent of the total calories; then finally after a return to the original diet. The low

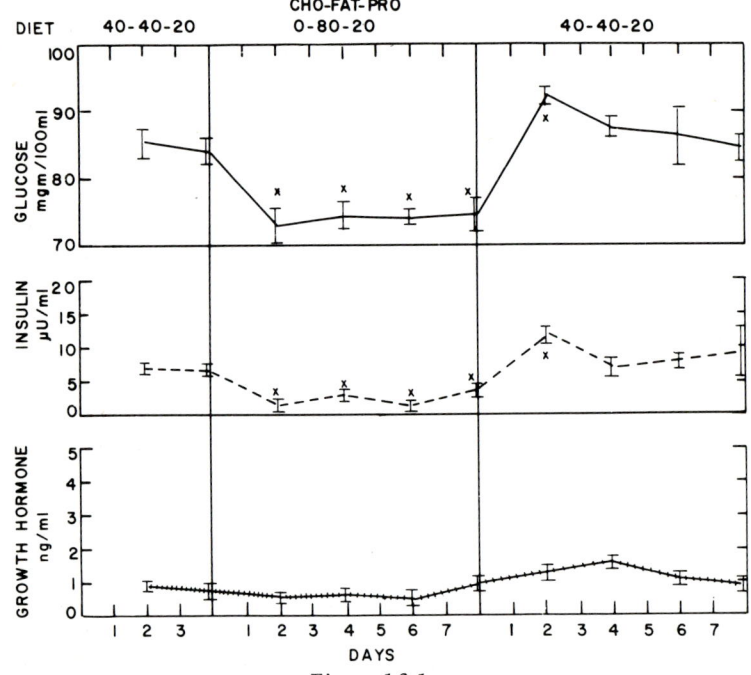

Figure 16.1

The mean fasting plasma glucose, insulin and growth hormone concentrations in five normal weight subjects consuming isocaloric diets of varied carbohydrate and fat content. The composition of each diet is expressed as per cent of total calories consisting of carbohydrate (CHO), fat and protein (PRO). x indicates significant changes ($p < 0.05$) from the initial diet phase.

carbohydrate diet was associated with a transient decrease in fasting glucose concentrations and a small but definite decrease in fasting plasma insulin. Intravenous and oral glucose tolerance both decreased slightly but without any significant change in the glucose-stimulated insulin response. In a second experiment, in which subjects were fed the same control diet followed by a formula diet containing only fat and protein with no carbohydrate, the decrease in fasting plasma glucose and insulin was more marked (Fig. 16.1). Plasma insulin decreased from a mean of 7.3 μU/ml during the control phase to 1.9 μU/ml during the carbohydrate-free diet. This was associated with a slight decrease in intravenous glucose tolerance but no significant change in the glucose stimulated insulin response. Following reinstitution of the control diet, a rebound of both glucose and insulin was observed with values slightly higher than the original basal values.

Thus it is clear that in both lean and obese subjects the carbohydrate content of the diet influences fasting plasma insulin and glucose concentrations. However, the changes induced by diet are greater in obesity when the initial fasting insulin concentrations are high.

The effect of the carbohydrate content of the diet on glucose tolerance is somewhat less clear. Since the classic work of Himsworth (1933), it has been known that carbohydrate loading improves and carbohydrate restriction impairs glucose tolerance in normal subjects.

In the studies of obese subjects by Grey & Kipnis (1971) no significant effect of high and low carbohydrate diets on glucose tolerance could be detected although the insulin secretory response to oral glucose was less following the period of restricted carbohydrate intake. Brunzell *et al* (1971), on the other hand, have found that in a mixed group of normal subjects and mild diabetics, high carbohydrate intake (85 per cent of calories as carbohydrate compared to 45 per cent in the control study) resulted in improved glucose tolerance and a decrease in the fasting plasma insulin concentration without any changes in glucose stimulated insulin secretion.

Because of these conflicting reports, and the question of the role of dietary carbohydrate in the genesis of hyperinsulinaemia and insulin resistance in obesity, we undertook three different experiments in an attempt to dissociate the effects of antecedent diet from the effects of change in body weight and adipose cell size. They are described below.

Varied Carbohydrate intake and Weight Reduction in Spontaneous Obesity

In the first experiment the metabolism of forearm muscle *in vivo* and of adipose tissue *in vitro* was studied in two obese subjects fed isocaloric low and high carbohydrate diets, both before and after reduction to normal weight (Horton et al, 1972). Initially, the subjects were fed isocaloric diets containing either 85 or 250 g of carbohydrate/M^2 for periods of three weeks each. Glucose tolerance, forearm muscle metabolism and adipose tissue metabolism were studied in each diet phase. The subjects were then reduced to normal weight during a six to nine month period during which they were fed a balanced formula diet containing 600 calories per day. Following weight reduction, the initial studies were repeated during a second weight maintenance phase on low and high carbohydrate diets. Initially both subjects were moderately obese with an increased percentage of body fat and large adipose cells. Reduction to normal weight was associated with a parallel decrease in cell size and no change in their estimated total cell number. The metabolic changes associated with weight reduction and altered carbohydrate intake were consistently the same in both subjects.

The glucose and insulin responses during the four oral glucose tolerance tests done on subject C.E. are shown in Figure 16.2. At both weights the high carbohydrate diet was associated with improved glucose tolerance and lower plasma insulin responses. When one compares the studies done before and after weight reduction on

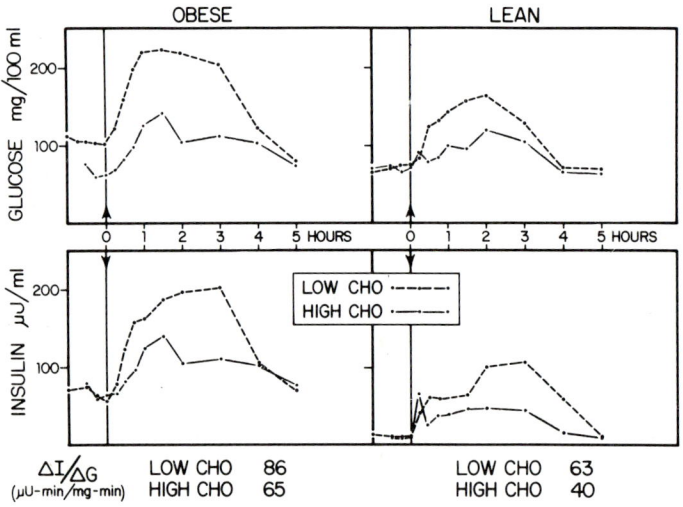

Figure 16.2
The effects of weight reduction and altered carbohydrate content of the diet on plasma glucose and insulin concentrations during oral glucose tolerance tests in subject C.F. Glucose dose = 40 g/M^2.

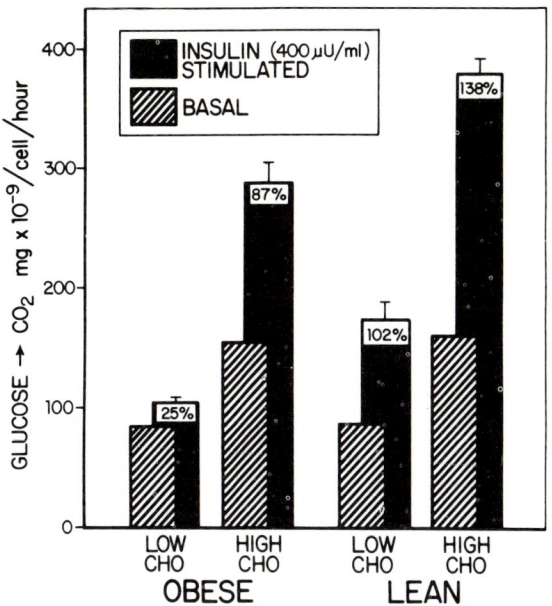

Figure 16.3
The effects of weight reduction and altered carbohydrate content of the diet on glucose oxidation by adipose tissue pieces *in vitro* for subject C.E.

the same diet, it is apparent that weight loss was also associated with improved glucose tolerance and a smaller insulin response. Thus, both weight reduction and high carbohydrate feeding appear to have increased the sensitivity of the tissues to the action of insulin.

To correlate simultaneous changes in adipose tissue and muscle metabolism two parallel experiments were done. First, both basal and insulin stimulated glucose metabolism were studied in adipose tissue pieces and, second, forearm muscle metabolism was studied using the forearm perfusion technique of Andres *et al* (1956).

Figure 16.3 shows the effect of weight loss and altered carbohydrate intake on glucose oxidation by adipose tissue *in vitro*. At either weight the high carbohydrate diet was associated with a significant increase in the basal rate of glucose oxidation. On the other hand, weight reduction, when studied with the subject on comparable diets, had no effect on the basal rate. The effect of insulin, 400 μU/ml, in the incubation medium was also studied. When the subject was obese, the high carbohydrate diet resulted in an increase in insulin responsiveness of the tissue either when expressed as an increase in the absolute rate of glucose oxidation or as a percentage increase above the basal rate. The same effect of high carbohydrate intake was seen after weight reduction. When the responses to insulin are compared with the subject on the same diet before and after weight reduction, the adipose tissue in the obese state was relatively less responsive to insulin than it was in the lean state. Thus, obesity *per se* appears to be associated with insulin resistance in adipose tissue and high carbohydrate feeding appears to improve insulin sensitivity rather than decrease it.

Using the forearm perfusion technique, we also studied glucose uptake by muscle under basal conditions and in response to the intra-arterial infusion of insulin at a rate of 100 µU/min/kg. The mean fasting arterial glucose concentration was higher in the obese state and there was a marked elevation of both the fasting plasma insulin concentrations and the insulin:glucose ratio, indicating a state of marked insulin resistance. Weight reduction resulted in a moderate decrease in blood glucose concentrations and a marked decrease in mean plasma insulin from 51.6 to 6.2 µU/ml. There was a concomitant decrease in the insulin:glucose ratio from 54 to 10. No effect of dietary carbohydrate content on either the arterial insulin concentration or the insulin:glucose ratio could be demonstrated.

The uptake of glucose by forearm muscle before and after insulin infusion is shown in Figure 16.4. Under basal conditions (30-60 min) glucose uptake was very small when the subject was obese despite markedly increased arterial insulin concentrations. This in contrast to

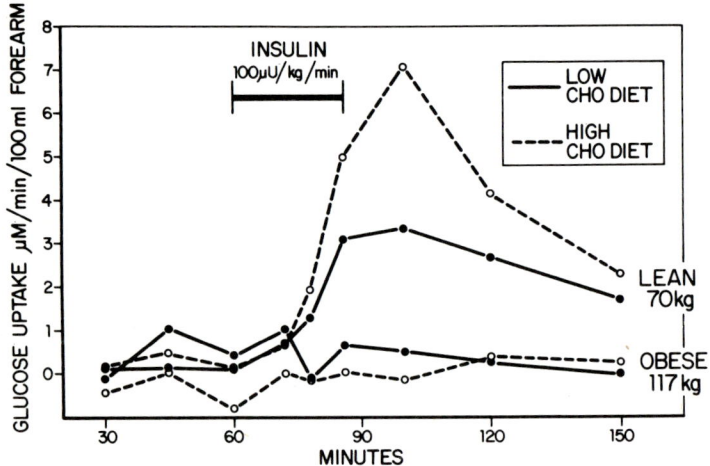

Figure 16.4

The effects of weight reduction and altered carbohydrate content of the diet on basal and insulin-stimulated glucose uptake by forearm muscle in subject C.E.

an increased basal glucose uptake previously reported in obese subjects by Rabinowitz & Zierler (1962) using the same technique. In our study, no significant difference was found in the basal rate of glucose uptake before and after weight reduction. There was, however, a very striking difference in the response to insulin infusion. Despite increasing arterial insulin concentrations up to 400-500 µU/ml, no increase in glucose uptake occurred in either of the two forearm studies done when the subject was obese. After weight reduction, insulin infusion resulted in an eight- to ten-fold increase in glucose uptake which is identical to that of normal weight controls. In addition, after weight reduction the response to insulin was greater while the patient was taking the high carbohydrate diet, suggesting that insulin sensitivity in muscle as well as in adipose tissue is increased by carbohydrate loading.

This study demonstrates that it is possible to separate the metabolic effects which are associated primarily with changes in body weight and adipose tissue mass from those which are associated with changes in the immediately preceeding carbohydrate content of the diet. It does not exclude, however, possible long-term effects of antecedent carbohydrate intake consumed over a period of many weeks or months.

The data indicate that obesity itself, independent of prior carbohydrate intake, is associated with hyperinsulinaemia and insulin resistance in adipose tissue and skeletal muscle. Reduction to normal weight and body composition is associated with a reduction of fasting insulin concentrations to normal and complete restoration of insulin sensitivity in both tissues. Short-term high carbohydrate feeding, on the other hand, is associated with improved glucose tolerance and increased sensitivity of peripheral tissues to insulin action, effects opposite to those attributed to obesity.

Effects of Varied Carbohydrate Intake and Weight Gain in Experimental Obesity.

In order to investigate further the question of whether or not insulin resistance and other changes which occur in experimental obesity are due to factors associated with adipose cell enlargement or are related to an increase in the carbohydrate content of the antecedent diet, two further studies have been completed (Sims *et al,* 1973).

In the first study, referred to as the *variable carbohydrate:fat study,* isocaloric diets were taken for two periods of three weeks each period to and following an average gain in weight of 20 per cent (Sims *et al,* 1973). Either 100 or 300 g of carbohydrate/M^2 was given in random sequence during the two test periods at each weight, the intake of protein was kept constant, and the diets were made isocaloric with fat. During the period of gain in weight the subjects increased total caloric intake by increasing all elements of the diet and maintained normal physical activity.

In the second study, referred to as the *constant carbohydrate study,* the intake of carbohydrate and protein was kept constant throughout and weight gain was induced by the progressive addition of fat to the diet. The basal diet, without fat supplement, contained 1800 kcal/M^2 with 40 per cent of the calories as carbohydrate, 20 per cent as protein and 40 per cent as fat. After the subjects had gained 19 to 23 per cent above their initial weight, the total caloric and fat intake was adjusted to maintain constant weight during the final four-week test period. The data from both studies were subjected to analysis of variance in which the order of the diets and other variables were taken into consideration.

In the variable carbohydrate:fat study, the intention was to dissociate the effects of antecedent carbohydrate intake from the effects of weight gain on plasma insulin concentrations, glucose metabolism, adipose tissue metabolism *in vitro* and other parameters previously studied in experimental obesity. The changes in fasting plasma insulin and intravenous glucose tolerance are shown in Table 16.2. At either level of weight there was a significant increase in the fasting plasma insulin concentration and the fasting insulin:glucose ratio associated with the diet containing the high carbohydrate:fat ratio. This is consistent with the previously reported findings of Grey & Kipnis (1971) on the effects of isocaloric high- and low-carbohydrate diets on fasting plasma insulin in spontaneously obese subjects. The intravenous glucose tolerance was improved by the high carbohydrate diet at both weights. Oral glucose tolerance was improved when the subjects were studied on the high carbohydrate diet at initial weight, but no significant dietary effect was observed when the subjects were obese. When studies done with similar diets are compared, the fasting insulin concentration was also increased in association with weight gain. Intravenous glucose tolerance was not significantly different, however, and an effect of gain in weight in decreasing oral glucose tolerance was observed only when the men were studied on the high carbohydrate:fat diet. These data suggest that a high carbohydrate intake plays at least as great a role as weight gain in elevating fasting plasma insulin concentrations but that, unlike obesity, it results in improved rather than decreased glucose tolerance.

Further evidence to support this hypothesis is gained from the

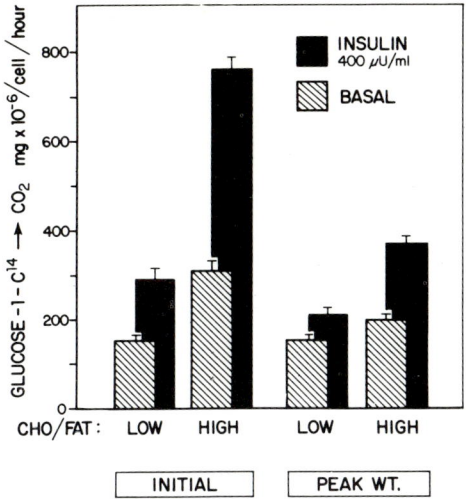

Figure 16.5
The effects of weight gain and altered carbohydrate: fat ratio in the diet on basal and insulin stimulated glucose oxidation by adipose tissue *in vitro*.
(Sims *et al*, 1973) (reproduced by permission of Academic Press, Inc.).

studies of glucose oxidation by adipose tissue pieces *in vitro* for the previously mentioned subjects. Figure 16.5 shows the mean basal and insulin-stimulated (400 μU/ml) rates of glucose-1-^{14}C oxidation to $^{14}CO_2$. An initial weight, the high carbohydrate:fat diet was associated with an increase in both the basal glucose oxidation rate and the response to insulin. After weight gain the same relative effect of the high carbohydrate:fat diet was seen, but the insulin responsiveness was blunted when compared to the parallel studies done at the initial weight. These findings are similar to those observed in spontaneous obesity as described above.

The question whether the hyperinsulinaemia and insulin resistance seen in experimental obesity is a carry-over from the high carbohydrate intake during the period of weight gain is best answered by the second study in which only dietary fat was increased to achieve the increase in weight. In our initial studies, in which the intake of all elements of the diet were increased during the period of weight gain, the fasting plasma insulin concentration was increased approximately 50 per cent. Oral glucose tolerance was diminished, the insulin response to glucose was increased and growth hormone secretion was suppressed. In the subjects who gained weight by increasing dietary fat only, the mean fasting plasma insulin concentration increased 64

Table 16.2

Changes in plasma insulin and intravenous tolerance associated
with gain in weight and change in the dietary carbohydrate/fat ratio[a]

Diet Ratio	Baseline	After gain in weight	
	Fasting plasma insulin ($\mu U/ml$)		
Low carbohydrate/fat	6.8 ± 0.8	8.3 ± 1.0	**
High carbohydrate/fat	8.3 ± 1.1 *	13.1 ± 2.3	
	Fasting insulin:glucose ratio		
Low carbohydrate/fat	0.10 ± 0.01	0.13 ± 0.03	***
High carbohydrate/fat	0.13 ± 0.01 *	0.19 ± 0.03	
	Intravenous glucose tolerance (K^b)		
Low carbohydrate/fat	2.03 ± 0.57	2.42 ± 0.71	**
High carbohydrate/fat	3.06 ± 0.61 NS	2.84 ± 0.84	

[a] $p < 0.1$*; $p < 0.05$**; $p < 0.01$***

[b] Glucose disappearance rate

per cent from 9.2 ± 0.7 to 15.1 ± 1.5 $\mu U/ml$ ($p < 0.01$). This was associated with a slight but significant increase in fasting plasma glucose from 70 ± 2 to 75 ± 3 mg/100 ml ($p < 0.05$). The glucose, insulin and growth hormone responses to oral glucose are illustrated in Figure 16.6. There was a significant decrease in the oral glucose tolerance associated with an increased insulin response similar to that seen in our previous studies. It is of interest, however, that no suppression of the growth hormone response occurred. This supports the findings of Merimee & Rabin (1973) that a dietary effect in suppressing growth hormone secretion appears to be related primarily to a high carbohydrate intake and not to the total calories ingested. It is possible that suppression of growth hormone secretion in obesity is a function of the associated high carbohydrate intake and not secondary to the enlarged adipose tissue mass as has been generally assumed.

The development of hyperinsulinaemia and insulin resistance in

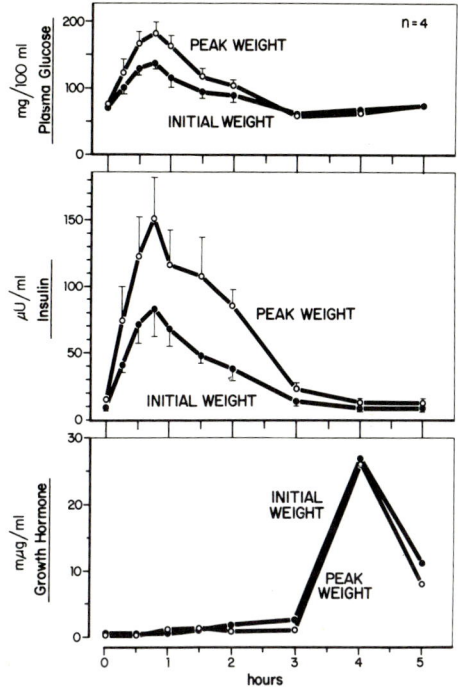

Figure 16.6
The mean (± S.E.) plasma glucose, insulin and growth hormone concentrations during oral glucose tolerance tests in four normal subjects before (closed circles) and after (open circles) gain in weight by increasing dietary fat only.

this group was confirmed further in a variety of ways. The mean glucose disappearance rate (K) during intravenous glucose testing decreased from 1.7 ± 0.12 to 1.2 ± 0.22 mg/100ml/min ($p < 0.05$) despite a significant increase in the insulin response (Fig. 16.7). The plasma insulin response following the ingestion of a beef meal containing 1 g protein/kg body weight was also increased despite the fact that some of the subjects did not consume the entire test meal at peak weight. The plasma glucose concentration changed only slightly during this test and does not account for the marked increase in insulin secretion observed at peak weight (Fig. 16.8).

In our earlier studies of forearm metabolism in experimental obesity induced by increasing all elements in the diet (Horton *et al*, 1970) we found that basal glucose uptake by muscle was unchanged, but that the response to the intra-arterial infusion of insulin was markedly blunted after gain in weight in four of the five subjects studied. In addition, Felig & coworkers (1971) measured the

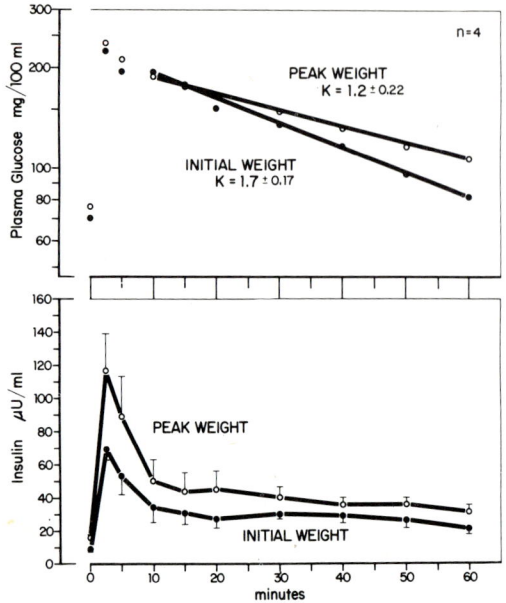

Figure 16.7
The mean glucose disappearance rate (K) and plasma insulin concentrations during intravenous glucose tolerance tests (25 g glucose I.V.) in four normal subjects before (closed circles) and after (open circles) gain in weight by increasing dietary fat only.

balances of 16 individual amino acids across forearm muscle and found that the arterial concentrations of six specific insulin-sensitive amino acids were increased after weight gain, that this was associated with increased release of those amino acids from muscle in the basal state and that the effect of insulin in inhibiting their release was diminished. Thus, the development of insulin resistance in muscle, as well as in adipose tissue, was demonstrated following weight gain in normal subjects and is similar to that seen in spontaneous obesity (Rabinowitz & Zierler, 1962).

To evaluate further whether or not peripheral insulin resistance develops in association with gain in weight without any increase in dietary carbohydrate, forearm muscle metabolism was studied in the four subjects who gained weight by increasing only fat in their diet (Fig. 16.9). Before weight gain, basal glucose uptake and the response to intra-arterial insulin infusion were the same as we have found in normal controls. After gain in weight, the basal glucose uptake was slightly but not significantly higher than that observed at initial weight. The response to insulin infusion was markedly blunted

ENDOCRINE AND METABOLIC ALTERATIONS 245

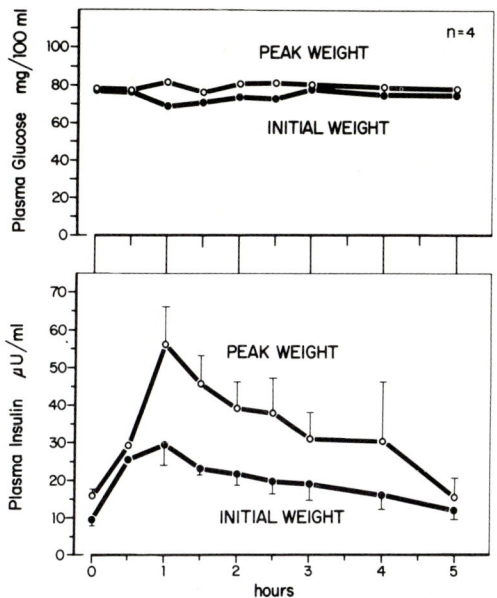

Figure 16.8
The mean plasma glucose and insulin concentrations following a beef meal (1 g protein/kg) in four normal subjects before (closed circles) and after (open circles) gain in weight by increasing dietary fat only.

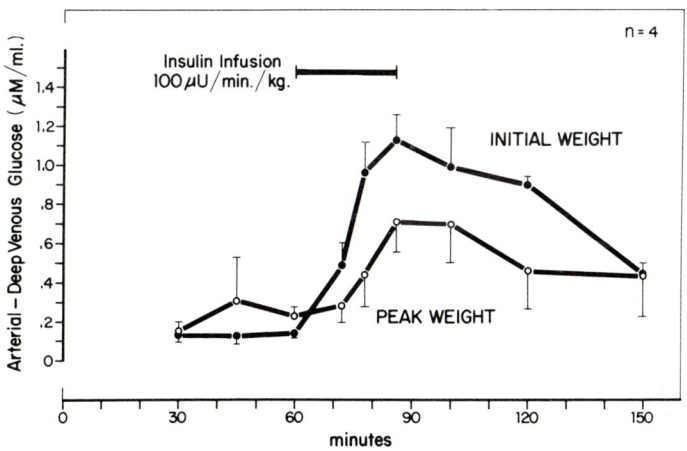

Figure 16.9
Comparison of mean (± S.E.) basal and insulin-stimulated arterial-deep venous glucose concentration differences across forearm muscle in four normal subjects before (closed circles) and after (open circles) gain in weight by increasing dietary fat only.

however, with only a three-fold increase in glucose uptake in contrast to the nine- to ten-fold increase which occurred before weight gain. Thus, decreased sensitivity of muscle to insulin action also developed in these subjects following weight gain without any increase in carbohydrate intake.

CONCLUSION

These studies have demonstrated that hyperinsulinaemia and insulin resistance involving both muscle and adipose tissue can be induced in normal subjects who overeat and gain weight and can be reversed in spontaneously obese subjects by caloric restriction and weight reduction. Since the changes in experimental obesity occur regardless of whether the increased calories are provided as a mixture of carbohydrate, protein and fat or as fat alone, we have concluded that the development of hyperinsulinaemia and insulin resistance is not a specific effect of a high dietary carbohydrate intake as has been suggested in the past. A dietary mechanism for the development of hyperinsulinaemia has not been excluded, however. It is still possible that a high intake of fat may act as a direct stimulus of insulin secretion or that an increase in the total caloric intake may provide a relative excess of carbohydrate and amino acid substrates which in turn could result in chronic β-cell stimulation.

Likewise, the reversal of hyperinsulinaemia and insulin resistance by weight reduction in subjects with spontaneous obesity may be secondary to the restriction of total calories rather than of carbohydrate specifically.

The other possibility is that the development of hyperinsulinaemia in obesity may be the result of a primary decrease in the sensitivity of peripheral tissues to insulin action completely independent of the antecedent diet. The study by Salans *et al* (1968) of massively obese patients before and after weight reduction suggested that enlargement of the adipocyte with lipid stores leads to insulin resistance. There is now evidence that a deficiency of insulin receptors in several tissues including adipocytes, thymocytes and liver cell membranes may exist in some forms of obesity in man and animals and that this deficiency may be altered by weight reduction (Kahn *et al,* 1973).

It is clear, however, that factors other than adipose cell size influence the degree of insulin resistance in obesity. In the present studies we have demonstrated that short-term feeding of a high carbohydrate:fat diet is associated with improved glucose tolerance and increased sensitivity of peripheral tissues to insulin, effects opposite to those associated with the development of obesity.

Finally, it should be emphasized that the fact that hyperinsulinaemia and insulin resistance can be induced in normal subjects by weight gain and reversed in obese subjects by weight reduction does not mean that these changes are secondary to the level of dietary intake and body weight in all forms of obesity. There may be as many syndromes of obesity in man as there are in experimental animals, and in some of these hyperinsulinaemia or peripheral insulin resistance may be an aetiological factor.

Acknowledgements

We are indebted to Catherine Armstrong, B.S., Brenda Meyer, B.S. and Maureen O'Connell, B.S., for expert technical assistance in the laboratory; to Mrs. Vivian Ho, research dietitian, for control of the experimental diets; to Mabel Hills, R.N. and the nursing staff of the Clinical Research Center for conduct of the experimental protocols; and to Mrs. Elizabeth Birchenough for expert secretarial assistance with the manuscript.

REFERENCES

ANDRES, R., CADER, G. & ZIERLER, K.L. (1956) The quantitatively minor role of carbohydrate in oxidative metabolism by skeletal muscle in intact man in the basal state. Measurements of oxygen and glucose uptake and carbon dioxide and lactate production in the forearm. *J. Clin. Invest.*, 35, 671.

BJÖRNTORP, P., DE JOUNGE, K., SJÖSTRÖM, L. & SULLIVAN, L. (1970) The effect of physical training on insulin production in obesity. *Metabolism*, 19, 631.

BRAY, G.A. (1970) The myth of diet in the management of obesity. *Am. J. Clin. Nutr.*, 23, 1141.

BRUNZELL, J.D., LERNER, R.L., HAZZARD, W.R., PORTE, D.Jr. & BIERMAN, E.L. (1971) Improved glucose tolerance with high carbohydrate feeding in mild diabetes. *N. Eng. J. Med.*, 284, 521.

DANFORTH, E.Jr. (1971) Hormonal interrelationships in response to carbohydrate-free isocaloric diets in normal man. *Diabetes*, 20, supple. 1, 343.

FELIG, P., HORTON, E.S., RUNGE, C.F. & SIMS, E.A.H. (1971) Experimental obesity in man: Hyperaminoacidaemia and diminished effectiveness of insulin in regulating peripheral amino acid release. *Annual Meeting of the Endocrine Society*, June 24-26, 1971.

GOLDMAN, R.F., HAISMAN, M.F., BYNUM, G., SALANS, L.B. DANFORTH, E.Jr., HORTON, E.S. & SIMS, E.A.H. (1974) Experimental obesity in man. VI. Metabolic rate in relation to dietary intake. Fogarty International Conference on Obesity, October 1973 (in press).

GREY, N. & KIPNIS, D.M. (1971) Effect of diet composition on the hyperinsulinaemia of obesity. *N. Eng. J. Med.*, 285, 827.

HINSWORTH, H.P. (1933) The physiological activation of insulin. *Clin. Sci.*, 1, 1.

HIRSCH, J. & KNITTLE, J.L. (1970) Cellularity of obese and nonobese human adipose tissue. *Fed. Proc.*, 29, 1516.

HORTON, E.S., DANFORTH, E. Jr., SIMS, E.A.H. & SALANS, L.B. (1972) Correlation of forearm muscle and adipose tissue metabolism in obesity before and after weight loss. *Clin. Res.*, 20, 548.

HORTON, E.S. RUNGE, C.F. & SIMS, E.A.H. (1970) Forearm metabolism in human experimental obesity. *J. Clin. Invest.*, 49, 45A.

KAHN, C.R., SOLL, A.H., NEVILLE, D.M. Jr., GOLDFINE, I.D., ARCHER, J.A., GORDEN, P. & ROTH, J. (1974) The insulin receptor in obesity and other states of altered insulin sensitivity. Fogarty International Conference on Obesity, October 1973 (in press).

KALKHOFF, R.K., GOSSAIN, V.V. & MATUTE, M.L. (1973) Plasma glucagon in obesity. Response to arginine, glucose and protein administration. *N. Eng. J. Med.*, 289, 465.

KALKHOFF, R.K., KIM, H.J., CERLETTY, J. & FERROW, C.A. (1971) Metabolic effects of weight loss in obese subjects: Changes in plasma substrate levels, insulin and growth hormone responses. *Diabetes*, 20, 83.

KARAM, J.H., GODSKY, G.M. & FORSHAM, P.H. (1963) Excessive insulin response to glucose in obese subjects as measured by immunochemical assay. *Diabetes*, 12, 197.

MERIMEE, T.J. & RABIN, D. (1973) A survey of growth hormone secretion and action. *Metabolism*, 22, 1235.

PAULSEN, E.P. & LAWRENCE, A.M. (1968) Glucagon hypersecretion in obese children. *Lancet*, 2, 110.

PERLEY, M.J. & KIPNIS, D.M. (1967) Plasma insulin responses to oral and intravenous glucose: Studies in normal and diabetic subjects. *J. Clin. Invest.*, 46, 1954.

RABINOWITZ, D. (1970) Some endocrine and metabolic aspects of obesity. *Ann. Rev. Med.*, 21, 241.

RABINOWITZ, D. & ZIERLER, K.L. (1962) Forearm metabolism in obesity and its response to intra-arterial insulin. Characterization of insulin resistance and evidence for adaptive hyperinsulinism. *J. Clin. Invest.*, 41, 2173.

SALANS, L.B., KNITTLE, J.L. & HIRSCH, J. (1968) The role of adipose cell size and adipose tissue insulin sensitivity in the carbohydrate tolerance of human obesity. *J. Clin. Invest.*, 47, 153.

SIMS, E.A.H., DANFORTH, E. Jr., HORTON, E.S., BRAY, G.A. GLENNON, J.A. & SALANS, L.B. (1973) Endocrine and metabolic effects of experimental obesity in man. *Recent Prog. Horm. Res.*, 29, 457.

SIMS, E.A.H. & HORTON, E.S. (1968) Endocrine and metabolic adaptation to obesity and starvation. *Am. J. Clin. Nutr.*, 21, 1455.

SIMS, E.A.H., HORTON, E.S. & SALANS, L.B. (1971) Inducible metabolic abnormalities during development of obesity. *Ann. Rev. Med.*, 22, 235.

WISE, J.K., HENDLER, R. & FELIG, P. (1973) Evaluation of alpha-cell function of infusion of alanine in normal diabetic and obese subjects. *N. Eng. J. Med.*, 288, 487.

DISCUSSION

Dr. Ashwell. Dr. Björntorp (chapter 12) suggested that insulin resistance in obese subjects appears first in the muscles and results in high circulating insulin concentrations. Does Dr. Horton have any experimental data to confirm this?

Dr. Horton. The question whether hyperinsulinaemia comes first and insulin resistance is secondary to it, or insulin resistance comes first and hyperinsulinaemia is secondary, has plagued everyone.

Many workers consider that chronic stimulation of the pancreatic β-cell results in hyperinsulinaemia, and that peripheral insulin resistance is merely an adaptive phenomenon secondary to chronic exposure to high insulin concentrations.

This is the view which I favour. In some of our studies we attempted to find out whether high carbohydrate intake is the primary stimulus to the β-cell, or whether other substrates may act as stimuli. The experiments where weight gain was produced merely by increasing dietary fat, still do not exclude substrate as the primary stimulus to the β-cell and it may be the total calorie intake which is important. If excessive amounts of fat, or a relative excess of carbohydrate or aminoacids, are fed this may stimulate the β-cell.

Insulin resistance is shared not only by muscle and adipose tissue but also by the liver. All of these tissues become resistant to insulin—it is not correct or possible to say that one becomes resistant sooner than another. I believe it is the hyperinsulinaemia which comes first.

Dr. Lewis. My colleagues and I have conducted a small number of studies in which we have produced weight gain in lean, normal young men by a dietary supplement of 1,000 calories daily, of a composition similar to that in their previous diet. There was no change either in plasma cholesterol or triglyceride concentrations. However, when we gave 1,000 calories in the form of mixed carbohydrate there was a striking rise in tryglyceride and fall in cholesterol concentrations. Has Dr. Horton made similar observations?

Dr. Horton. In our original studies in which we increased all elements of the diet, a significant increase in both cholesterol and triglyceride concentrations were found. However, they remained within normal limits. We were interested to discover that free fatty acid concentrations were lower at peak weight than previously.

In subsequent studies in which we gave diets containing either a high or a low proportion of carbohydrate it was again found that the triglyceride concentrations were slightly higher on the former intake. Free fatty acid concentrations were lower on the diet with a higher proportion of carbohydrate. Thus, we believe that the original depression of free fatty acids was secondary to high carbohydrate intake and not to the weight gain itself.

In our most recent studies in which we have achieved weight gain by increasing dietary fat, the fat had a P:S ratio of 5:1 and was given mostly as corn oil disguised in a wide variety of ways. We found a slight decrease in cholesterol concentrations which we attributed to the high P:S ratio of the extra dietary fat. The changes in triglyceride concentrations have not been analysed yet, in this group.

Dr. Carlstrom. Are there any differences between the obese, the lean and the diabetic subjects with regard to the uptake of free fatty acids during your bilateral forearm experiments?

Mr. Whichelow. We have data for obese and lean subjects but they are a little conflicting because men and women appeared to behave differently when they were obese, but not when they were lean. There was a release of free fatty acids from the tissues after glucose. We have no data from diabetics.

Mr. Miller. I think we should refer to a low proportion of carbohydrate in a diet. The absolute amount in a low carbohydrate high calorie diet could be proportionally more than the absolute amount in a high carbohydrate low calorie diet.

Has Dr. Horton found any metabolic difference between the 'hard gainers' and the 'easy gainers'?

Dr. Horton. Your comment on terminology is relevant: the so-called low carbohydrate diets have contained $85g/M^2$ of carbohydrate. Since the individuals concerned were approximately $2\ M^2$, that is 170g carbohydrate intake which is in a low normal range. It is not a truly restricted carbohydrate intake and provides about 25% of the total calories.

We have not yet been able to determine where the excess calories go in these hard and easy gaining individuals. The requirement of $2700\ cal/M^2$ in order to maintain weight was a surprisingly high figure, and unfortunately, we do not have well controlled metabolic data for them. We have made more detailed measurements in other groups who gained weight on a high fat diet. They gained quite efficiently, so we do need to repeat the experiments using a mixed diet.

Dr. Galton. Dr. Horton, the number of fat cells did not increase during your overfeeding studies. You took this as evidence of stability of the adult adipose cell number. The weight gains were only 10 to 15 per cent; the increase in body fat could have been accommodated by already existing fat cells. Have you looked at individuals grossly overweight as a result of overfeeding? What occurred to their fat cell number.

Dr. Horton. The range of weight gain in all our subjects has been from 10 to about 30 per cent. No one gained more.

These are relatively short-term experiments of six to nine months. We have no data on the effect of overfeeding and maintained weight gain for one, two or five years in an individual.

One other problem is the Hirsch & Gallien technique which has been used for the estimation of cell size and number, since it is likely to have missed very small primordial fat cells.

Our estimates of cell number, measured at the beginning of the experiment, after weight gain and finally after reduction in weight, show no change. Whether long-term overfeeding in the adult could result in new cell formation remains uncertain.

Professor Adedevoh. Hyperinsulinaemia has been reported in East Africa and in Nigeria in normal populations when standards for Europeans are used. In your studies individuals were fed a high proportion of carbohydrate in their diet and high fat diets and the relative increase in insulin concentrations were up to 50 per cent for the high fat diet group. I would be interested to know what is the relationship between the insulin concentrations for the high carbohydrate and the high fat groups--or, if you have performed the two experiments in the same individual, how do they compare.

Dr. Horton. If the insulin concentrations are compared after weight gain in those who have gained by a high carbohydrate intake or a mixed diet and those gaining by a high fat diet, there is no difference in the hyperinsulinaemia. If, in a given individual, the effect of a 'low carbohydrate' diet or a 'high carbohydrate' diet, is compared at a given weight, there is a slight difference. With higher carbohydrate intake, the insulin concentrations are three to five $\mu U/ml$ higher than the values produced during lower carbohydrate intake. This has not been a constant finding in people with spontaneous obesity who we have studied.

Professor Wynn. I should like to comment about the 'easy' and 'hard gainer' since it seems to me tremendously important in relation to the understanding of obesity and the converse situation of constitutional thinness.

In my metabolic ward, I often have three or four very obese individuals who are easy gainers, and one or two people recovering from severe weight loss, often anorexia nervosa, who tend to be hard gainers. The hard gainers can be extremely mystifying; it is possible for a woman under thirty not to gain weight on 6,000 calories a day, although she is confined to her room or her bed for many weeks. We know that she is receiving the calories because metabolic studies have been conducted. For her to gain weight, she needs to receive amounts of testosterone sufficient to produce concentrations equivalent to those circulating in males.

Dr. Horton. I also have studied several young women with anorexia nervosa and I have found the opposite; they seem to be adapted metabolically to their low calorie intake. We have observed weight maintenance on intakes as low as 500 or 600 Kcal/day, with basal metabolic rates of minus 20 to minus 30 per cent. As these individuals have been re-fed they have gained weight in proportion to their calorie intake. We carry out re-feeding very gradually, starting with 1,000 Kcal/day, increasing by increments of 200 or 250 Kcal at intervals of a few days, until they are receiving 2,000 to 2,400 Kcal/day. With that approach, weight gain seems to be efficient.

17. A Preventive Programme for Obesity Control

Five-year follow-up on the success of an educational endeavour to influence physical activity and diet among 13 year old girls.

JOHANNA T. DWYER and J. MAYER

In the mid-1960s our laboratory undertook an obesity prevention and control programme in conjunction with the city schools in a suburb of Boston. The programme was conducted in the upper elementary and early secondary (junior high) schools of the community. It consisted of three hourly classes per week, in addition to two regular physical education classes, especially designed to increase physical activity among the obese and to impart nutrition education and psychological support for students who were, or apparently becoming, obese. The programme was available for two years free of charge to all who were judged obese in four out of the five junior high schools in the suburb. At least on a short-term basis, the programme was effective, and obesity was reduced among the participants (Seltzer & Mayer, 1970).

However, since obesity is a chronic condition, it is necessary to evaluate the effects of intervention not only over the short-term but also the long-term. The purpose of the present study was to investigate obesity status in one of these classes five years later, with particular attention to any resulting differences between those obese who had participated in the programme and those who had not, and to evaluate the special characteristics of the non-obese who had become obese in the succeeding five years.

In 1970 we undertook a follow-up survey of the girls in the 1965, 7th Grade classes who were originally approximately 13 years of age. They were re-examined in 1970 during their last year of secondary school (12th Grade) at approximately 17 years of age. We wished to observe progress and detect differences between girls who had been in the programme and those who had not with respect to physical measurements, nutrition knowledge and attitudes towards obesity and obesity prevention programme.

MATERIALS AND METHOD

POPULATION

The population consisted of all girls in the 1970 graduating year of the senior high schools from a middle class suburb of Boston, Massachusetts, who had been enrolled in that public school system five years before. The obesity control programme was initiated late in 1965, so baseline data on height-weight status for most of the children were expected to be available prior to the programme.

One hundred adolescent girls had been judged obese in 1965 on the basis of a Wetzel* (1940) grid rating of A-4 or above and the Seltzer-Mayer (1965) triceps skinfold criteria for obesity. They were informed of their eligibility for the obesity prevention and control programme and invited to join it in the autumn of that year. Fifty-eight of them (programme) participated for five to 18 months in the voluntary obesity control programme conducted in their schools. The remaining 42 subjects (non-programme) either failed to volunteer, dropped out of the programme or were in the non-participating school.

The other 580 girls in the 1965 class were considered to be non-obese on the same objective criteria.

Height-Weight Records

Height and weight from kindergarten to 12th Grade were abstracted from the health records for all the girls. These measurements had usually been taken by physical education teachers or school health personnel. Unfortunately after the 10th Grade in one school the measurements had been abandoned, so that records for the later years were incomplete.

Nutrition Knowledge Questionnaire

An objective test consisting of 57 items geared to the practical rather than the academic type of general nutrition knowledge was administered to the subjects (Dwyer *et al*, 1973). Questions dealt specifically with weight control. Sample items include the following: 'Alcohol furnishes more calories than sugar'; 'You can lose weight by eating foods providing fewer calories, or by exercising more than usual, or both'. The test was taken by the subjects while they were waiting to be measured. Subjects were supervised so that each respondent's answers would be her own. They were allotted the full class period, 45 minutes, for the test, although most of the subjects

---

* The Wetzel grid is a semilogarithmic chart allowing a log plot of weight against height.

took only 30 minutes to complete it. A perfect score on the test was 57.

Food Habits and Activity Questionnaire

Subjects were also asked to complete a questionnaire dealing with their attitudes and reported behaviour in relation to exercise modification, perceptions of obesity and of the obesity control programme. Most of the questions involved simple yes/no responses but space was provided for any additional comments the subject might have.

RESULTS

FOLLOW UP

Table 17.1 shows the completeness of the follow-up effort and current status with respect to obesity in 1970. Sixty-three percent of the former programme obese, 45 per cent of the non-programme obese and 54 per cent of the non-obese were measured; 57 per cent of the girls in the 1965 class were measured again. Despite extensive efforts to locate and measure those who were absent from the physical education classes in the school the final number followed up

Table 17.1
Obesity in 17 year old girls originally obese at the age of 13

Method of assessment in 17 year old	OBESE+ N=100*		NON-OBESE N=580*
	Programme N-58*	Non-programme N=42*	
Obese by:			
Triceps	21	14	40
Wetzel	22	11	46
Both	17	9	24
Non-obese by:			
Triceps	15	5	274
Wetzel	14	8	228
Both	19	10	282
Total measured	36	19	314
Lost to Follow-up:			
Moved	7		122
Not measured	15	14	122

+ Obese as determined by both Wetzel grid and triceps skinfold criteria
* N refers to the number in each group at age 13.

256 OBESITY SYMPOSIUM

Table 17.2

Original mean anthropometric measurements of selected adolescent girls when aged 13

	FORMERLY OBESE								NEWLY OBESE at age 17 N = 40		LEANEST at age 17 N = 27	
	Programme N = 30		Non-programme N = 17		Total N = 47							
	x	S.E.	x	S.E.	x	S.E.			x	S.E.	x	S.E.
Age (yrs)	13.3	0.1	13.2	0.1	13.3	0.1			13.0	0.2	13.2	0.1
Stature (cm)	155.9	2.01	157.2	1.84	156.7	0.91			153.3	1.72	150.7	1.41
Weight (kg)	58.8	1.28	56.7	1.72	58.0	1.03			51.6	1.35	39.6	0.04
Triceps skinfold (mm)	24.6	1.17	25.7	0.79	25.0	0.80			—		—	
Ponderal Index	12.2	0.09	12.4	0.11	12.3	0.09			12.7	0.06	13.4	0.08
Biepicondylar diameter (mm)	61.0	0.58	—		—				—		—	
Wrist breadth (mm)	49.6	0.44	—		—				—		—	
Hand Index *	442	4	—		—				—		—	

* $\dfrac{\text{hand length}}{\text{hand breadth}} \times 100$

x = mean

S.E. = standard error

was low, partly perhaps because the subjects' response to our request to be measured was voluntary and partly because 24 per cent of the students measured in 1965 had moved from the suburb. In order to assess the effect of a selection or volunteer bias among those obese who were followed up, a comparison was made between the 1965 measurements of those who were measured in 1970 with those who could not be measured. It did not reveal any systematic differences. Nevertheless, this does not definitively eliminate the possibility.

PREVALENCE OF OBESITY

In 1965, obesity was defined as a height-weight ratio of A-4 or above, on a Wetzel grid for the spring measurement of the year, plus a triceps skinfold measurement in excess of the Seltzer-Mayer (1965) criteria (22 mm for girls of 12 years of age or 23 mm for those of 13 years) in the autumn prior to the beginning of the programme. On this basis, 14 per cent of the girls in 1965 were defined as obese.

In 1970 obesity was considered to be present when the triceps skinfold equalled or exceeded the appropriate age Seltzer-Mayer criterion of 28 mm. The larger standard measurement reflects the normal increase in fat tissue with pubertal growth in the female. From this triceps criterion alone, 20 per cent of those measured were defined as obese in 1970 (Table 17.1). From the Wetzel grid alone, 21 per cent would be declared obese. If both the triceps and the Wetzel grid criteria were used, 14 per cent would be declared obese.

Those who had participated in the programme in 1965-66 were as likely to be obese in 1970 as those eligibles who had not done so (Table 17.1).

Forty subjects who had not been classified as obese in 1965 were found to be obese in 1970. For purposes of further discussion, these subjects will be termed the 'newly obese'.

Anthropometric Measurements

Table 17.2 presents the 1965 anthropometric measurements when available prior to the programme, for those subjects who were formerly obese subjects and who were remeasured in 1970. At the start, programme and non-programme obese did not differ with respect to age, stature, weight or triceps skinfold measurement, but the programme obese were more lateral as judged by their lower ponderal indices. In contrast to these formerly obese, the newly obese subjects were shorter, lighter and less lateral in 1965.

Table 17.3 presents the changes over five years among the various groups of subjects. No significantly different changes in triceps skinfold measurements, weight or stature were observed between

Table 17.3

Changes in anthropometric measurements among groups of adolescent girls

	N	Triceps Skinfold mm		Weight kg		Stature cm	
		x	S.E.	x	S.E.	x	S.E.
FORMERLY OBESE at age 13							
Programme							
Successes	12	−1.8	1.52	+5.8	1.84	+5.1	1.20
Failures	18	+4.6	1.42	+9.3	1.83	+4.1	0.77
Total	30	+2.0	1.17	+7.9	1.34	+4.5	0.66
Non-Programme							
Successes	4	−3.8	2.32	+3.4	2.52	+2.5	1.24
Failures	13	+3.2	1.37	+7.1	1.69	+3.7	0.72
Total	17	+1.5	1.36	+6.3	1.44	+3.7	0.58
Total							
Successes	16	−2.3	1.26	+5.2	1.50	+4.8	0.93
Failures	31	+3.9	0.99	+8.4	1.27	+3.9	0.53
NEWLY OBESE at age 17	40	—		+14.0	1.21	+7.8	0.84
LEANEST at age 17	27	—		8.6	1.22	+10.0	1.15

x = mean

S.E. = standard error

programme and non-programme obese, although in both groups mean changes were upward. In comparison to all of the formerly obese, the newly obese had gained more weight and height.

Among the programme and non-programme obese, some subjects succeeded in reducing their relative obesity and others did not. Subjects were classified as 'successes' if they had succeeded in becoming non-obese by the age appropriate Seltzer-Mayer triceps criterion and 'failures' if they had not. Table 17.3 reports their progress.

The 'successes' (e.g. those who had brought their obesity under control) had actually reduced their triceps skinfolds over the five years. They had significantly lower skinfold measurements, had experienced less weight gain and a slightly but not significantly greater gain in stature than had the failures. The newly obese might also be considered 'failures' since they had all become obese during adolescence. It was they who had gained most weight and stature of all those found to be obese in 1970.

Table 17.4 presents the anthropometric measurements of the subjects in 1970. As might be expected, the formerly obese who had succeeded in their weight reduction efforts were lighter, had lower triceps skinfold measurements and higher ponderal indices but did not appear to differ in their bony measurements or in stature.

In comparison to the newly obese, the failures among the formerly obese were shorter but did not differ appreciably in bony measurements nor were they heavier or more lateral.

Height-Weight Records

A number of investigators have suggested that menarche occurs earlier in obese girls (Frisch & Revelle, 1969; Tanner, 1962; Zacharias *et al*, 1970). The pubertal growth spurt in height, which closely coincides with the onset of menarche, is preceeded in females by a period of fat deposition (Tanner, 1962). Borjeson (1964) has suggested that the fat increase continues after the year of maximum growth and then declines in later adolescence. He further suggests that therapeutic efforts would best be directed to periods of decrement in storage of fat. Moreover, Frisch & Revelle (1971) have suggested that a critical weight may be the trigger which initiates the adolescent growth spurt in some way. Thus it was of interest to obtain some information on the timing of pubertal events in the population studied.

Unfortunately, data on age of menarche was not available, but in lieu of this, it was hoped that the year of maximum growth in height might yield some information on the onset of puberty among the

Table 17.4

Mean anthropometric measurements of selected groups of girls
(mean 17.8 years)

	FORMERLY OBESE at age 13						NEWLY OBESE at age 17		LEANEST at age 17	
	Successes: Nonobese at age 17		Failures: Obese at age 17		Total					
	$N = 16$		$N = 31$		$N = 47$		$N = 40$		$N = 27$	
	x	S.E.	x	S.E.	x	S.E.	x	S.E.	x	S.E.
Stature (cm)	161.3	1.55	160.8	1.05	160.9	0.86	162.9	0.72	160.7	1.07
Weight (kg)	62.4	1.26	66.8	0.48	65.3	1.08	65.8	1.18	48.3	1.04
Triceps skinfold (mm)	20.4	0.91	30.1	0.73	26.6	0.95	29.3	0.60	10.0	0.20
Biepicondylar diameter (mm)	60.1	0.73	60.0	0.55	60.1	0.44	60.5	0.45	58.2	0.60
Wrist breadth (mm)	48.2	0.67	49.2	0.39	48.9	0.35	49.2	0.42	47.8	0.04
Hand index	431	4	430	4	431	3	429	3	427	4
Ponderal index	12.3	0.11	12.0	0.09	12.1	0.06	12.2	0.06	13.4	0.07

x = mean
S.E. = standard error

various groups of girls. Accordingly, height-weight records on all of the obese subjects were analysed to ascertain the year of maximum growth in height.

Table 17.5 presents the results for all who were formerly obese in 1965, as well as for the newly obese (those who became obese after 1965). The formerly obese tended to experience the year of maximum growth in height earlier than the newly obese ($p < 0.05$).

ATTITUDES TOWARD FOOD AND OBESITY

Twenty-nine of the formerly obese subjects and 25 of the newly obese subjects completed a questionnaire on their food habits and attitudes toward obesity and the programme. Since this was a very small number of respondents, only clear differences between groups will be mentioned.

Table 17.5

School grade in which obese adolescent girls experienced maximum growth in height

	MAXIMUM INCREASE IN HEIGHT OCCURRED IN:						
	3rd or 4th Grade		5th or 6th Grade		7th or 8th Grade		Total
	N	Per cent	N	Per cent	N	Per cent	N
Formerly obese at age 13	12	25	28	61	7	14	47
Newly obese at age 17	2	7	16	62	8	31	26

Seventy-six per cent of the obese subjects affirmed that they had had a weight problem in the past and 79 per cent believed they had one at present. More of the formerly obese than of the newly obese said that their first weight problem occurred before ten years of age.

Regardless of an earlier or later onset of obesity or obesity since the 7th Grade, over half of the subjects claimed that they themselves had first decided they had a weight problem. The next most frequent response was parents, followed by family physician among the formerly obese and friends among the newly obese.

One question on which the formerly obese and the newly obese differed was: 'Has anyone in the school system ever told you that you had a weight problem?'. Among the formerly obese, 48 per cent indicated that they had been told by someone in the school system, while only 12 per cent of the newly obese had been so informed. It was most frequently the physical education teacher, the school physician or the school nurse who had mentioned their weight problem to them, although some subjects reported that it had been other teachers and adults in the school.

Obese subjects were asked where they received their guidance in weight control. Almost three-quarters of the subjects relied upon themselves for guidance, sometimes coupled with other sources of advice, such as parents, their family physician, friends and diet clubs, in that order of frequency.

Subjects emphasized dieting to solve their weight problems. Seventy-three per cent of the obese subjects were currently on a diet, another 33 per cent claimed that they dieted from time to time, and the others used various ways of cutting down on food from time to time. No subject reported that she ate whatever she wanted whenever she wanted it.

The major problem subjects had in dieting were, in rank order: snacking, binge and urge eating, holidays, weekends, eating away from home, desserts, choice of foods and portion size. Their most common dieting efforts were to take smaller portion sizes, consume fewer snacks and eliminate certain foods from the diet. Modifications of meal number or size were less common.

As might be expected, a high proportion of the subjects reported that other members of their families had weight control problems.

Sixty-one per cent of the respondents believed that increased physical activity was extremely or very important in weight control. However, very few of them had actually continued vigorous physical activity once the school programme had stopped.

The major reasons listed by the subjects for their lack of physical activity included the following in rank order: 'no time to do so' (given by more than 40 per cent of the subjects), 'no facilities to do so', 'do not enjoy', 'no one to do it with', 'feel awkward'. If they did make an effort to increase physical activity in order to help control their weight, most of these subjects preferred to do so by increasing independent activities rather than school connected activities.

Finally, when their views were solicited on the obesity prevention and control programme, 63 per cent of the subjects felt that schools should have such a programme. Of those who had not joined the programme when it was available, roughly a third were sorry now that they had not done so. Among the favourable remarks for the obesity control programme were: 'Through proper instruction, weight can be controlled', 'I need to relearn exercise and eating patterns and this might help', 'Exercise is good when losing weight', 'Perhaps I could have learned to prevent my constant gain of weight if I had joined the programme; I haven't learned on my own yet'.

Typical of the negative comments were the following: 'I was able to control my weight on my own', 'I can't imagine myself being successful in a flab lab', 'My peers looked down on those in the 'fat' class'.

NUTRITION KNOWLEDGE TEST

Since the obesity prevention and control programme had involved nutrition education of a general nature, it was thought that differences might exist between programme and non-programme participants some years later. Table 17.6 presents the data relating to this question. Neither former membership in the programme nor success in weight reduction seemed to be associated with a difference in score. The nutrition knowledge of the obese, at least as measured by this test, was not significantly different from all subjects in the class.

Table 17.6

12th Grade girls
Scores for nutritional knowledge

	N	Mean Score (± S.E.)
FORMERLY OBESE		
Programme		
Successes	8	31 (± 2.6)
Failures	12	33 (± 2.0)
Total	20	33 (± 1.6)
Non-Programme	4	34 (± 2.0)
Successes	4	34 (± 2.0)
Failures	9	29 (± 3.6)
Total	13	30 (± 2.6)
Total		
Successes	12	32 (± 1.8)
Failures	21	32 (± 1.7)
NEWLY OBESE AT AGE 17	27	31 (± 1.5)
ALL OBESE AT AGE 17	48	32 (± 1.0)
LEANEST AT AGE 17	20	28 (± 1.8)
ALL SUBJECTS IN CLASS	299	31 (± 0.4)

Note: maximum possible score was 57

However, their scores were higher than those of the leanest subjects in the sample.

DISCUSSION

PREVALENCE OF OBESITY AND ANTHROPOMETRIC FINDINGS

Obesity has negative connotations in American society today, particularly among adolescents (Bullen et al, 1963; Dwyer et al, 1969; Dwyer et al, 1970; Dwyer & Mayer, 1968; Monello & Mayer, 1963). This fact, plus the uncertain prognosis in the treatment of obesity during this age period and the ease with which temporary fattening during puberty is confused with early onset of a more permanent condition, makes it mandatory that adolescent girls be truly obese before labelling them as such. In planning the obesity control programme it was thought that false positives would be kept to a minimum by use of both height-weight ratios and skinfold measurements as objective criteria of obesity.

The Wetzel grid criterion was used for the initial screen of students in the class. It was followed up by skinfold measurements on all those height-weight ratios that were above A-4. The triceps measurement identifies fewer children as being obese than do weight-for-height ratios such as the Wetzel grid weight-for-age standards, and more children than does visual assessment (Rauh & Shumsky, 1969). Thus the prevalence of obesity will largely depend upon the type of measurement and cut-off point adopted.

Unfortunately, none of these criteria are as good as required. The Wetzel grid is constructed on a log-scale with height and weight data plotted against one another. Some of the difficulties of various weight-for-height ratios of this type have recently been documented by Florey (1970) and Newens & Goldstein (1972). Briefly stated, the Wetzel criterion at best is a poor measure of adiposity. Such a weight to height relationship treats muscularity, the contribution of bone to weight and adiposity in an equivalent manner. It may overselect large children as obese when in fact they are stocky or simply developmentally advanced and underidentify slower growing children who have excessive development of adipose tissue. Moreover, crossing over from channel to channel is common; it is the general trajectory of growth rather than a given point measurement which is most satisfactory in identifying the obese. While the Wetzel grid is easier to read than charts which plot the two measurements separately, it is less sensitive in detecting growth trends since it is based on an undefined cross-sectional sample, rather than a longitudinal sample of the same children from age to age. It thus tends to obscure individual differences.

Visual assessment usually correctly identifies the frankly obese and those who are strongly endomorphic in their body conformation, but it has several shortcomings. It tends to classify those 'stocky' children who are mesomorphic endomorphs as non-obese, since these tend to be mistaken for simply muscular children. Males are also declared to be obese less frequently than females, since girls at all ages have a more visible pattern of fat deposition. Further, it may under-identify obesity in the case of younger children and over-identify fat older children. Preadolescent children from nine to 12 years of age often present a slender appearance even when they are quite fat since they are usually long-legged. After about the age of 12 in girls or 14 in boys, the body becomes more lateral due to growth of the trunk and lessened growth of the legs. This broadening is often confused with obesity, even among trained observers visual methods possess the obvious disadvantage of varying from person to person since they are subjective in nature.

Only children who have or are likely to develop larger than average fat components of weight are of interest for obesity control programmes.

Undoubtedly, if one is to use subcutaneous fat measurement to make inferences about total body adiposity, the method used by Durnin & Rahaman (1967) utilizing the sum of a number of sites is preferable to a single depot measurement. Unless meticulous attention is paid to technique, errors are easily made in triceps skinfold measurements, as Ruiz and coworkers (1971) have recently shown. Ruffer (1970) has suggested that the Seltzer-Mayer triceps skinfold criteria for obesity may overlook some small individuals who are in fact obese for their body size and he suggests that, at the extremes, fatness is not independent of stature. Rauh & Shumsky (1968, 1969) have been highly critical of the standard. Many of their comments relate to the separate issue of methodological difficulties in using a single site triceps measurement as any more than a gross screening tool (which was, after all, the only use recommended by the authors). No satisfactory practical substitute is offered and the utility of combining triceps measurements with height-weight data is overlooked entirely, although this has always been the method of choice in our own investigations.

We are satisfied that all of those identified as obese in 1965 were in fact obese. In addition to the estimates of height, weight and triceps skinfold reported here, serial measurements were taken at three-monthly intervals during the programme. Also a paediatrician with extensive experience in the investigation of obesity evaluated each child periodically. Moreover, the subsequent status of the subjects as ascertained in 1970 suggests that most of those judged to be obese were in fact still obese five years later. Those who were not obese reported that in most instances rather strenuous efforts had been made to achieve weight reduction.

It was disappointing that few differences were noted between the prevalence of obesity of former programme participants and non-participants in the 1970 follow-up. The low success rates are similar to those reported on long-term follow-up of treatment by other investigators of obese children of approximately the same age (Haase & Hosenfeld, 1956; Hammar *et al*, 1971; Lloyd *et al*, 1961; Mossberg, 1948).

Perhaps some children whose obesity was of a borderline nature (e.g. Wetzel criterion negative, triceps criterion positive, or *vice versa*) were not identified in 1965. Some of these girls may have been missed in the screening because of the importance attached to keeping false positives as few as possible. Prime suspects for overlooked borderline cases are those who were found to be newly obese in 1970. The use of single height-weight ratios followed by triceps skinfold measurements to corroborate the presence of obesity may have biased us towards selecting the taller and developmentally advanced obese child whilst eliminating the smaller obese child. While it is likely that some of the newly obese in 1970 did have obesity of pubertal origin, others may have already been obese by 1965. The fact that they were smaller and less developmentally advanced in 1965 than those who were classified as obese suggests that some of them were obese in 1965 and overlooked. This points to the dangers of using height-weight ratio as the initial screening tool for determining obesity. While obesity is always represented by excessive adipose tissue, it is only sometimes reflected by weights which are grossly above the norm. Yet it is weight-for-height tables which girls of this age are most likely to use as confirmation of their obesity (Dwyer *et al*, 1969).

Borjeson (1962), Cheek *et al* (1970), Forbes (1964) and others have suggested that there may be two types of obesity in childhood. One type is characterized by advanced development, infantile onset and increased height as well as increased lean body mass. The other is more likely to be associated with excess weight due only to excess fat, with normal bone age, body length and a history of obesity dating from childhood. In our study, the former type was probably well identified; more cases of the latter may have been overlooked and appeared as the newly obese in 1970.

While our failure to identify all of those in the 7th Grade who later became obese is disturbing from the methodological standpoint, the question of what could have been done to treat them successfully even if they had been identified is even more problematic. Preventive and curative efforts seem to be only moderately successful and the long-term results for treatment or cure are dismal. In view of the very real psychological difficulties many adolescents experience after being 'officially' labelled as obese, caution on borderline cases is warranted. At the same time, the emergence of a substantial number of newly obese points to the need for continuous monitoring of fatness and growth throughout the school years, so that clearly deviant patterns can be recognized and treated as early as possible. The developmental aspects of disorders of weight have been well documented at this time of life by Borjeson (1962, 1964), Crisp *et al* (1970), Heald (1965) and Mullins (1958).

It should be noted that the stature and weight of the group of obese girls in 1970 was lower, although not significantly so, than measurements on girls of the same age who were obese in these same schools in 1967. The variation may be attributable to differences in sampling and variations between anthropometrists.

Height-Weight Records

Ascertainment of the year of maximum growth gave a gross indication of the relative physiological age of the subjects. The newly obese seemed to be somewhat slower to mature than those girls who had been obese in the 7th Grade. Several workers have reported that the obese mature earlier as a group than do the non-obese (Frisch & Revelle, 1969; Tanner, 1962; Zacharias *et al,* 1970).

Attitudes Toward Food and Obesity, and Knowledge of Nutrition

Most of the obese subjects were clearly aware of their obesity and had been for several years. None of them reported that they were eating *ad libitum*. Unfortunately perhaps for the utility of their efforts, most of them were engaging in self-prescribed diet. While their overall knowledge of nutrition on the objective test was higher than that of the leanest subjects, it may not have been sufficient to allow them to make the logical decisions about their food intakes which those who must restrict their appetite are forced to do constantly. Perhaps more effective nutrition education would improve the efficiency of their efforts to monitor calorie intake.

CONCLUSION

As might be expected, an hourly exercise programme three days a week for five to 18 months during school hours did not have sufficient impact on sedentary, obese 13 year old girls. Lasting habits of increased physical activity sufficient to lead to measurable improvements in weight control were not learned. However, the exercise programme did have some short-term beneficial effects both on fatness and fitness.

As many workers have demonstrated, it is in the use of leisure time that the obese girl is most strikingly inactive in comparison with her peers (Corbin & Fletcher, 1968; Durnin, 1971). Therefore it is necessary to have not only a school day which includes more physical activity but also a generally more active life style. Changes in mode of life and changes in diet take time and effort. Judging from students' reactions this method of treating obesity did not appear, at least in retrospect, to be onerous or unpleasant to most of the girls. However, increased physical activity both in and out of school are probably requisites to progress and success. School programmes of longer duration, begun earlier in life and conducted at more frequent intervals, might be expected to have more lasting effects.

Acknowledgements

The research reported in this chapter was supported in part by the Maternal and Child Health Service Training Grant, Grant Number AM 02839 from the National Institutes of Health, and the Fund for Research and Teaching, Nutrition Department, Harvard School of Public Health.

Our gratitude is due to our former colleague, Dr. Berverly A. Bullen, of Sargent College, Boston University for her help in the initial study in 1965 as well as in the planning of the 1970 study. Miss Anne Maxwell, M.S. and Miss Joan Hamilton, B.S. performed the anthropometric measurement survey in 1970. Miss Helene D. Breivogel, Director of Girls' Physical Education in the Newton, Massachusetts public school system was most helpful in arranging for the follow-up study. Miss Janet Pilz, A.B. provided clerical help and Miss Kathryn Dowd, A.B. editorial assistance in preparing the manuscript.

REFERENCES

BORJESON, M. (1962) Overweight children. *Acta Paediat. Scand.*, suppl. 132.
BORJESON, M. (1964) Overweight in Swedish school children in *Symposia of the Swedish Nutrition Foundation II. Occurence Causes and Prevention of Overweight.* Ed. Blix, G. p.18. Uppsala: Almquist & Wiksells.
BULLEN, B.A., MONELLO, L.F., COHEN, H. & MAYER, J. (1963) Attitudes toward physical activity, food and family in obese and nonobese adolescent girls. *Amer. J. Clin. Nutr.*, 12, 1.
CHEEK, D.B., SCHULTZ, R.B., PARRA, A. & REBA, R.C. (1970) Overgrowth of lean and adipose tissues in adolescent obesity. *Pediat. Res.*, 4, 268.
CORBIN, C.B. & FLETCHER, P. (1968) Diet and physical activity patterns of obese and nonobese elementary school children. *Res. Quart. Amer. Assoc. Health Phys. Ed. & Rec.*, 39, 922.

CRISP, A.H., DOUGLAS, J.W., ROSS, J.M. & STONEHILL, E. (1970) Some developmental aspects of disorders of weight. *J. Psychosom. Res.*, 14, 313.

DURNIN, J.V.G.A. (1971) Physical activity by adolescents. *Acta Paediat. Scand.*, 217, 133.

DURNIN, J.V.G.A. & RAHAMAN, M.M. (1967) Assessment of the amount of fat in the human body from measures of skinfold thickness. *Brit. J. Nutr.*, 21, 681.

DWYER, J.T., FELDMAN, J.J. & MAYER, J. (1971) The social psychology of dieting. *J. Health & Soc. Behav.*, 11, 269.

DWYER, J.T., FELDMAN, J.J., SELTZER, C.C. & MAYER, J. (1969) Body image in adolescents: attitudes toward weight and perception of appearance. *J. Nutr. Ed.*, 1, 14.

DWYER, J.T. & MAYER, J. (1968) Psychological effects of variations in physical appearance during adolescence. *Adol.*, 3, 353.

DWYER, J.T., ORR, R. & MAYER, J. (1973) Knowledge of practical aspects of nutrition among professionals and laymen. Unpublished manuscript. Boston.

FLOREY, C. Du V. (1970) The use and interpretation of ponderal index and other weight for height ratios in epidemiological studies. *J. Chronic Dis.*, 23, 93.

FORBES, G.B. (1964) Lean body mass and fat in obese children. *Pediatrics*, 34, 308.

FRISCH, R.E. & REVELLE, R. (1969) The height and weight of adolescent boys and girls at the time of peak velocity of growth in height and weight: longitudinal data. *Human Biol.*, 4, 536.

FRISCH, R.E. & REVELLE, R. (1971) Height and weight of girls and boys at the time of initiation of the adolescent growth spurt in height and weight and the relationship to menarche. *Human Biol.*, 43, 140.

HAMMER, S.L. CAMPBELL, V. & WOOLEY, J. (1971) Treating adolescent obesity: Long range evaluation of previous therapy. *Clin. Pediat. (Phil)*, 10, 46.

HAASE, K.E. & HOSENFELD, H. (1956) Zur fettsucht im kindesalter. *Z. Kinderheilk.*, 78, 1.

HEALD, F.P. (1965) The relationship between obesity in adolescence and early growth. *J. Pediat.*, 67, 35.

LLOYD, J.K., WOLFF, O.H. & WHELAN, W.S. (1961) Childhood obesity: a long term study of height and weight. *Brit. Med. J.*, 2, 145.

MONELLO, L.F. & MAYER, J. (1963) Obese adolescent girls: an unrecognized minority group. *Amer. J. Clin. Nutr.*, 13, 35.

MOSSBERG, H.A. (1948) Obesity in children: a clinical-prognostical investigation. *Acta Pediat.*, 35, suppl. 2.

MULLINS, A.G. (1958) Prognosis in juvenile obesity. *Arch. Dis. Childh.*, 33, 307.

NEWENS, E.M. & GOLDSTEIN, H. (1972) Height, weight and assessment of obesity in children. *Brit. J. Prev. Soc. Med.*, 26, 33.

RAUH, J.L. & SCHUMSKY, D.A. (1968) An evaluation of triceps skinfold measures from urban school children. *Human Biol.*, 40, 263.

RAUH, J.L. & SCHUMSKY, D.A. (1969) Relative accuracy of visual assessment of juvenile obesity. *J. Amer. Dietet. Assoc.*, 55, 459.

RUFFER, W.A. (1970) Two simple indices for identifying obesity compared. *J. Amer. Dietet. Assoc.*, 57, 326.

RUIZ, L., COLLEY, J.R. & HAMILTON, P.J. (1971) Measurement of triceps skinfold thickness. An investigation of sources of variation. *Brit. J. Prev. Soc. Med.*, **25**, 165.

SELTZER, C.C. & MAYER, J. (1965) A simple criterion of obesity. *Postgrad. Med.*, **38**, A101.

SELTZER, C.C. & MAYER, J. (1970) An effective weight control programme in a public school system. *Am. J. Pub. Hlth*, **60**, 679.

TANNER, J.M. (1962) *Growth at Adolescence.* Oxford: Blackwell.

WETZEL, N.C. (1940) The Wetzel grid for evaluating physical fitness. Cleaveland, Ohio: NEA Service Inc.

ZACHARIAS, L., WURTMAN, R.J. & SCHATZOFF, M. (1970) Sexual maturation in contemporary American girls. *Amer. J. Obstet. Gynecol.*, **108**, 85.

18. The Low-Carbohydrate Diet

JOHN YUDKIN

The twin objectives in devising a diet for the treatment of obesity are that it should be effective in removing excess fat and that it should become a permanent eating habit.

As to the first, weight loss will occur when energy intake is sufficiently restricted. This restriction may be more than expected, because of the possible adaptation of the overweight person to an abnormally high energy intake, and the possible adaptation of the person losing weight to an abnormally low energy intake. But there is no doubt that there is an intake of energy for each overweight individual below which loss of excess fat is inevitable.

As well as being low in energy the diet must also be capable of becoming permanent. I know of no evidence that it is of advantage to introduce a temporary 'crash diet' to ensure rapid loss before introducing the diet that will be needed to maintain that loss.

A diet that becomes a permanent eating pattern must fulfil several criteria. It must be nutritionally adequate, it must be palatable, it must be simple, it must be sociable and it must not be expensive. A diet that meets these criteria as well as being low in energy is the low-carbohydrate diet.

The principle of this diet is that the individual restricts his carbohydrate intake to about 60 g/day, but does not consciously restrict the protein or fat in his diet. Some individuals find it possible to achieve adequate weight control with a carbohydrate intake of 100 g/day or even a little more. In practice, the patient is told to avoid food and drink containing added sugar, and to use simple tables to restrict foods containing starch and other assimilable carbohydrates in order to give him the prescribed carbohydrate intake. For the purpose of this diet, one has to include alcohol in the carbohydrate count.

LOW ENERGY, HIGH NUTRIENTS

Nutritional adequacy is often overlooked in the prescription of many diets for weight reduction. It shows a lack of nutritional competence on the part of the doctor to stress almost exclusively that his patient should restrict energy. It shows a high order of negligence to carry this to the extent of stressing the relative energy content of foods without reference to their nutrient content. It is this attitude that is responsible for the unrealistic approach to childhood obesity, telling the mother to restrict milk and ignore the orange drink or cola, or the dilution with sugar of the already nutrient-poor breakfast cereal.

The fact is that most foods that are high in carbohydrates are also relatively low in nutrients. The most obvious example is sugar (sucrose) which contains no nutrients whatsoever. Thus, foods and

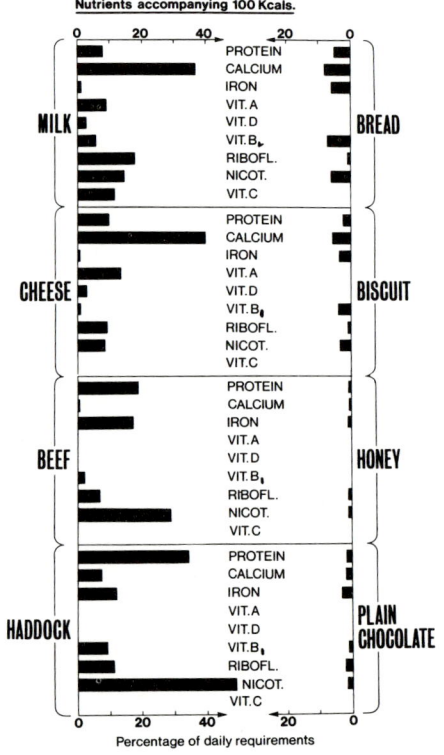

Figure 18.1
Comparative nutrient content of carbohydrate-poor and carbohydrate-rich foods.
Columns express percentage of recommended intakes for women, of nine selected nutrients, provided by 100 Kcal portions of the foods.

drinks that are rich in sugar will be relatively poor in nutrients in proportion to the energy they supply. These include soft drinks, confectionery, most cakes and biscuits, ice cream and made-up desserts.

Virtual elimination of these items from the diet is enough to reduce carbohydrate intake to an effective level. More often, it is necessary also to restrict other sources of carbohydrates, especially starch. This implies a restriction on such foods as bread, rice, pasta and potatoes.

The limited allowance of carbohydrate should be taken largely as fruit and milk. Not only do they contribute an important supply of nutrients, but they contribute greatly to the palatability of the diet, both directly and by increasing the possible range of prepared dishes.

The principle that, in general, foods rich in carbohydrates are poor in nutrients is illustrated in Figure 18.1. This shows the quantity of several nutrients that accompany 100 Kcalories.

I have made an assessment of the nutrient intake of persons both before and after the adoption of the low carbohydrate diet. This showed firstly that apparently unlimited protein and fat, when carbohydrate is restricted, is an amount of protein and fat not significantly different from that consumed on the diet previously taken (Table 18.1). As a result, there is a reduction of energy intake equivalent to the reduction in the carbohydrate intake.

Table 18.1
Calorific constitutents in low-carbohydrate diet

	Normal Diet	Low-Carbohydrate Diet	Difference
PROTEIN (g)	(77)	(80)	(+3)
	84	83	−1
FAT (g)	(122)	(109)	(−23)
	124	105	−19
CARBOHYDRATE (g)	(206)	(65)	(−141)
	216	67	−149

(Figures in parantheses - Yudkin & Carey 1960
Other figures - Stock & Yudkin 1970)

MYTHS ABOUT THE LOW-CARBOHYDRATE DIET

During the last 10 or 12 years, much has been written about the low-carbohydrate diet. Books and articles written for the lay press have often been presented as if some extraordinary new discovery has been made about metabolic processes. These claims have no scientific validity and their chief consequence has been to antagonize the medical and nutritional establishment. The members of the establishment in turn have failed to distinguish between what people in fact eat from what it is supposed that they eat; they also fail to distinguish between a low-carbohydrate diet and a carbohydrate-free diet. Thus, they have criticized the low-carbohydrate diet as being high in protein and high in fat, as leading to prolonged and pronounced ketosis, increase in blood cholesterol and increase in blood uric acid, and as lacking in calcium, ascorbic acid and a number of other nutrients.

As we have seen, the diet is not high in protein or fat. The reason for supposing that it is derives from the belief that 'as much as you like' is the same as 'a large amount'. The fact is that deliberate restriction of carbohydrate leads to automatic limitation of protein and fat to about their previous levels. Of course the proportion of these dietary components is increased, since the total food intake is reduced. It is perhaps for this reason that concern has been expressed in regard to the fat component, since it has been common to regard the percentage of fat in the diet as a major factor determining the concentration of blood cholesterol.

There is an increasing belief that we have paid far too much attention to cholesterol concentration as a possible hazard to health. Be that as it may, it is highly implausible that a given amount of fat that is harmless when energy intake is excessive becomes harmful when this excess is corrected by a reduction in the intake of sugar and starch.

Consider a typical diet that provides 100 g protein, 100 g fat and 300 g carbohydrate each day. This yields 2500 Kcal (10.5 MJ) of which 900 Kcal (3.7 MJ) or 38 per cent come from fat. Now let us reduce the energy content by about one-third by reducing the carbohydrate intake to 100 g. This diet will now provide 1700 Kcal (7.1 MJ) instead of 2500 Kcal (10.5 MJ), and although the amount of fat has not been altered, it will now provide just over 50 per cent of the total energy. Is it seriously to be supposed that, by taking no sugar in his tea or coffee, choosing soda water as a mixer instead of tonic water and doing without toast and marmalade for breakfast, a man endangers his life through a mathematical formula that calculates his unchanged fat intake as a percentage?

There is indeed some evidence that a diet that is devoid of carbohydrate does lead to hypercholesterolaemia; it of course also leads to a significant degree of ketosis. But an increase of blood cholesterol or of blood uric acid does not occur when as little as 50 g of carbohydrate are taken and ketosis, if it does occur, is negligible

(Table 18.2). This is not surprising, since it is accepted that a carbohydrate intake that provides at least 15 per cent of the energy content of the diet is adequate to prevent ketosis; Evans and her colleagues (1974) have shown that the diet has always provided more carbohydrate than this.

Table 18.2
Blood and urine tests on eight young women consuming low-carbohydrate diet

	Normal Diet	Low-Carbohydrate Diet
Plasma cholesterol mg/100 ml	203	197
Plasma triglyceride mg/100 ml	95	95
Plasma uric acid mg/100 ml	3.2	3.4
Urinary N, g/24 h	11.5	12.3

None of the differences were statistically significant ($p > 0.05$)

Ketone bodies: traces found in 11 out of 32 24-h samples collected on four separate days during a period on low-carbohydrate diet.

(from Evans *et al*, 1974)

NUTRIENT CONTENT OF THE LOW-CARBOHYDRATE DIET

Here let me add a personal note as to why I believe that the low-carbohydrate diet is the most suitable diet, not only for weight control but for general nutritional health and well-being. It seems to be increasingly evident that the more we diverge from the mode of living that man has slowly adopted over millions of years of evolution, and the more rapidly we do so, the more likely we are to suffer ill effects. This is now clear in relation to our increasing sedentariness, the adverse reactions to drugs that one had imagined were quite free from side effects, and in relation to the accumulation of harmful substances in our environment. This does not imply that we should now stop living in cities, abandon the motor car and television, move into caves in the countryside, give up agriculture and revert to hunting and gathering our food. Nor do I mean that we must start buying our foods only from the health food store, and try to live on honey, yoghourt, sesame seeds and bread made from compost-grown stone-ground wheat.

However, I do suggest that, in so far as it is possible in an industrialized and urbanized community, we are likely to do better nutritionally if we eat the sorts of foods that were eaten by our pre-Neolithic ancestors. Fortunately, man has always been omnivorous, so that he can choose from a very wide variety of foods. But he should, as far as possible, choose foods that are recognizably those that would have been available to him from his hunting and gathering. This does not preclude foods that are preserved by methods such as canning, freezing or dehydration, but it does suggest that we may not be physiologically or biochemically adapted to made-up foods. A moment's consideration shows that the majority of these made-up foods are those that are rich in sucrose, which we now consume in far greater quantities than did our forebears. There is even evidence that, as a species, man is not fully adapted to made-up foods rich in starch, such as bread, although this is less evident since they have been an important part of his diet for an appreciably longer time than has sucrose.

I am afraid that these views will be found unacceptable to the conventional nutritionist. Any suggestions that all is not well with the foods now available in the affluent society, and with the way we choose them, is apt to be regarded as a declaration of adherence to the large and increasing army of food cranks. Nevertheless, I sincerely believe that we have for too long accepted that any direction in which food production and preparation goes, especially if it increases the choice and palatability of our diet, is likely to be nutritionally desirable.

Let us return to the nutrient content of the low-carbohydrate diet.

It transpires that the nutritional value of the low-carbohydrate diet is in most respects better, and in no respect worse, than the equicaloric diet obtained by general food restriction (Table 18.3). But it is common for obese patients to be told that the best way for them to lose weight is simply to eat less than they have been doing; to eat the same foods in the same proportion as before but not so much. One way then of assessing the low-carbohydrate diet is to compare its nutrient content with that of a diet in which the same caloric reduction of about 33 per cent is achieved by an overall decrease of the habitual diet. Clearly, this will result in a reduction of all the nutrients by the same amount, that is, by one-third.

The low-carbohydrate diet is a diet that will reduce superfluous adiposity, but it will not need to be changed when this has been done. Although there has been little work in which this has been studied in a range of people with varying requirements and showing varying degrees of obesity, personal observation indicates that, when

Table 18.3
Nutrients in Low-Carbohydrate diet

	Normal Diet	Low-Carbohydrate Diet
VITAMIN A (mg)	3.06	3.10
VITAMIN D (mg)	5.0	7.7
THIAMINE (mg/1000 Kcal)	0.49	0.60
RIBOFLAVIN (mg/100 Kcal)	0.71	1.12
NICOTINAMIDE (mg/1000 Kcal)	5.61	7.04
ASCORBIC ACID (mg)	70	75
CALCIUM (mg)	1070	980
IRON (mg) - TOTAL	12.8	11.7
- ANIMAL SOURCES	6.8	8.6

carbohydrate is limited, food intake tends to adjust itself to energy requirements over a fairly wide range. It is important to stress this when the diet is used to treat obesity, since it underlines the important point that the diet is intended as a new but permanent pattern of eating and not simply as a cure for obesity, to be abandoned when an acceptable loss of weight is achieved. It is also my own belief, as I have indicated, that this diet is desirable for most people, including children, for purely nutritional reasons. Its adoption by children would help to prevent obesity both in childhood and in later life.

PALATABLE, BUT NOT IRRESISTIBLE

Not everyone will be able to answer in the way Zsa-Zsa Gabor did when asked what she usually had for breakfast: 'Caviare and champagne, of course! What else is there?' But it is true that today most people can choose to eat or drink from a very wide range of foods. It can be accepted that their diet will largely be foods and drinks that they consider to be the most palatable. However, one of the main reasons for an excessive caloric intake is that people over-indulge in foods and drinks which are difficult to resist because they are extremely palatable, and increasingly so with the widening variety of new foods and drinks. Moreover, even a casual inspection shows that these are mostly carbohydrate-rich snacks which are of low nutrient content but of high energy value.

It follows from these considerations that any change in diet, whether for energy restriction or for any other reason, will inevitably be less attractive than is the freely chosen diet hitherto consumed. The acceptability of the new diet will depend on a number of factors: chiefly the personality of the individual, but also on the incentive that is inherent or that can be encouraged or evoked. Although the new diet must of necessity be less acceptable than is the habitual diet, it is more likely to be accepted if its palatability is made as high as possible. One of the major virtues of the low-carbohydrate diet is that it allows free choice, both qualitatively and quantitatively, from foods such as meat, fish, cheese, eggs, butter, cream and leafy vegetables. In addition, it strongly recommends that part of the carbohydrate ration should be in the form of milk and fruit, which add appreciably to palatability and, especially in relation to milk, to nutrient supplies.

People will not adhere to a diet that insists on an inflexible eating pattern that is very different from that of the rest of the family, or that cannot reasonably well be followed in a restaurant or at a party. It is claimed that people like the rigidity imposed by some dietary regimes. But I cannot believe that it is useful—and it may even be argued that it is dishonest—to suggest as some slimming groups do that it is essential for the control of obesity that one eats liver once a week, fish five times a week, eggs and cheese for breakfast or lunch but not for supper, until recently it was also suggested that tomatoes and green beans were not fattening in the evening, although they were fattening at breakfast or lunch time.

A DIET TO LIVE WITH

Certainly a rigid diet must make it difficult for the ordinary busy housewife to fit her dietary requirements into the family eating pattern. On the other hand, there is no difficulty in sharing the wide range of carbohydrate-free items in the low-carbohydrate diet, and simply avoiding the sugar in tea or coffee, the soft drinks and the desserts, and restricting the consumption of bread, pasta and other starch-rich foods.

The low-carbohydrate diet is simpler to calculate than is the calorie-counted diet. The latter requires a knowledge of the energy value of every item of food and drink. The low-carbohydrate dieter needs to know the carbohydrate content only of those foods that contain carbohydrate. As we saw, the foods without carbohydrate comprise not only the total range of meats and poultry and fish and cheese but also eggs, butter and leafy vegetables.

It is often said that the low-carbohydrate diet is costly, and thus is not practicable for a large number of persons. This is almost always not true. The truth is that meat need not necessarily be fillet steak, nor the fish salmon or the cheese Camembert or Stilton. Secondly, people frequently do not realize how much they are spending on the carbohydrate-rich confectionery, cakes, biscuits and drinks that they consume. It is not uncommon for these items to account for a quarter or even more of the food budget. Thirdly, many of those that seem reluctant to spend money on a highly nutritious diet seem quite willing to spend it on some of the useless foods and gadgets that are claimed—often quite falsely—to help them to become slim.

THE REGULATION OF FOOD INTAKE

The fact that a limitation of dietary carbohydrate results in an automatic limitation of total food intake has implications in relation to the mechanisms that regulate food intake. Much of what has been written on this subject assumes that the regulation is concerned entirely with matching energy intake against a given energy expenditure. There is now strong evidence that to some extent it is also possible to adjust expenditure to a given intake.

As regards the regulation of intake itself, experience with the low carbohydrate diet indicates that this involves not only the energy content of the food consumed, but also the nature of the food consumed. First, there is the specific factor of palatability. We rarely pay sufficient attention to the fact, well known to laymen, that people eat more food if it is highly palatable, and less if it is unpalatable. It so happens that many of the most attractive, almost irresistible, foods are those that are rich in carbohydrate, especially sugar. The individual who has had a splendid and more than adequate dinner can be tempted to eat meringue glacé or chocolate soufflé without difficulty. Again, it cannot be denied that we often eat sweet snacks because we enjoy the taste, and not because we are in need of additional energy. As for sweetened drinks, these may be taken because of thirst but this need for fluid rarely coincides with a need for more energy.

In regard to drinks, it should here be pointed out that the large and increasing consumption of soft drinks may well be caused by a degree of habituation, if not addiction, to caffeine. The cola drinks contain this drug, and much of the demand for these drinks, I am convinced, comes about because of the stimulation it produces. It is to me extraordinary that parents who would refuse to give their young children tea or coffee have no hesitation in allowing them to consume cola drinks, or the widely advertized glucose drinks, which also contain significant quantities of caffeine.

But many carbohydrate-rich foods, especially those that are rich in starch rather than in sugar, cannot be said to have a high degree of palatability for most people. It seems then that these foods do not produce satiety as readily as do the foods rich in protein or fat. This is perhaps more readily evident if we consider the situation of an obese person who had lost weight on this diet. He is by definition eating to satiety on a diet containing perhaps 70 g of carbohydrate a day, together with 100 g protein and 100 g of fat; this will give some 1600 Kcal (6.7 MJ) a day. If he now reverts to his previous diet, he will again eat to satiety, but with perhaps 250 g of carbohydrate though with no more protein or fat. Thus he will now be satiated with 2300 Kcal (9.6 MJ) rather than his former 1600 Kcal (6.7 MJ).

It is clear from these observations that the intake of food is not determined solely by its energy content.

CONCLUSION

The low-carbohydrate diet is not the only possible diet for weight reduction or control. Certainly there are some obese people who can lose weight by reducing their fat intake or by counting calories. What is claimed for the low-carbohydrate diet are such qualities as its high nutritional value, its ease of calculation and its compatability with the rest of the family's eating habits. For many people this combination makes it the diet of choice.

REFERENCES

EVANS, E., STOCK, M. & YUDKIN, J. (1974) The absence of undesirable changes during consumption of the low carbohydrate diet used for the treatment of obesity. *Amer. J. Clin. Nutr.* In press.

STOCK, M. & YUDKIN, J. (1970) Nutrient intake of subjects on low carbohydrate diet used in the treatment of obesity. *Am. J. Clin. Nutr.*, 23, 948.

YUDKIN, J. & CAREY, M. (1960) The treatment of obesity by the 'high fat' diet: the inevitability of calories. *Lancet*, 2, 939.

19. Further Follow Up Experience After Prolonged Therapeutic Starvation

CATHERINE J. CAMPBELL, I. W. CAMPBELL, J. A. INNES,
J. F. MUNRO and ANNE L. NEEDLE

Bloom (1959) subjected nine obese patients to a short period of in-patient starvation. He noted that five continued to lose weight during a follow up period from two to nine months, and suggested that therapeutic fasting was a worthwhile procedure. Since then considerable information has been accumulated concerning the metabolic and other immediate consequences of fasting the obese. Starvation is an effective method of weight reduction, but it involves lengthy periods of hospitalization and is not without risk. Its widespread use can only be justified if there is a pressing need for temporary weight loss or if it can be shown that the long term results are superior to those obtained by conventional treatment. A critical review of those disappointingly few series which report follow up results would suggest that short periods of starvation (i.e. up to four weeks) are of limited permanent value either at the time of initial referral to hospital, or in patients with refractory obesity (Munro, 1973). Our previous experience, however, had suggested that prolonged in-patient starvation might be of greater permanent value if patients were reduced to within 25 per cent in excess of their ideal weight (Munro *et al*, 1970). We now describe the follow up experience in 75 patients with refractory obesity.

PATIENTS AND METHODS

All the patients had previously attended the obesity clinic, but had failed to lose weight. They had expressed the desire to be admitted for starving and said that they were prepared to remain in hospital until reduced to within 25 per cent in excess of their ideal weight. There were 48 women, average age 29 years (range 15 to 57) and 27 men, average age 30 years (range 14 to 53). Five patients discharged themselves within a week or so of admission and have been excluded from further analysis. The mean weight of the remaining 45 women was 75.3 per cent in excess of ideal (range 41 to 141 per cent), and that of the remaining 25 men was 75.5 per cent in excess of ideal (range 45 to 123 per cent). The patients were admitted to two hospitals both of which provide good rehabilitative facilities which they were encouraged to use. After a short assessment period they commenced the starvation regime. Initially, if specifically requested a low calorie carbohydrate restricted meal was provided, and many took one such meal a week. Subsequently this offer was withheld. The emphasis, however, was on trust rather than supervision and many admitted to periodic 'cheating'. In all other respects the regime previously described was followed (Munro *et al*, 1970).

At the completion of fasting, patients were refed in hospital for four to seven days, and were offered further dietary advice. During follow up the policy was to see them at intervals of four weeks or less. They were given every encouragement to lose weight and they and their close relatives had the opportunity of attending a monthly 'group' session held for patients during and following starvation. Many were treated with anorexiant drugs and nine were refered for psychiatric treatment. 11 underwent further short periods of out-patient starvation and four were re-admitted for starvation, one on two separate occasions. Thus the 70 patients were treated with a total of 75 'episodes'.

The following criteria were applied to evaluate follow up results:

Default - default from the clinic within 12 months of discharge and without subsequent reattendance

Failure - regain of > 15 kg or of > 50 per cent of total weight loss during starvation

Modified success - regain of 10 to 15 kg or of 33 to 50 per cent total weight loss during starvation

Success - weight regain of less than 10 kg and less than 33 per cent of weight loss

Patients in whom follow up was available for at least 12 months, but who thereafter failed to attend, were classified as 'success', 'modified success' or 'failure', with subsequent default. When a patient failed to attend they were personally written to and were sent not less than three further appointments.

Patients have been subdivided into groups according to sex, per cent in excess of ideal weight at time of admission, and to whether or not they reduce to within 25 per cent in excess of ideal weight at the completion of fasting. The results are presented accordingly.

Table 19.1

Mean weight loss (kg) during therapeutic starvation with range, related to percentage excess of ideal weight on admission

Percentage excess of ideal weight on admission	Female	Male
40–59	14.7 (2.0–27.0)	24.8 (16.0–39.0)
60–79	24.8 (14.0–36.0)	27.0 (13.0–46.0)
80–99	36.8 (28.0–43.0)	37.0 (21.0–46.0)
100 or over	47.7 (27.0–72.0)	57.6 (38.0–77.0)
Mean	27.4 (2.0–72.0)	33.1 (16.0–77.0)

RESULTS

During a mean fast of 14 weeks the overall mean weight loss was 29.6 kg. The mean weight changes in the various sub groups are shown in Table 19.1. Only 39 of the 75 patients, including four of the 12 most severely obese, were starved to within 25 per cent in excess of ideal weight (Table 19.2).

Following discharge 12 patients defaulted within one year. Of these one died in a road traffic accident and eight are known to have left the district. A further six have defaulted after at least 12 months follow up and 24 other patients were lost at some stage of follow up, but have subsequently reattended. The mean period of follow up was 28.2 months (12–64 months) and during this time there has been a mean weight change from 28.2 per cent in excess of ideal weight (range 7 to 83 per cent) to 62.7 per cent (range zero to 137 per cent). The follow up results of the various sub groups are presented in Tables 19.3 and 19.4.

In all, 39 episodes are deemed failures and 24 patients are now in excess of their preadmission weight. Some of the failures regained weight extremely rapidly, irrespective of whether or not they had reduced to within 25 per cent in excess of ideal weight (Figs. 19.1 and 19.2). Others managed to maintain their discharge weight for a considerable time only to regain. This was often associated with default (Fig. 19.3), but sometimes it occurred for other reasons. For example, one man, a main line engine driver, had been seen regularly

Table 19.2

Relationship between percentage excess of ideal weight on admission and ability to reduce to within 25 per cent of ideal in male and female patients

MALE			FEMALE		
% excess weight on admission	% excess weight on discharge		% excess weight on admission	% excess weight on discharge	
	Less than 25	More than 25		Less than 25	More than 25
40–59	6	0	40–59	8	4
60–79	7	6	60–79	10	11
80–99	1	3	80–99	3	4
100 +	3	2	100 +	1	6
TOTAL	17	11	TOTAL	22	25

Table 19.3

Follow up results of 47 episodes of therapeutic starvation in female patients related to percentage excess of ideal weight at admission and discharge

% excess weight on admission	40–59		60–79		80–99		100 and over		TOTAL	
% excess weight on discharge	<25	>25	<25	>25	<25	>25	<25	>25	<25	>25
DEFAULT	1	1	2	2	1	0	0	1	4	4
SUCCESS	2/1*	0	1/1+	3	0	0/1+	0	0	3/2	3/1
FAILURE	3	3	4	4	2	3	1	4	10	14
MODIFIED SUCCESS	1	0	1/1x	2	0	0	0	1	2/1	3

* Default at 24 months
+ Default at 18 months
x Default at 12 months

Table 19.4

Follow up results of 28 episodes of therapeutic starvation in male patients related to percentage excess of ideal weight at admission and discharge

% excess weight on admission	40–59		60–79		80–99		100 and over		TOTAL	
% excess weight on discharge	<25	>25	<25	>25	<25	>25	<25	>25	<25	>25
DEFAULT	1	0	1	0	0	1	0	1	2	2
SUCCESS	1	0	1/1*	2	0	1	0/1+	0	2/2	3/0
FAILURE	4	0	2	4	1	1	2	1	9	6
MODIFIED SUCCESS	0	0	2	0	0	0	0	0	2	0

* Default at 12 months
+ Default at 18 months

during a follow up period of 36 months without significant regain in weight. He was then seen by a doctor unfamiliar with his problem and discharged from further attendance. Although the error was detected and corrected he began to eat compulsively in order, he said, to demonstrate to the doctors the importance of his regular attendance (Fig. 19.4).

Eight episodes have been classified as 'modified successes' though one has occurred in a patient who subsequently defaulted. 'Modified

Ⓘ = Ideal weight
+ 25% = 25% in excess of ideal weight

Ⓐ = admission for
Ⓓ = discharge from } in-patient starvation

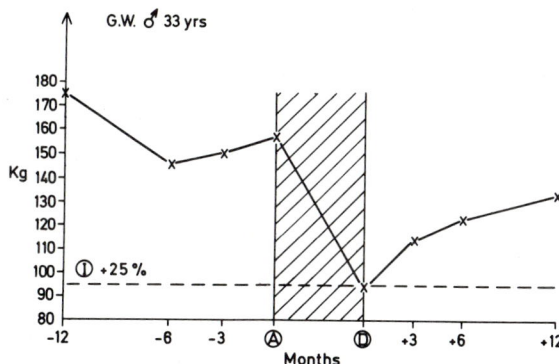

Figure 19.1

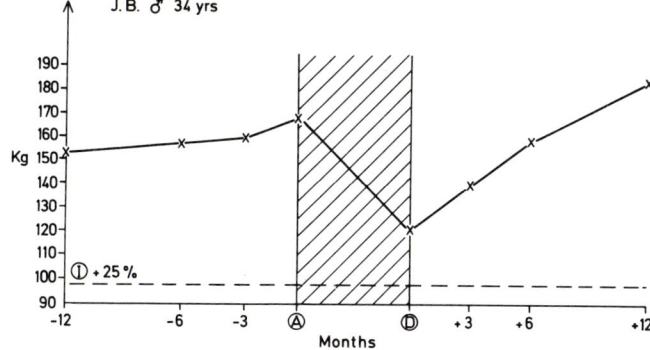

Figure 19.2

288 OBESITY SYMPOSIUM

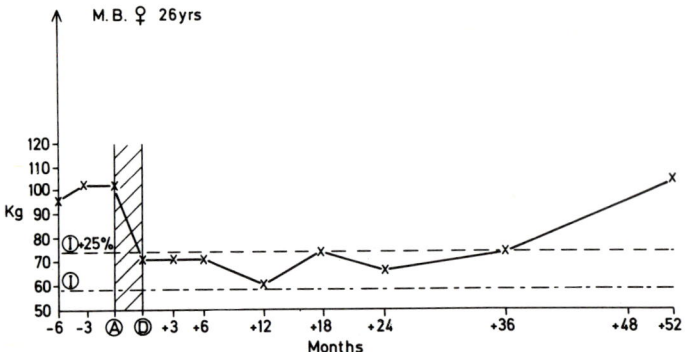

Figure 19.3

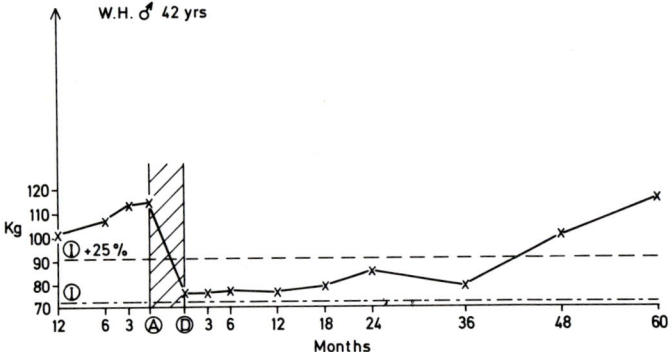

Figure 19.4

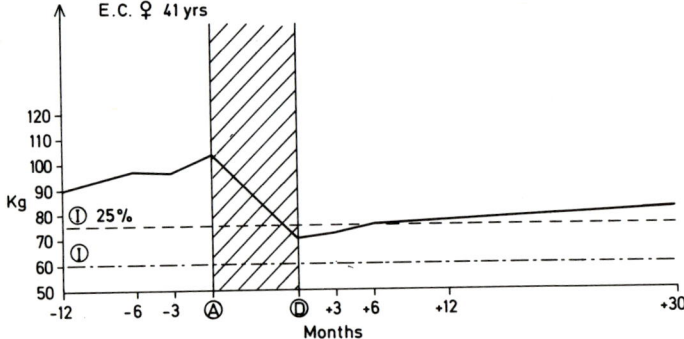

Figure 19.5

success' was obtained in five patients who reduced to within 25 per cent in excess of their ideal weight (Fig. 19.5).

Of the 16 'successes' five have now been lost to follow up and their present status is therefore uncertain. Six of the 11 patients still attending were discharged while more than 25 per cent in excess of their ideal weight (Fig. 19.6), the remainder having reduced to within that weight (Fig. 19.7).

Two of the patients admitted twice reduced on both occasions to within 25 per cent in excess of their ideal weight only to regain weight rapidly (Fig. 19.8). One is now struggling to keep her weight within 100 kg compared with the prestarvation weight of 162 kg and is a 'modified success' (Fig. 19.9). The fourth who has been admitted on three separate occasions regained weight rapidly following the

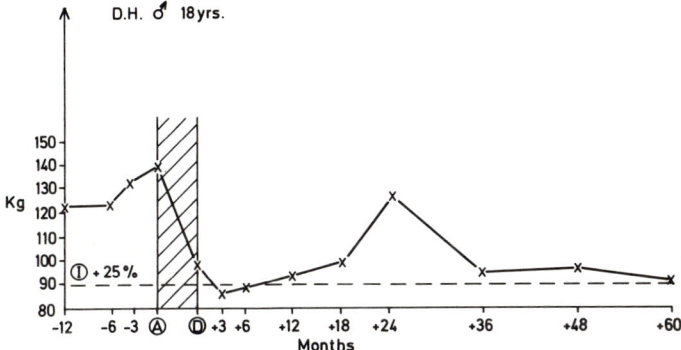

Figure 19.6

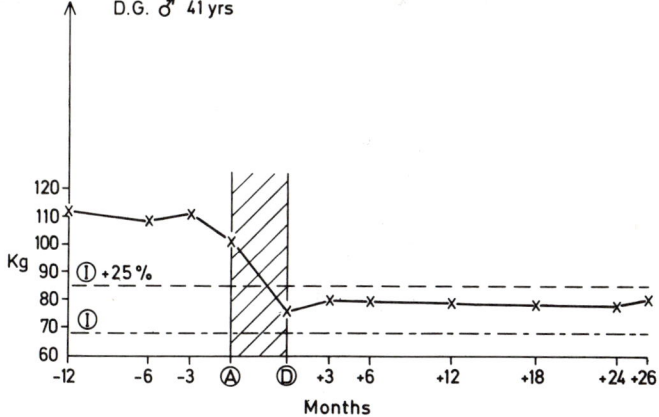

Figure 19.7

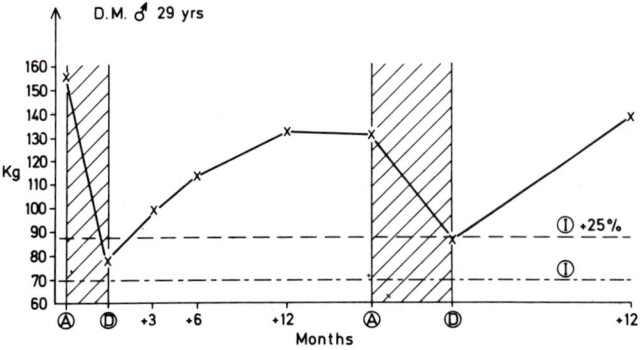

Figure 19.9

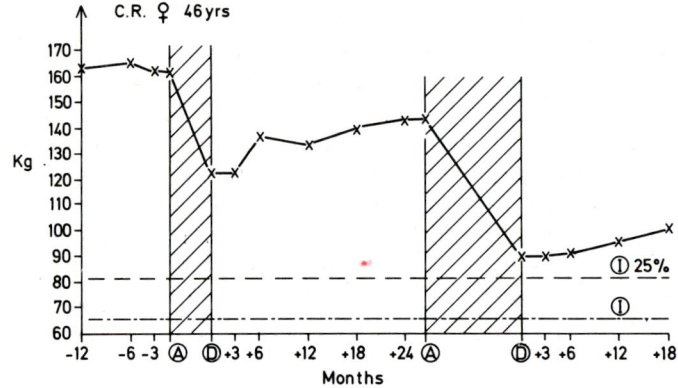

Figure 19.8

second admission, but did much better with his last period of starvation and is also classified as a 'modified success'.

DISCUSSION

The overall results are clearly disappointing in that two thirds of the patients followed up for 12 months or more have been classified as failures and that more than one third have actually regained all the weight lost. Moreover, although those patients at present classified as 'successes' or 'modified successes' are maintaining a steady weight, the incidence of failure increases with length of follow up. This is especially true during the first 12 months and reports of follow up for such short periods are of very limited value. The results for men and women appear to be similar and suggest that the most over-weight patients are least likely to succeed. However, the initial per cent in excess of ideal weight is of no clear predictive value. We have failed to substantiate the previous impression that the ability to reduce to within 25 per cent of ideal weight was associated with increased prospects of long term success. Long term success, however, is closely correlated with regular attendance at the follow up clinic and only two patients are known to have kept their weight down despite prolonged lapse of follow up. A proportion of patients who regained weight rapidly admitted on careful enquiry that although superficially their eating habits had been reformed they continued to eat excessively, but in secret.

It is important to remember that all the patients were 'failures' before admission and the primary reason for selection had been their inability to respond satisfactorily to conventional treatment despite regular supervision at an obesity clinic for a period of at least one year. All were considered to be suffering severely, either physically or psychologically, from their morbid obesity. Thus, for the small proportion of successes a mean weight change of −27 kg at a mean follow up of 27 months represents a worthwhile achievement. Success, however, cannot be solely gauged in terms of weight reduction and many who regained weight have no regrets. Ten patients, only two of whom were defined as successes, have had 12 elective operations including hiatus hernia repair, cholecystectomy and total hip replacement. Nine have married since starvation and among the women there have been six pregnancies including one full term delivery in a previous habitual aborter. Eleven patients have employment that they previously could not have had. It follows that the distinction between success and failure is necessarily arbitrary.

Therapeutic starvation would be better justified if patient selection could be improved but at present the long term sequelae of the alternative form of radical therapy, bypass surgery, are uncertain. The current policy is to offer surgery only to selected patients who have regained weight following starvation.

SUMMARY

Seventy five patients were admitted for 80 periods of prolonged in-patient starvation. Five took their own discharge within two weeks of admission and 12 defaulted from follow up within 12 months of discharge. The others have all be followed up for periods of between 12 and 64 months. Thirty nine episodes have been classified as failure, eight as modified success and 16 successes. Success was associated with regular attendance at follow up, but could not be otherwise predicted. A number of other patients obtained tangible benefit from starvation despite subsequent regain in weight.

Acknowledgements

We wish to thank the many other doctors, the nurses and other staff involved in the care of these patients.

REFERENCES

BLOOM, W.L. (1959) Fasting as an introduction to the treatment of obesity. *Metabolism*, 8, 214.

MUNRO, J.F. (1973) The Management of Obesity. *Brit. J. Hosp. Med.*, 10, 8.

MUNRO, J.F., MacCUISH, A.C., GOODALL, J.A.D., FRASER, J. & DUNCAN, L.J.P. (1970) Further experience with prolonged therapeutic starvation in gross refractory obesity. *Brit. Med. J.*, 4, 712.

20. A Review of the Medicinal Treatment of Obesity

PAMELA D. SAMUEL and W. BURLAND

"O, that this too too solid flesh would melt, thaw and resolve itself into a dew!" (Hamlet I, ii. 129).

Most early methods of treating obesity had scant scientific basis and there appears to have been little interest in the adverse effects of overweight and the aesthetic value of weight reduction until the beginning of the twentieth century. Thomas Dutton in his book 'Obesity—Its Cause and Treatment', published in 1896, stated that 'quite a host of quack nostrums are advertised... These nostrums... are composed of strong salts, as iodide of potassium, purges and the *Fucus Vesiculosus*, ... To say the least of them, they are altogether unscientific, and in many cases are positively injurious'.

The only treatment with any scientific basis used at this time was thyroid extract (Anders, 1898). Other hormone preparations were used twenty to thirty years later; pituitary extracts and sex and adrenal hormones were all reported to have been used (Williams, 1926). As recently as 1954, human chorionic gonadotrophin has been claimed to be effective in the treatment of obesity (Simeons, 1954). There are, however, as many trials which claim efficacy as those which claim inefficacy (Carne, 1961; Craig *et al.*, 1963; Gusman, 1936; Lebon, 1961; Somar, 1959).

THYROID HORMONE

Recent clinical trials with the thyroid hormones have also produced evidence for and against their efficacy as a treatment for obesity (Goodman, 1969; Gordon *et al.*, Hollingsworth, 1970; Rabinowitz & Myerson, 1967; Sabeh, 1965). The calorigenic effect of thyroid hormone is preceded by a lag phase. This has led to the belief that metabolic transformations of thyroid hormone necessarily precede induction of its ultimate metabolic action. The response can be prevented by inhibitors of protein or nucleic acid synthesis, suggesting that at least some of the calorigenic effect of thyroid hormone is an increased energy requirement for protein synthesis and enhanced synthesis of various enzymes including those of the glycerol phosphate cycle. It is generally agreed that the effect of physiological doses of thyroxine is disappointing. Pharmacological doses on the other hand produce good weight loss (Gwinup and Poucher, 1967) and there is little evidence of tolerance to this effect. However, thyroxine administration results in a corresponding depression in endogenous thyroxine production with consequent problems on withdrawal of the drug (Garrow, 1973). As Gwinup and Poucher have stated, the use of therapeutic doses of thyroid analogues in the treatment of obesity merely substitutes one clinical entity—thyrotoxicosis—for another—obesity.

DINITROPHENOL

Also of historical interest is another metabolic 'stimulant', dinitrophenol. This was introduced into clinical medicine for the purpose of treating obesity in 1933 (Tainter *et al.*, 1933). Other nitrocompounds have similar metabolic actions when their two nitro groups appear in the meta position. The action of dinitrophenol and related compounds is to increase oxidative metabolism and therefore heat production, chiefly by direct peripheral action. These compounds stimulate endogenous oxygen uptake and inhibit phosphorylation in intact living cells and homogenates (Simons, 1953). The increase in metabolism involves fat primarily and there is little increase in the metabolism of protein or carbohydrate. In clinical use the drug produced good weight losses but difficulties in standardizing individual doses were experienced (Rabinowitz & Fowler, 1934). The toxicity of the drug, however, vastly outweights its therapeutic value as an anti-obesity agent (Masserman & Goldsmith, 1934) and it is no longer used.

COMPOUNDS ALTERING INTESTINAL ABSORPTION

Many substances produce a loss in weight by reducing absorption of food. These are not generally used therapeutically as anti-obesity agents but clinical trials have shown their efficacy. Oral doses of neomycin in man produce moderate malabsorption of fat, protein, carbohydrate and some minerals and vitamins (Dobbins *et al.*, 1968; Hvidt, 1963). Tetracycline, kanamycin, polymyxin and bacitracin may also produce malabsorption in man (Falloon *et al.*, 1966; Powell *et al.*, 1962). Goldsmith *et al.* (1960) showed in man that kanamycin and neomycin act by reducing the reabsorption of bile acids so bringing about steatorrhoea and weight loss. Similarly, cholestyramine binds cholic acid in the intestinal lumen resulting in steatorrhoea and subsequent weight loss. Clinical trial in obese women, however, has shown cholestyramine to be unacceptable because the calorific deficit produced is small and weight loss would only result from long-term treatment measured in years (Campbell *et al.*, 1970). Malabsorption of other components of the diet may be due to morphological alterations of the intestinal mucosa (Dobbins, 1968). Indomethacin (Kendall, 1971), colchicine and para-aminosalicylic acid also produce malabsorption, but none of these effects are of therapeutic value in the treatment of obesity.

DIURETICS

Diuretics are often used by physicians to reduce the weight of obese patients. Initial weight loss is rapid due to loss of water but after diuretics are stopped, even though a reducing diet is maintained, body weight increases due to repletion of body water. Clinical trial of diuretics in the treatment of obesity has shown them to be of little value (Bunge, 1971).

BILE

It has been suggested that bile acids have a direct action on appetite suppression (Bray & Gallagher, 1968).

Cholecystokinin

In this connection it has been shown that rats with gastric fistulae, who frequently consume more than do control animals, respond to intraperitoneal injections of cholecystokinin by profoundly reducing their food consumption (Smith, 1974). Similar effects have been noted when the sulphated octapeptide of cholecystokinin was used. Gastrin and secretin in similar situations had no effect. It is of interest that neither secretin nor gastrin stimulate the flow of hepatic bile whereas cholecystokinin, secreted from the duodenal mucosa into the circulation in response to food, stimulates bile flow by contracting the gall bladder (Hally & Lloyd, 1968).

BIGUANIDES

Obese diabetic patients treated with metformin or phenformin show a weight loss (Clarke & Duncan, 1968; Duncan et al., 1968; Patel and Stowers, 1964). This weight loss was attributed to the anorexigenic effect of biguanides. However, animal data have indicated that weight loss is not due to a reduction in food intake and experiments in man showed that in two groups of patients receiving 1,250 Kcalories daily, those who were given phenformin lost 20 per cent more weight than those on diet alone (Pederson, 1965). Pederson attributes this to reduction in the amount of body water which may be related to a decrease in carbohydrate metabolism and an increase in fat metabolism (Pederson and Olsen, 1968). Clinical trials which have compared the efficacy of biguanides in obese non-diabetic patients have been contradictory. Hart & Cohen (1970) conducted a double blind cross over trial of phenformin against placebo in obese non-diabetic subjects and showed that although weight losses were marginally greater on phenformin, the differences were not significant. Strong & Lawson (1970) showed similar results with metformin in a trial in which fenfluramine gave significant weight loss. However, Munro et al., (1969) showed that in seventy-seven patients treated for sixteen weeks with metformin or phenformin or identical placebos, there was a statistically significant difference between the weight loss of control and treated groups, but no difference between the two biguanides. Other controlled clinical studies have shown that biguanides impair intestinal absorption of glucose (Czyzyk et al., 1968) and xylose (Berchtold et al., 1969). Stowers & Bewsher (1969) showed that phenformin produced a greater weight loss than could be due to an anorectic effect and reduction in caloric intake alone. Basal metabolic rate and respiratory quotient were not significantly altered and nitrogen excretion was not increased. It was concluded that the excess calories must have been lost in the faeces. The efficacy of the biguanides in the treatment of obese non-diabetics is not satisfactorily proven or accepted.

This treatment is only commonly used in obesity associated with diabetes.

BULK FILLERS

Both methyl cellulose and guar gum act as bulk fillers by swelling in the stomach after ingestion. The distension of the stomach is said to reduce appetite. It has been found that methyl cellulose preparations swell relatively slowly and are unlikely to reach their full bulk before leaving the stomach (Drug. Ther. Bull., 1970). They are thus better laxatives than anorexiants. Yudkin (1959) found that relatively large doses of methyl cellulose given with diet produced a better weight loss than diet alone. In refractory obese patients lower doses produced little weight loss as compared to placebo or phenmetrazine (Duncan et al, 1960). There have not, as yet, been any clinical trials to show the true efficacy of guar gum.

THE PHENYLETHYLAMINES

Amphetamine and Related Compounds

In 1939 Nathanson reported that amphetamine (Fig. 20.1) reduced appetite in man and it was reported to be effective in the management of obesity (Lesses & Myerson, 1938). Harris and coworkers (1947) demonstrated that loss of weight in dogs and man was due primarily to a reduction in food intake. Subjects kept on a constant calorie diet and given amphetamine did, however, show a weight loss; this was attributed to increased energy expenditure due to restlessness. Aldesberg & Mayer (1949) showed that amphetamine

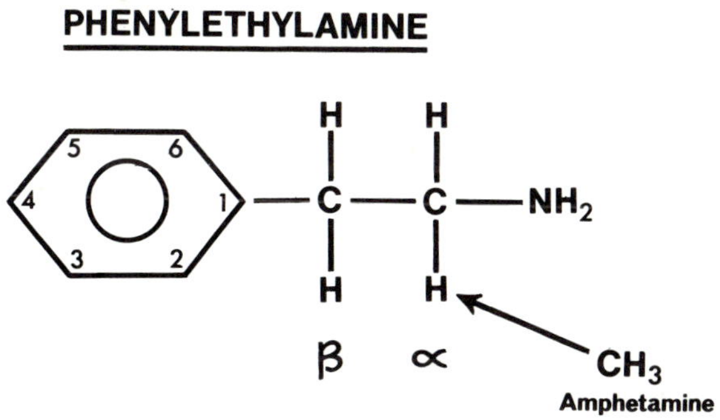

PHENYLETHYLAMINE

Figure 20.1

sulphate was effective in increasing weight loss in obese patients. However, they found that the effect of treatment was reduced with time and that stimulation and tolerance occurred. Patients tended voluntarily to increase the dose, implying that larger doses were needed in order to maintain anorexia and the feeling of well-being.

Gold (1945) had previously reviewed the use of amphetamine in the treatment of obesity and had drawn attention to the disadvantages, principally its stimulant properties and the risk of dependence. He emphasized the need for compounds with more selective action.

Recent chemical and pharmacological research has therefore been orientated towards the finding of phenylethylamine derivatives (Fig.

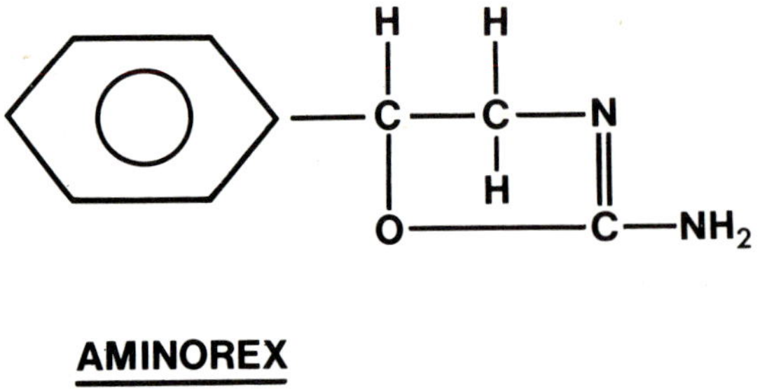

AMINOREX

Figure 20.2

20.1) which, whilst retaining the anorectic effect of amphetamine, have a reduced central stimulant effect. The structural chemistry necessary to maintain high anorectic activity of the phenylethylamine derivatives has been defined (Beregi *et al*, 1970; van de Schoot *et al*, 1962). They are as follows: that the chain between the amino group and the ring is restricted to two carbon atoms, that the binding of amino to a secondary carbon atom may be required, that substitution in the other position leads to loss of activity and that the introduction of substitutents on the amino group is allowed, although large substitutents result in a decrease or loss of activity. Figs. 20.1 to 20.8 show phenylethylamine compounds which have been used or are in clinical use in the U.K., U.S.A. and other parts of the world.

These compounds usually contain a methyl group in the α position of the chain. Experiments have shown that substitution of a methyl group in this position leads to a three-fold reduction in central stimulant properties and a halving of anorectic effect (Holm *et al.*, 1960).

The anorectic effect of amphetamine and its related compounds is mediated through inhibition of the activity of the lateral hypothalamus and a resultant suppression of food intake (Blundell & Lesham, 1973; Grossman, 1967).

Aminorex

The chemical structure of aminorex is shown in Fig. 20.2. The compound differs from amphetamine in that it has a ring structure in the side chain. Early clinical studies indicated that it was an effective anorectic agent (Hadler, 1967; Sandoval *et al.*, 1971; Wood & Owen, 1965). In 1968 it was found that aminorex was associated with an increased incidence of pulmonary hypertension (Follath *et al.*, 1971) and it was withdrawn from use. Early rat pharmacology had failed to demonstrate this side effect (Lancet, 1971). Although no other phenylethylamine derivatives have demonstrated this adverse effect, the Committee on Safety of Medicines, in the United Kingdom, ask practitioners to report any cases of pulmonary hypertension which occur whilst patients are undergoing therapy with appetite suppressant drugs.

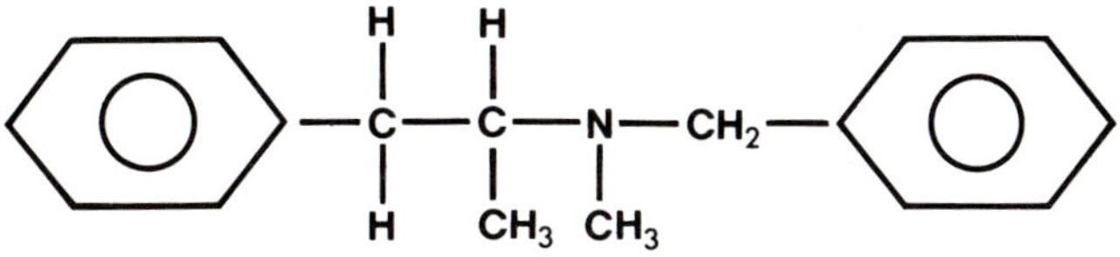

BENZPHETAMINE

Figure 20.3

Benzphetamine

The structure of benzphetamine is shown in Figure 20.3. Simkin & Wallace (1960) showed that benzphetamine was significantly better than placebo in producing weight loss in obese patients; side effects did not appear to be significantly greater during treatment. They also showed it to be similar to amphetamine in weight reducing properties and side effects (Simkin & Wallace, 1961). Schapiro & Bogran (1960) showed benzphetamine to be superior to phenmetrazine in weight reducing properties; side effects were similar, although dry mouth and malaise were more frequent with phenmetrazine. Similar results were obtained by Poindexter (1960) who showed that amphetamine and phenmetrazine produced similar weight losses but that benzphetamine was superior. Both benzphetamine and phenmetrazine caused fewer side effects than amphetamine. Patel & coworkers (1963), however, showed a significantly greater weight loss with amphetamine, benzphetamine or phenmetrazine when compared

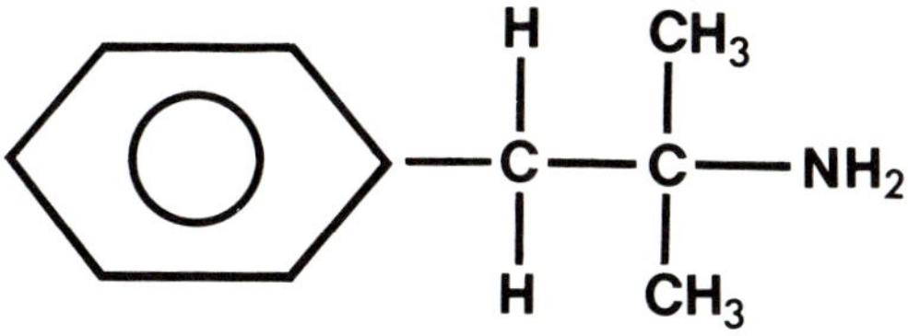

PHENTERMINE

Figure 20.4

with placebo, but no significant difference between treatments. Insomnia, mood elevation, over-stimulation and nervousness were reported with all three compounds.

Phentermine

Phentermine (Fig. 20.4) has been found to cause less stimulation of the central nervous system than amphetamine. However, its ability to raise blood pressure, increase cardiac contractile force and heart rate, and to cause cardiac arrhythmias in dogs is similar to amphetamine (Lawlor *et al.*, 1969).

Acute doses of phentermine have been shown to reduce hunger and caloric intake in man (Silverstone, 1972). Clinical trial has demonstrated that phentermine and amphetamine produce similar weight losses (Leriche, 1960) and that intermittent therapy is as effective as continuous therapy (Munro *et al.*, 1969). Steel *et al.* (1973) confirmed the therapeutic benefit of intermittent treatment but, although clinically appreciable central nervous system stimulation to phentermine was not encountered, 20 per cent of patients noted sleeplessness and a similar number felt more energetic.

Phenmetrazine

Phenmetrazine hydrochloride was first synthesized by Thoma & Wick in 1954. The compound is a phenylethylamine derivative containing an oxazine ring (Fig. 20.5).

Phenmetrazine was reported to have little effect on the cardiovascular and central nervous system (Thoma & Wick, 1954). It was first shown to be clinically successful in the treatment of obesity during trials in France and Germany (Alexandre, 1955; Berneike, 1955; Bleckman & Solus, 1955; Canadell, 1955; Pulch, 1955).

An early clinical evaluation of phenmetrazine in 140 obese patients showed it to be a reliable anorexigenic agent. Good weight losses were reported, although the increment of weight loss fell with time. The side effects were stimulation and excitation although to a lesser extent than previously seen in amphetamine treated patients (Nathanson, 1956; Phear, 1959).

Controlled double blind studies have confirmed that phenmetrazine produces a significant weight loss in obese patients (Duncan *et al.*, 1960; Hampson *et al.*, 1960) and is effective in the treatment of obese children (Rendle-Short, 1960).

Phenmetrazine is not without undesirable side effects. Addiction may lead to euphoria and toxic psychotic illness indistinguishable from amphetamine psychosis or alcoholic hallucinations (Bethel, 1957; Evans, 1959; Kahan & Mullins, 1958; Silverman, 1959).

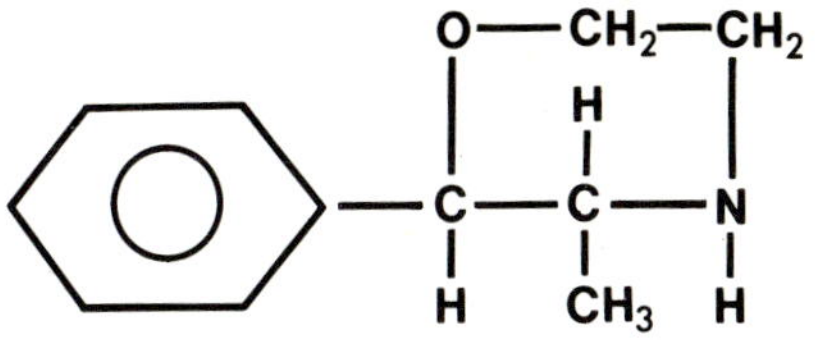

PHENMETRAZINE

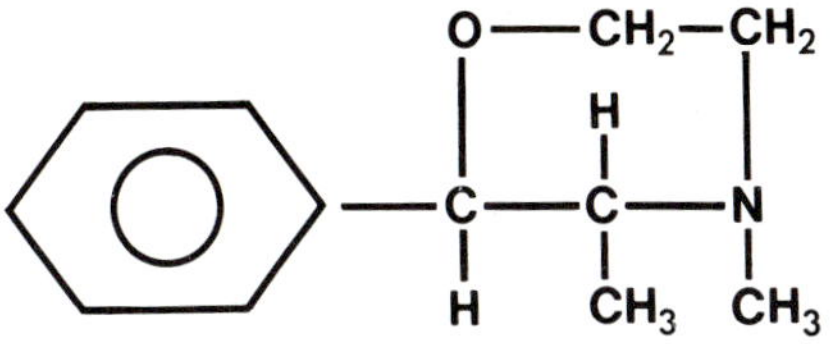

PHENDIMETRAZINE

Figure 20.5

Phendimetrazine

Phendimetrazine differs from phenmetrazine by the presence of a second methyl group on the nitrogen of the amino group (Fig. 20.5). Pharmacologically, it is reported to have similar effects to phenmetrazine with regard to central stimulation and appetite suppression. However, its effects on the cardiac and respiratory systems in dogs and cats differ from phenmetrazine (Stegen *et al.*, 1960). Phenmetrazine has a pressor effect and causes tachycardia and tachypnoea, and induces changes in the electrocardiogram. None of these changes was seen with phendimetrazine. Double blind clinical trials have shown that the compound brings about significant losses in body weight (Cass, 1961; Naumann, 1962; Ressler & Schneider, 1961; Le Riche & Van Belle, 1962). In obese diabetics, weight loss was reported but there was no effect on blood glucose attributable to phendimetrazine (Runyan, 1962). In all these studies the side effects which occurred were dry mouth, sleeplessness and mood elevation. Mydriasis was noted in five patients (Le Riche & Van Belle, 1962).

Diethylpropion

Diethylpropion is a tertiary phenylethylamine and contains a $=O$ group in the β position of the side chain (Fig. 20.6). In 1959 Martin reported that in rats it reduced food intake without causing central nervous system stimulation. No deleterious effects on blood pressure,

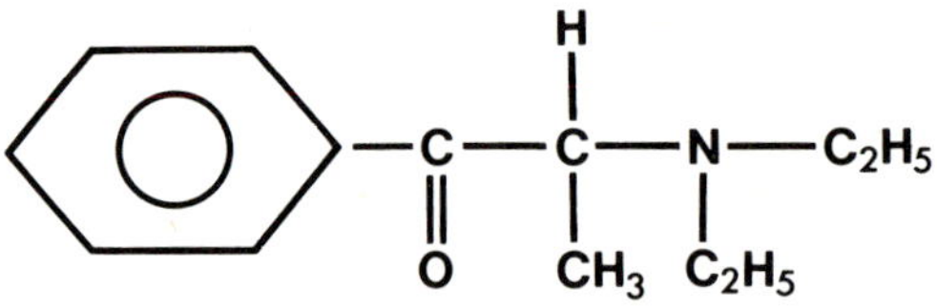

DIETHYLPROPION

Figure 20.6

pulse, respiration or the electrocardiogram were reported after the intravenous injection of diethylpropion to patients with essential hypertension, early congestive cardiac failure, post-cerbrovascular accident, coronary artery disease or angina pectoris (Alfaro et al., 1960).

Results from early clinical trials indicated that diethylpropion was an effective weight reducing agent with few side effects (Ravetz, 1959). One of the first controlled clinical investigations was a double blind cross over study on obese diabetic patients. A weight loss of more than 1 kg per month was reported in a significantly greater number of patients taking diethylpropion than in those taking placebo (Illig & Illig, 1959).

A study carried out by Decina & Taryol (1960) showed weight loss in thirteen of fifteen patients treated with diethylpropion and seven of thirteen patients treated with placebo. In this and other studies side effects were mild; restlessness, dry mouth and constipation were most frequently reported but significant differences in weight loss between diethylpropion treated and placebo treated obese patients were observed (Andelman et al., 1967; Cunningham, 1963; Rosenberg, 1961; Schneeberg, 1961; Seaton et al., 1961).

In a study by Silverstone and coworkers in 1968, diethylpropion was reported to reduce hunger. However, it also caused restlessness and dryness of mouth. Together with the observations of Smart et al (1967), who showed evidence of increased critical flicker frequency with diethylpropion, it was indicated that the compound has some central stimulant properties in man.

The effects of diethylpropion were reduced after ten weeks of treatment, according to Bose (1969) and Seaton et al (1961). Intermittent therapy has been shown to be successful (Le Riche et al., 1967; Silverstone & Solomon, 1965) although continuous therapy gave a slightly but significantly greater weight loss. A more recent clinical trial of the compound used continuously for twenty-four weeks showed that a significantly better weight loss was obtained with diethylpropion than with placebo and its effectiveness remained evident for twenty-four weeks (McKay, 1973).

Diethylpropion has been shown to be effective in overweight associated with pregnancy (Boileau, 1968; Jordon et al., 1961; Silverman et al., 1971), in patients who have obesity associated with cardiovascular disease (Evanselista, 1968), angina pectoris (Russek, 1966), or diabetes mellitus (Illig & Illig, 1959; Fineberg, 1961; Silverstone & Buckle, 1966; Williams, 1968) and in obese children (Everly Jones, 1962). Dependence has been reported by Clein and Benardy (1962) and by Jones (1968).

Halogen Substitution in the Benzene Ring

Anorexigenic action can be separated from stimulant properties if the aromatic ring is made to contain halogen substituents. This was shown originally by Holm and coworkers (1960) who produced a para-chloro derivative (chlorphentermine) and para and ortho-bromo derivatives which had appetite suppressant properties similar to amphetamine but lacked the central stimulant activity prominent with the latter compound. At about the same time it was shown that trifluoro methyl substitution at the para position produced a compound with anorectic action but with little or no central stimulation effect (Leonard et al., 1961; Weisman, 1960). The meta–CF_3 derivative was found to be always associated with high anorectic activity (Beregi et al., 1970).

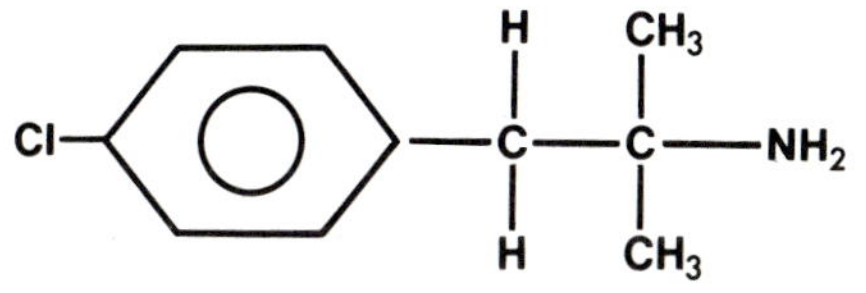

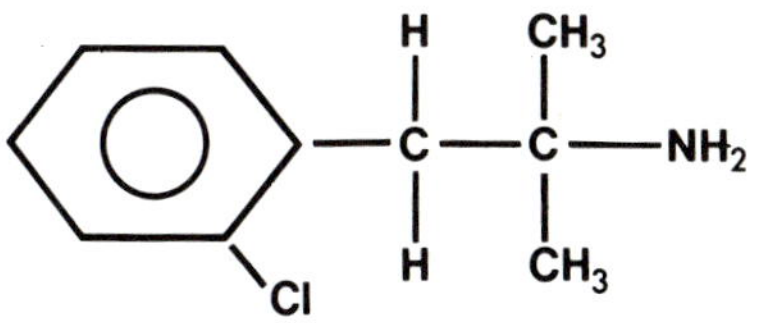

Figure 20.7

Chlorphentermine

Chlorphentermine is a phenylethylamine derivative which contains a chloride in the four position of the benzene ring (Fig. 20.7). Pharmacological studies have shown it to reduce food intake and body weight in rats to an extent comparable with that of amphetamine and other anorexgenic compounds. These studies also showed that spontaneous activity, which is an indicator of central stimulant effect, was unaffected by chlorphentermine but increased by amphetamine (Holm et al., 1960).

Early clinical evaluation showed the compound to be a satisfactory anorectic agent. The reported side effects were principally a dry mouth, nausea and vertigo. Some patients actually complained of lack of central stimulation (Boxer et al., 1961; Vague, 1964). Double blind studies have shown it to cause significant weight losses in obese patients (Berry, 1965; Jackson and Whyte, 1965; Levin et al., 1963; Lucy & Hadden, 1962; Tricket & Weir, 1968). Restlessness and insomnia were not reported. Seaton and his coworkers (1964) stated that chlorphentermine produced a similar weight loss to that of phenmetrazine, diethylpropion and amphetamine and that tolerance to the anorectic effect of the drug developed after an average of six weeks' treatment. Fineberg (1962) compared chlorphentermine with amphetamine in a six-week cross over study; weight losses were similar. Amphetamine produced central stimulation, whereas drowsiness, weakness and dizziness, were noted with chlorphentermine. Chlorphentermine proved effective in the treatment of obese adolescents (Rauth & Lipp, 1968) and in the treatment of postpartum obesity (Duckman & Chen, 1968).

Chlortermine

Rodos (1969) reported on the clinical effect of this ortho-chloro substituted compound (Fig. 20.7) which in all other respects seems to resemble chlorphentermine.

Fenfluramine

Fenfluramine has a fluorine substitution in the benzene ring (Fig. 20.8). Trifluoromethyl substitution in the ring structure of phenylethylamine brought about an effect similar to that produced by chlorphentermine (Leonard et al, 1961; Weisman & Schneider, 1960). When CF_3 is substituted in the 3 position, the resultant secondary amine (fenfluramine) was found to have anorectic properties without evidence of central nervous stimulation. It seemed rather to have mild central sedative properties and to be without pressor effects (Beregi et al, 1970; Le Douarec & Schmitt, 1964). Depression

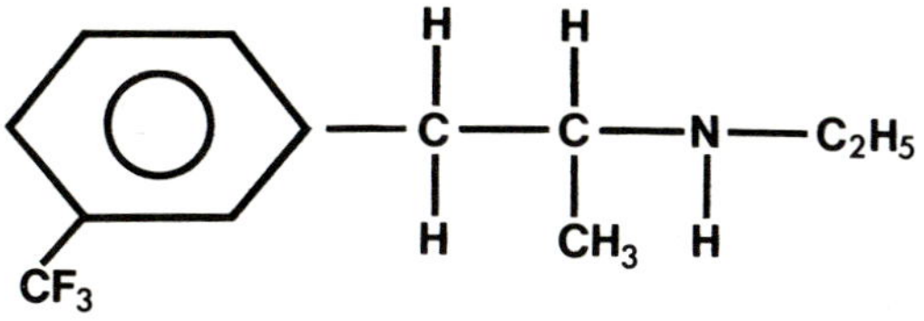

FENFLURAMINE

Figure 20.8

of food intake in animals is mediated by a direct action on the lateral hypothalamus but unlike amphetamine and other related agents the action of fenfluramine is mediated via tryptaminergic mechanisms (Bizzi et al, 1970; Blundell & Leshem, 1973; Funderbunk et al, 1971).

Early clinical studies showed that the drug was an effective appetite suppressant in man (Bernard & Duriez, 1963; Brousselle et al, 1963; Poire et al, 1966; Recordier et al, 1963; Spence & Medvei, 1966). The main side effects are sedation, gastrointestinal symptoms, especially diarrhoea, dizziness and dry mouth. Depression on withdrawal has been reported (Steel & Briggs, 1972). Double blind studies have shown fenfluramine to be effective in the treatment of obese patients (Brodbin & O'Connor, 1968; Duncan et al., 1965; Hooper, 1972; Munro et al., 1969; Traherne, 1965). Steel et al., (1973) have recently demonstrated that it remained effective for nine months during continuous treatment. Clinical trials have shown the drug to be effective in the treatment of obesity associated with hypertension (Bolodeoku et al., 1972; Waal-Manning & Simpson, 1969) and in anxiety where its central sedative properties are valuable (Gaind, 1969), in obese diabetics (Dykes, 1973; Turtle et al., 1971), and in obese children (Bacon & Lowry, 1967; Lorber & Greenwood, 1971; Rayner, 1971).

Gottestam & Gunne (1971) found that fenfluramine had no central stimulant effect in amphetamine dependent subjects. This confirmed evidence submitted by Hawks (1970), Jones (1971) and Woodard (1970). Hill & Turner (1967) found no change in critical flicker frequency (CFF) in man after fenfluramine; in fact, the compound abolished the increase in CFF caused by amphetamine (Turner, 1971). Abuse of fenfluramine has been reported (Levin, 1972, a, b): however, the 'abusers' were drug dependent servicemen, all but one of whom were already using cannabis. Gluckman (1973), studying rats trained to self-injection techniques, reported that fenfluramine was not reinforcing in animals trained on other compounds, and in contrast to some other medicines tested, including amphetamine and diethylpropion, rats trained on fenfluramine did not tend to self-administer the compound.

In 1966, Duhault & Boulanger showed that fenfluramine has a lipid mobilizing effect in the rat; this was later demonstrated in man (Mace *et al.,* 1972; Pawan, 1969). *In vitro* studies have indicated that fenfluramine may also block triglyceride synthesis (Galton & Wilson, 1971). In man fenfluramine has been shown to increase the uptake of glucose into muscle (Butterfield & Whichelow, 1968; Turtle & Burgess, 1973). *In vitro* studies have also shown that fenfluramine causes an increase in glucose uptake into isolated skeletal muscle in the presence of insulin. It is believed that most of the effect of fenfluramine is mediated through its anorexigenic action; how much of the weight loss in obese patients is due to metabolic effects remains unknown. Fenfluramine has recently been extensively reviewed by Burland (1974).

NON-PHENYLETHYLAMINE ANORECTIC AGENTS

Mazindol

Mazindol is not a phenylethylamine derivative, yet it has appetite suppressant properties. It is at present available in the United States of America.

Mazindol is an imidazo–isoindole. Its chemical structure is shown in Fig. 20.9. It is a synthetic tricyclic compound, chemically known as 5-hydroxy-5-p-chlorophenyl–2, 3–dihydro–5H–imidazo (2, 1-a) isoindole.

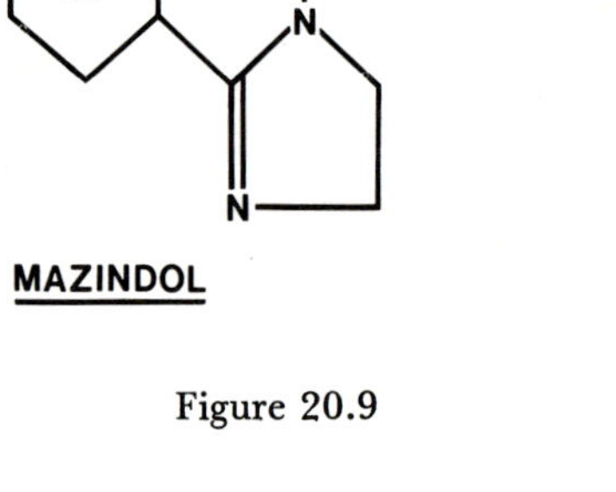

MAZINDOL

Figure 20.9

The compound has been shown to produce central nervous stimulation and anorexia in monkeys (Gogerty et al., 1968). Doses which produce anorexia, however, are well below those which cause central stimulation. A preliminary clinical trial of mazindol showed it to be similar in its effect to amphetamine with regard to appetite suppression (de Felice et al., 1969). The side effects were central stimulation, which was qualitatively different from that produced by amphetamine, and at higher doses tachycardia occurred. Hadler (1972) showed mazindol to cause a greater weight loss than placebo. However, systolic blood pressure and pulse rate were found to rise. The main side effects were insomnia, dizziness and dry mouth.

Goldrick & coworkers (1973) have shown that the weight loss produced by mazindol and fenfluramine are similar over a sixteen-week period. The side effects produced by mazindol were agitation, mental stimulation and insomnia, usually being troublesome only during the first two weeks.

In a double blind study of mazindol on amphetamine dependent subjects, Gottestam & Gunne (1972) found that it was placed between placebo and amphetamine when the subjects rated its similarity to amphetamine. The central stimulant effect of the drug differed little from placebo, whereas amphetamine produced a significantly different central stimulant effect.

CONCLUSIONS

The anorectic compounds remain the medicinal treatment of choice in obesity. They have acknowledged drawbacks. These are principally that some may cause central stimulation. However this property has been quantitatively reduced by modification of the phenylethylamine structure. It has almost been excluded at therapeutic dose levels by chlorine substitution in the benzene ring in chlorphentermine, and exchanged for mild sedation by addition of a trifluoro methyl group in the C-3 position in the ring in the case of fenfluramine. Central stimulation leading to mood elevation potentially leads to abuse, dependance and addiction. Until recently it has been believed that the pharmacologically induced anorexia is short-lived and can only be maintained by increasing doses, so leading to excessive central stimulation with the risks previously mentioned. Published evidence by McKay (1973) on diethylpropion, and Steel et al. (1973) on fenfluramine, for example, have disproved this since the compounds were found to be effective for 24 and 36 weeks without any increase in dosage.

Side effects other than those referred to above are a further problem though not a hazard to life. Dry mouth and gastrointestinal upsets do occur.

Whilst the search for more precise and safe medicinal agents continues and whilst the results from other treatments remain unsatisfactory, these compounds will remain in frequent and widespread use.

REFERENCES

ADLESBERG, D. & MAYER, M.E. (1949) Results of prolonged medical treatment of obesity with diet alone, diet and thyroid preparations and diet and amphetamine. *J. Clin. Endocrin.*, 9, 275.
ALEXANDRE, C. (1955) Preliminary study of a new stimulant (A-66) in the treatment of obesity. *Presse med.*, 63, 1122.
ALFARO, R.D., GRACANIN, V. & SCHLUETER, E. (1960) A clinical pharmacologic evaluation of diethylpropion. *J. Lancet (USA)*, 80, 526.
ANDELMAN, M.B., JONES, C. & NATHAN, S. (1967) Treatment of obesity in underprivileged adolescents. *Clin. Paed.*, 6, 327.
ANDERS, J.M. (1898) *Textbook of the Practice of Medicine*. p. 1221. London: Kebman Publishing Co. Ltd.
BACON, G.E. & LOWRY, G.H. (1967) A clinical trial of fenfluramine in obese children. *Curr. Therap. Res.*, 2, 626.
BERCHTOLD, P., BOLLI P., ARBENZ, U. & KEISER, G. (1969) Intestinale absorptions storung infolge Metforminbehandung (Zur Frage der Wirkungsweise der Biguanide). *Diabetologia*, 5, 405.
BEREGI, L.G., HUGON, P., LEDOUAREC, J.C., LAUBIE, M. & DUHAULT, J. (1970) Structure-activity relationships in CF_3 substituted phenylethylamines In *Amphetamines and Related Compounds*, Ed. Costa, E. & Garattini, S. p.21. New York: Raven Press.
BERNARD, J.G. & DURIEZ, J. (1963) The treatment of obesity with trifluethamine, the new anorectic. *Sem. Hop. Paris*, 39, 229.
BERNEIKE, K.H. (1955) Further studies on the medical treatment of obesity with Preludin. *Med. Klin.*, 50, 494.
BERRY, R.L. (1965) Obesity treatment of complicated and uncomplicated cases with chlorphentermine hydrochloride. *Indust. Med. Surg.*, 34, 490.
BETHEL, M.F. (1957) Toxic psychosis caused by Preludin. *Brit. Med. J.*, 1, 30.
BIZZI, A., BONACCORSI, A., JESPERSEN, S., JORI, A. & GARATTINI, S. (1970) Pharmacological studies on amphetamine and fenfluramine. In *Amphetamines and Related Compounds*, Ed. Costa, E. & Garattini, S., p. 577 New York: Raven Press.
BLUNDELL, J.E. & LESHAM, M.B. (1973) Disassociation of the anorexic effects of fenfluramine and amphetamine following intrahypothalamic injection. *Brit. J. Pharmacol.*, 47, 183.
BOLODEOKU, J.O., ADADEVOH, B.K. & PALMER, E.O. (1972) Therapeutic effect of fenfluramine (Ponderax) in obese Nigerians—weight reducing and hypotensive properties. *Nigerian Med. J.*, 2, 199.
BOILEAU, P.A. (1968) Control of weight gain during pregnancy: use of diethylpropion hydrochloride. *Applied Therapeutics*, 10, 763.
BOSE, A. (1969) Low calorie intake in post operative convalescence. Trial with diethylpropion as an adjunct. *Clin. Trial.*, 6, 167.

BOXER, E. (1961) Chlorphentermine. *Practitioner*, **187**, 216.
BRAY, G.A. & GALLAGHER, T.F. (1968) Suppression of appetite by bile acids. *Lancet*, **1**, 1066.
BRODBIN, P. & O'CONNOR, C.A. (1967) A double blind clinical trial of an appetite depressant, fenfluramine, in general practice. *Practitioner*, **198**, 707.
BROUSSOLE, P., ROSIER, Y. & GANDIN, F. (1963) A new anorexiant. *Annal. Med. Pract. Soc.*, **234**, 34 & 39.
BUNGE, H.C. & HUNECKE, I. (1971) Treatment of obese patients with diuretics. *Dtsch. Z. Verdau Stoffwechselkr.*, **31**, 17.
BURLAND, W.L. (1974) A global review of experience with fenfluramine. Fogarty International Center Conference on Obesity, N.I.H. Bethesda. To be published.
BUTTERFIELD, W.J.H. & WHICHELOW, M.J. (1968) Fenfluramine and muscle glucose uptake in man. *Lancet*, **2**, 109.
CAMPBELL, U.D., JUHL, E. & QUAADE, F. (1970) Treatment of obesity with cholestyramine. *Nord. Med.*, **84**, 1628.
CANADELL, J.M. (1955) Preludin in the treatment of obesity *Boll. Inst. Pat.* **10**, 164.
CARNE, S. (1961) The action of chorionic gonadotrophin in the obese. *Lancet*, **2**, 1282.
CASS, L.J. (1961) Evaluation of phendimetrazine bitartrate as an appetite suppressant. *Canad. Med. Ass. J.*, **84**, 1114.
CLARKE, B.F. & DUNCAN, L.J.P. (1968) Comparison of chlorpropamide and metformin treatment on weight and blood glucose response of uncontrolled obese diabetics. *Lancet*, **1**, 123.
CLEIN, L.J. & BENADY, D.R. (1962) Case of diethylpropion addiction. *Brit. Med. J.*, **2**, 456 (letter).
CRAIG, L.S., RAY, R.E., WAXLER, S.H. & MADIGAN, H. (1963) Chorionic gonadotrophin in the treatment of obese women. *Amer. J. Clin. Nutr.*, **12**, 230.
CUNNINGHAM, G.L.W. (1963) Diethylpropion in the treatment of obesity. *J. Coll. Gen. Pract.*, **39**, 347.
CZYZYK, A., TAWECKI, J., SANDOWSKI, J. & PONIKOWSKA, I. (1968) Effect of biguanides on intestinal absorption of glucose. *Diabetes*, **17**, 492.
DECINA, L. & TANYOL, H. (1960) Treatment of obesity with a new anorexiant, diethylpropion without special stress on diet. *New York State J. Med.*, **60**, 2702.
DE FELICE, E.A., BRONSTEIN, S. & COHEN, A. (1969) Double blind comparison of placebo and a new appetite suppressant on obese volunteers. *Curr. Res. Therap.*, **11**, 256.
DOBBINS, W.O., HERRERO, B.A. & MANSBACK, C.M. (1968) Morphologic alterations associated with neomycin induced malabsorption. *Amer. J. Med. Sci.*, **255**, 63.
DRUG AND THERAPEUTIC BULLETIN (1970) Nilstim and other methyl cellulose preparations as appetite suppressants. *Drug Ther. Bull.*, **8**, 92.
DUCKMAN, S., CHEN, W. & WEIR, J.H. (1968) Double blind evaluation of chlorphentermine hydrochloride versus placebo in postpartum weight control. *Curr. Therap. Res.* **10**, 619.
DUHAULT, J. & BOULANGER, M. (1966) Action de l'amphetamine et de certains de ses derives halogenes sur les metabolismes lipidique et glucidique. *J. Ann. Diabetol. De l'Hotel-Dieu*, p. 67.
DUNCAN, E.H., HYDE, C.A., REGAN, N.A. & SWEETMAN, B. (1965) A preliminary trial of fenfluramine in general practice. *Brit. J. Clin. Pract.*, **19**, 3.

DUNCAN, L.J., CLARKE, B.F. & MUNRO, J.F. (1969) The effect of biguanide treatment of bodyweight in diabetics and non-diabetics. *Postgrad. Med. J.*, 45, 13.

DUNCAN, L.J.P., ROSE, K. & MEIKLEJOHN, A.P. (1960) Phenmetrazine hydrochloride and methylcellulose in the treatment of 'refractory' obesity. *Lancet*, 1, 1262.

DUTTON, T. (1896) In *Obesity—Its Causes and Treatment*. p. 32, Ed. Kimpton, H. London and New York: Hirshfield Bros. Med. Publisher.

DYKES, J.R.W. (1973) The effect of a low calorie diet with and without fenfluramine, and fenfluramine alone on the glucose tolerance and insulin secretion of overweight non diabetics. *Postgrad. Med. J.*, 49, 314.

EVANS, J. (1959) Psychosis and addiction to phenmetrazin (Preludin). *Lancet*, 2, 152.

EVANSELISTA, I. (1968) Management of overweight patients with CVD: double blind evaluation of an anorectic drug—diethylpropion hydrochloride. *Curr. Therap. Res.*, 10, 217.

EVERLEY JONES, H. (1962) Trial of diethylpropion in the treatment of childhood obesity. *Practitioner*, 188, 229.

FALOON, W.W., PAES, I.C., WOOLFOLK, D., NANKIN, H., WALLACE, K. & HARO, E.N (1966) Effects of neomycin and kanamycin upon intestinal absorption. *Ann. N.Y. Acad. Sci.*, 132, 879.

FINEBERG, S.K. (1961) Obesity, diabetes and anorexigenics. *J.A.M.A.*, 175, 680.

FINEBERG, S.K. (1962) Evaluation of anorexigenic agents. Studies with chlorphentermine. *Amer. J. Clin. Nutr.*, 11, 509.

FOLLATH, F., BURKART, F. & SCHWEIZER, W. (1971) Drug induced pulmonary hypertension. *Brit. Med. J.*, 1, 265.

FUNDERBURK, W.H., HAZELWOOD, J.C., RUCKART, R.T. & WARD, J.W. (1971) Is 5-hydroxytryptamine involved in the mechanism of action of fenfluramine? *J. Pharm. Pharmacol.*, 23, 468.

GAIND, R. (1969) Fenfluramine (Ponderax) in the treatment of obese psychiatric out-patients. *Brit. J. Psychiat.*, 115, 963.

GALTON, D.J. & WILSON, J.P.D. (1971) The effect of drugs on lipogenesis from glucose and palmitate in human adipose tissue. *S. Afr. Med. J.*, 45, suppl. 19.

GARROW, J.S. (1973) Anti-obesity drugs. *Prescribers J.*, 13, 50.

GLUCKMAN, M.I. (1973) Differential self-injection behaviour produced by fenfluramine and other appetite inhibiting drugs, presented at the meeting of the Federation of American Societies for Experimental Biology.

GOGERTY, J.H., HOULITAN, W., GALEN, M., EDEN, P. & PENBERTHY, C. (1968) Neuropharmacological studies on a imidazo-isoindole derivative. *Fed. Proc.*, 27, 501.

GOLD, H. (1945) Clinical importance and uses. *Industrial & Engineering Chemistry*, 37, 117.

GOLDRICK, R.B., HAVENSTEIN, N. & WHYTE, H. (1973) Effects of caloric restriction and fenfluramine on weight loss and personality profiles of patients with long-standing obesity. *Aust. N.Z. J. Med.*, 3, 131.

GOLDSMITH, G.A., HAMILTON, J.G. & MILLER, O.N. (1960) Lowering of serum lipid concentrations: mechanisms used by unsaturated fats, nicotinic acid and neomycin. Excretion of sterols and bile acids. *A.M.A. Arch. Int. Med.*, 105, 512.

GOODMAN, N.G. (1969) Tri-iodothyronine and placebo in the treatment of

obesity. *Med. Ann. Dist. of Columbia*, 38, 658.
GOTTESTAM, G.K. & GUNNE, L.M. (1972) Subjective effects of two anorexigenic agents fenfluramine and AN448 in amphetamine-dependent subjects. *Brit. J. Addiction*, 67, 39.
GROSSMAN, S.P. (1967) Neuropharmacology of central mechanisms contributing to control of food and water intake. In *Handbook of Physiology*, Section 6, Volume 1, Ed. Code, C.F. & Heidel, W. p.287. Amer. Physiol. Soc., Washington.
GUSMAN, H.A. (1936) Endocrine Obesity. *Ohio State Med. J.* 32, 973.
GWINUP, G. & POUCHER, R. (1967) A controlled study of thyroid analogs in the therapy of obesity. *Amer. J. Med. Sci.*, 254, 416.
HADLER, A.J. (1967) Studies of aminorex a new anorexigenic agent. *J. Clin. Pharmacol.*, 7, 296.
HADLER, A.J. (1972) Mazindol, a new non-amphetamine anorexigenic agent. *J. Clin. Pharmacol.*, 12, 453.
HALLY, A.D. & LLOYD, S.M. (1968) *A Companion of Medical Studies, Vol. 1.* Ed. Passmore, R. & Robson, J.S. Oxford and Edinburgh: Blackwell.
HAMPSON, J., LORAINE, J.A. & STRONG, J.A. (1960) Phenmetrazine and dexamphetamine in the management of obesity. *Lancet*, 1, 1265.
HARRIS, S.C., IVY, A.C. & SEARLE, L.M. (1947) The mechanism of amphetamine-induced loss of weight: a consideration of the theory of hunger and appetite. *J.A.M.A.*, 134, 1468.
HART, A. & COHEN, H. (1970) Treatment of obese non-diabetic patients with phenformin. A double blind crossover trial. *Brit. Med. J.*, 1, 22.
HAWKS, D.V. (1970) Unusual effects of fenfluramine. *Brit. Med. J.*, 1, 238.
HILL, R.C. & TURNER, P. (1967) Fenfluramine and critical flicker frequency. *J. Pharm. Pharmacol.*, 19, 337.
HOLLINGSWORTH, D.R., AMATRUDA, I.I. & SCHEIG, R. (1970) Quantitative and qualitative effects of L-triiodothyronine in massive obesity. *Metabolism*, 19, 934.
HOLM, T., HUUS, I., KOPF, R., NEILSON, I.M. & PETERSEN, P.V. (1960) Pharmacology of a series of nuclear substituted phenyltertiary butylamines with particular reference to anorexigenic and central stimulating properties. *Acta Pharmacol. & Toxicol.*, 17, 121.
HOOPER, A.C. (1972) Comparison of fenfluramine (with *ad libitum* food intake) with 1,000 calorie diet in obesity. *J. Irish Med. Assoc.*, 65, 35.
HVIDT, S. & KJEIDSEN, K. (1963) Malabsorption induced by small doses of neomycin sulphate. *Acta Med. Scand.*, 173, 669.
ILLIG, A. & ILLIG, H. (1959) Wirkung bir adiposen diabetikern im doppeltblind versuch. *Medizinische Welt*, 1, 1077.
JACKSON, I.M.D. & WHYTE, W.G. (1965) Chlorphentermine SA in the treatment of obesity and the effect of weight loss on steroid excretion. *Brit. Med. J.*, 2, 453.
JONES, H.S. (1968) Diethylpropion dependence. *Med. J. Aust.*, 1, 267.
JONES, H.S. (1971) Fenfluramine used as a substitute for methyl amphetamines and dextramphetamines in the treatment of dependence on these drugs. *S. African Med. J.*, 45, suppl. 31.
JORDAN, M.J. & BADER, G.M. (1961) Use of diethylpropion combined with a supplement for safe and effective weight control in pregnancy. *Surgery*, 112, 663.
KAHAN, A. & MULLINS, A.G. (1958) Dangers of Preludin. *Brit. Med. J.*, 1, 1355.

KENDALL, M.J., NUTTER, S. & HAWKINS, C.F. (1971) Xylose test: effect of aspirin and indomethacin. *Brit. Med. J.*, 1, 533.

LANCET (1971), 2, 252 (Editorial)

LAWLOR, R.B., TRIVEDI, M.C. & YELONSKY, J.O. (1969) A determination of the anorexigenic potential of dl amphetamine d-amphetamine, l-amphetamine and phentermine. *Arch. Int. Pharmacodyn.*, 179, 401.

LEBON, P. (1961) Treatment of overweight with chorionic gonadotrophin. *J. Amer. Ger. Soc.*, 9, 11.

LE DOUAREC, J.C. & SCHMITT, J. (1964) Comparison pharmacologique de sept medicaments anorexigenes. *Therapie*, 19, 831.

LERICHE, H. (1960) A study of appetite suppressants in general practice. *Canad. Med. Assoc. J.*, 82, 467.

LE RICHE, W.H. & VAN BELLE, G. (1962) Study of phendimetrazine bitartrate as an appetite suppressant in relation to dosage, weight loss and side effects. *Canad. Med. Assoc. J.*, 87, 29.

LE RICHE, W.H. & CSIMA, A. (1967) A long acting appetite suppressant drug studied for 24 weeks in both continuous and sequential administration. *Canad. Med. Assoc. J.*, 97, 1016.

LEONARD, C.A., FUJITA, T., TEDESCHI, D.H. & FELLOWS, E.J. (1961) Neuropharmacology of dl-methyl-p-trifluromethyl phenethylamine hydrochloride. *Pharmacologist*, 3, 79.

LESSES, M.F. & MYERSON, A. (1938) Human autonomic pharmacology: benzedrine sulphate as an aid in treatment of obesity. *New Eng. Med. J.*, 218, 119.

LEVIN, A. (1972) The pattern of drug taking among drug dependent South African national servicemen. *S. African Med. J.*, 46, 1690.

LEVIN, A. (1972b) A comparison of patterns of drug abuse dependent young men in 1971 and 1970. *Geneeskunde*, 14, 245.

LEVIN, J., TRAFFORD, J.A.P., NEWLAND, P.M. & BISHOP, P.M.F. (1963) Chlorphentermine in the management of obesity. *Practitioner*, 191, 65.

LORBER, J. & GREENWOOD, N. (1971) The treatment of severe childhood obesity with fenfluramine. *S. African Med. J.*, 45, suppl. 40.

LUCEY, C. & HADDEN, D.R. (1962) Chlorphentermine. A new appetite suppressant. *Ulster Med. J.*, 31, 181.

MACE, P.M., MALCOLM, A.D., OUTAR, K.P. & PAWAN, G.L.S. (1972) Comparative effects of four anti-obesity agents on blood plasma lipids in man. *Proc. Nutr. Soc.*, 31, 14A.

MCKAY, R.H.G. (1973) Long term use of diethylpropion in obesity. *Curr. Med. Res. Opinion*, 1, 489.

MARTIN, G.J. (1959) A new anorexic agent, diethylpropion. Paper presented at the Sixth Spring Symposium on Overweight and Underweight at Michigan Acad. Gen. Prac. March 5th.

MASSERMAN, J.H. & GOLDSMITH, H. (1934) Dinitrophenol: its therapeutic and toxic actions in certain types of psychobiologic underactivity. *J.A.M.A.*, 102, 523.

MUNRO, J.F. (1973) Management of obesity. *Brit. J. Hosp. Med.*, 10, 7.

MUNRO, J.F., MACCUISH, A.C., MARSHALL, A., WILSON, E.M. & DUNCAN, L.J.P. (1969) Weight reducing effect of biguanides in obese non-diabetic women. *Brit. Med. J.*, 2, 13.

MUNRO, J.F., MACCUISH, A.C., WILSON, E.M. & DUNCAN, L.J.P. (1968) Comparison of continuous and intermittent anorectic therapy in obesity. *Brit. Med. J.*, 1, 352.

MUNRO, J.F., SEATON, D.A. & DUNCAN, L.J.P. (1966b) Treatment of refractory obesity with fenfluramine. *Brit. Med. J.*, 2, 624.
NATHANSON, M.H. (1939) The central action of beta-amino propylbenzene (Benzedrine). Clinical observations. *J. Amer. Med. Assoc.* 108. 528.
NAUMANN, D. (1962) Clinical studies of a new anorexiant. *Appl. Ther.*, 4, 550.
PATEL, N., MOCK, D.C. & HAGANS, J.A. (1963) Comparison of benzphetamine, phenmetrazine, d-amphetamine and placebo. *Clin. Pharm. & Ther.*, 4, 330.
PATEL, N. & STOWERS, J.M. (1964) Phenformin in weight reduction of obese diabetics. *Lancet*, 2, 282.
PAWAN, G.L.S. (1969) Effect of fenfluramine on blood lipids in man. *Lancet*, 1, 498.
PEDERSON, J. (1965) The effect of metformin on weight loss in obesity. *Acta Endocrinologica (Kbh)*, 49, 479.
PEDERSON, J. & OLESON, E.S. (1968) Observations on the mechanisms of increased weight loss during metformin administration in obesity. *Acta Endocrinologica (Kbh)*, 57, 683.
PHEAR, D. (1959) Phenmetrazine in the treatment of obesity. *Practitioner*, 183, 62.
POINDEXTER, A. (1960) Appetite Suppressant drugs: a controlled clinical comparison of benzphetamine, phenmetrazine, d-amphetamine and placebo. *Curr. Ther. Res.*, 2, 354.
POIRE, R., CRANCE, J.P. & ROMBACH, F. (1966) Three years of prolonged and controlled use of an anorectic (768 S or fenfluramine) in a psychiatric hospital environment without dietary changes and outside a cooperation context. *Ann. Med Nancy*, 5, 575.
POWELL, R.C., NUNES, W.T., HARDING, R.S. & VACCA, J.B. (1962) The influence of non-absorbable antibiotics on serum lipids and the excretion of neutral sterols and bile acids. *Amer. J. Clin. Nutr.*, 2, 156.
PULCH, M. (1955) Treatment of obesity with Preludin *Duetsches med. J.*, 6, 545.
RABINOWITZ, I.M. & FOWLER, A.F. (1934) Dinitrophenol. *Canad. Med. J.*, 30, 128.
RABINOWITZ, J.L. & MYERSON, R.M. (1967) The effects of triiodothyronine on some metabolic parameters of obese individuals. *Metabolism*, 16, 68.
RAUH, J.L. & LIPP, R. (1968) Chlorphentermine as an anorexigenic agent in adolescent obesity. Report of its efficacy in a double blind study of 30 teenagers. *Clin. Paed.*, 7, 138.
RAVETZ, E. (1959) Evaluation of anorexigenic products. Paper presented at Spring Symposium on Overweight and Underweight at Michigan Acad. Gen. Prac., March 5th.
RAYNER, P.H.W. (1971) Fenfluramine in childhood obesity. Clinical experience and effects of fenfluramine and weight loss on blood glucose, plasma insulin and plasma growth hormone. *S. African Med. J.* 45, suppl. 19 June.
RECORDIER, A.M., WAHL, M., JOUVE, G. & INGELSAKIS, A. (1963) Use of a new anorexigenic 768-S in the treatment of obesity. *Gazette medicale de France*, 70, 2585.
RENDLE-SHORT, J. (1960) Obesity in childhood: a clinical trial of phenmetrazine. *Brit. Med. J.*, 1, 703.
RESSLER, C. & SCHNEIDER, S.H. (1961) Clinical evaluation of phendimetrazine bitartrate. *Clin. Pharm. Ther.*, 2, 727.
RODOS, B.E., STEEN, B. & SVANBORG, A. (1970) Trial of an appetite

suppressant (Aminorex). *Lakartianingen*, 2, 1.
ROSENBERG, B.A. (1961) A double blind study of diethylpropion in obesity. *Amer. J. Med. Sci.*, 242, 201.
RUNYAN, J. (1962) Observations on the use of phendimetrazine a new anorexigenic agent in obese diabetics. *Curr. Ther. Res.*, 4, 270.
RUSSEK, H.I. (1966) Control of obesity in patients with angina pectoris: a double blind study with diethylpropion hydrochloride. *Amer. J. Med. Sci.*, 251, 461.
SABEH, G. (1965) Hydrocortisone and/or dessicated thyroid in physiologic dosage. *Metabolism.* 14. 603.
SANDOVAL, R.G., WANG, R.I.H. & RIMM, A.A. (1971) Body weight changes in overweight patients following an appetite suppressant in a controlled environment. *J. Clin. Pharmacol.*, 2, 120.
SCHAPIRO, M.M. & BOGRAN, N. (1960) Dietless weight loss with benzphetamine (Didrex[R]): a controlled comparison with phenmetrazine and placebo. *Curr. Ther. Res.*, 2, 233.
SCHNEEBERG, N.G. (1961) Clinical evaluation of diethylpropion (Tenuate) a new anorectic agent. *J. Albert Einstein Medical Centre*, 9 (1), 191.
SEATON, D.A., ROSE, K. & DUNCAN, L.J.P. (1964) Sustained action chlorphentermine in the correction of refractory obesity. *Practitioner*, 193, 698.
SILVERMAN, M. (1959) Subacute delirious state due to 'Preludin' addiction. *Brit. Med. J.*, 1, 696.
SILVERMAN, M. & OKUN, R. (1971) The use of an appetite suppressant (diethylpropion hydrochloride) during pregnancy. *Curr. Ther. Res.*, 13, 648.
SILVERSTONE, J.T. & BUCKLE, R.M. (1966) Obesity in diabetes. Some considerations of treatment. *Amer. J. Clin Nutr.*, 19, 158.
SILVERSTONE, J.T. & SOLOMON, T. (1965) The long term management of obesity in general practice. *Brit. J. Clin. Pract.*, 19, 395.
SILVERSTONE, J.T., TURNER, P. & HUMPERSON, P.L. (1968) Direct measurement of the anorectic activity of diethylpropion (Tenuate Dospan). *J. Clin. Pharmacol.*, 8, 172.
SIMEONS, A.T.W. (1954) The action of chorionic gonadotrophin in the obese. *Lancet*, 2, 946.
SIMONS, E.W. (1953) Mechanisms of dinitrophenol toxicity. *Biol. Rev.*, 28, 453.
SIMKIN, B. & WALLACE, L. (1960) A controlled clinical trial of benzphetamine (Didrex[R]) in the management of obesity. *Curr. Ther. Res.*, 2, 233.
SIMKIN, B. & WALLACE, L. (1961) A controlled clinical comparison of benzphetamine and D-amphetamine in the management of obesity. *Amer. J. Clin. Nutr.*, 9, 632.
SMART, J.V., SNEDDON, J.M. & TURNER, P. (1967) A comparison of the effects of chlorphentermine, diethylpropion and phenmetrazine on critical flicker frequency. *Brit. J. Pharmacol.*, 30, 307.
SMITH, G.P. (1974) in proceedings of Fogarty International Center Symposium on Obesity, N.I.H., Bethesda. To be published.
SOMAR, E. (1959) 40 day—550 calorie diet in the treatment of obese out patients. *Amer. J. Clin. Nutr.*, 7, 514.
SPENCE, A.W. & MEDVEI, V.C. (1966) Fenfluramine in the treatment of obesity. *Brit. J. Clin. Pract.*, 20, 12.
STEEL, J.M. & BRIGGS, M. (1972) Withdrawal depression in obese patients after fenfluramine treatment. *Brit. Med. J.*, 3, 26.

STEEL, J.M., MUNRO, J.F. & DUNCAN, L.J.P. (1973) A comparative trial of different regimens of fenfluramine and phentermine in obesity. *Practitioner*, 211, 232.
STEGEN, M.G., ZSOTER, T., TOM, H. & CHAOOEL, C. (1960) Pharmacologic and toxicologic studies on a new anorexigenic agent, phendimetrazine. *Toxicol. appl. Pharmacol.*, 2, 589.
STOWERS, J.M. & BEWSHER, P.D. (1969) Studies of the mechanism of weight reduction by phenformin. *Postgrad. Med. J.*, 45, 13.
STRONG, J.A. & LAWSON, A.A.H. (1970) Double blind cross over trial of fenfluramine and metformin in the treatment of obesity. In *Amphetamines and Related Compounds*, p. 673. Ed. Costa, E. & Garattini, S. New York: Raven Press.
TAINTER, M.L. STOCKTON, A.B. & CUTTING, W.C. (1933) Use of nitrophenol in obesity and related conditions. A progress report. *J.A.M.A.*, 101, 1472.
THOMA, O. & WICK, H. (1954) Uber einige Tetrahydro-1, 4-oxazine mit sympathico mimetrischen eigenschaften. *Arch. exper. Path. U. Pharmakol. Bd.*, 22, 540.
TRAHERNE, J.B. (1965) A clinical trial of fenfluramine. *Practitioner*, 195, 677.
TRICKETT, P.C. & WEIR, J.H. (1968) Clinical evaluation of chlorphentermine hydrochloride in a college population. *Pacific Medicine and Surgery*, 76, 35.
TURNER, P. (1971) Further studies on the human pharmacology of fenfluramine. *Suppl. S. African Med. J.*, 45, 19.
TURTLE, J. (1971) Current therapy of diabetes and its rationale. *Aust. N.Z. J. Med.*, 1, 13, suppl. 2.
TURTLE, J.R., BURGESS, J.A. & BAUCKHAM, S. (1971) The metabolic effects of fenfluramine 1. Forearm perfusion and intravenous infusion in normal subjects and therapeutic value as a hypoglycaemic agent in diabetes mellitus. *S. African Med. J.*, 45, suppl. 22.
VAGUE, J., TEITELBAUM, M. & MILLER, G. (1964) Clinical testing of an anorectic (chlorphentermine) presented in prolonged effect tablets. *Sem. Hop.*, 40, 1376.
VAN DER SCHOOT, J.B., ARIEUS, E.J., VAN ROSSUM, J.M. & HURKAMNS, J.A. (1962) Phenylisopropylamine derivatives structure and action. *Arzneimittel Forschung*, 12, 962.
WAAL MANNING, H.J. & SIMPSON, F.O. (1969) Fenfluramine in obese patients on various antihypertensive drugs. Double blind controlled trial. *Lancet*, 2, 1392.
WEISSMAN, A. & SCHNEIDER, J.A. (1960) Some anorectic and behavioural properties of p-trifluoro-methyl analogue of amphetamine. *Pharmacologist*, 2, 71.
WILLIAMS, L. (1926) *Obesity*. Oxford: University Press.
WILLIAMS, J. (1968) Trial of a long acting preparation of diethylpropion in obese diabetics. *Practitioner*, 200, 411.
WOOD, L.C. & OWEN, J.A. (1965) Clinical evaluation of a new anorexigenic drug, aminoxaphen, in obese diabetics. *J. New Drugs*, 5, 181.
WOODWARD, E. (1970) Clinical experience with fenfluramine in the United States. In *Amphetamines and Related Compounds*, Ed. Costa, E. & Garattini, S. p. 685. New York: Raven Press.
YUDKIN, J. (1959) The causes and cure of obesity. *Lancet*, 2, 1135.

21. Psychological Variables in the Control of Obesity

P. LEY, P. W. BRADSHAW, J. A. KINCEY, J. COUPER-SMARTT
and MARILYN WILSON

The experiments to be described were conducted as part of a larger programme of research aimed at finding practicable ways of improving communications between doctors and their patients. Part of this research is concerned with increasing patient satisfaction with communications from doctors especially in the hospital setting, and part with increasing the frequency with which patients follow advice given to them. Ley & Spelman (1967) and Ley (1972a) have shown that patients frequently fail to follow such advice. Evidence from these reviews is summarized in Table 21.1.

Ley & Spelman argued that non-compliance was due in part to failures in comprehension and memory on the part of the patient. Studies of patients understanding of what they are told have shown that there are many surprising gaps in comprehension (Boyle, 1970; Ley & Spelman, 1967; Ley et al, 1972; Riley, 1966). Research has also shown that patients frequently forget much of what they are told (Joyce et al, 1969; Ley, 1966, Ley, 1972a; Ley et al, 1973; Ley & Spelman, 1967). However it would be naive to suppose that if patients understood and remembered advice given to them they would all then follow it. Understanding and memory are necessary but not sufficient conditions for following advice.

There are a number of techniques developed by social and clinical psychologists which might be applicable to this problem. In order to assess their effectiveness it was necessary to find a condition which satisfied certain criteria. The condition should be of some clinical interest, common so that sufficient members will be available for experiment and capable of being measured objectively so that the effectiveness of persuasive communication variables can be assessed.

Simple obesity seemed to meet these requirements so it was decided to use the obese as subjects for some initial research on persuasive communication.

Table 21.1
A summary of studies of patients' compliance with medical advice

Type of advice	No. of studies	Patients who did not follow advice (per cent)		
		Range	Mean	Median
A. Medicine taking				
1 PAS and other T.B. drugs	20	8-76	37.5	35
2 Antibiotics	8	11-92	48.7	50
3 Psychiatric drugs	9	11-51	38.6	44
4 Other medicines— antacids, iron, etc.	12	9-87	47.7	47.5
B. Diet	11	20-84	49.4	45
C. Other advice e.g. child care, ante-natal care	8	30-79	54.6	51
D. All advice	68	8-92	44	44.4

(Ley, 1972a)

CLASSIFICATION VARIABLES

At the outset it is worth proposing a simple category system for the obese in relation to slimming procedures.

The first classification is concerned with whether or not there has been instigation to lose weight. Where instigation exists it is either self generated or generated by other people such as doctors and relatives. Where it is generated by other people it is possible for it to be accepted or rejected.

The second variable is concerned with the outcome of attempts to lose weight. Such attempts will be, or would be, either successful or unsuccessful.

Communications addressed to the obese can also be classified usefully into persuasive/motivational and technical advice. The persuasive/motivational communication is designed to instigate or increase motivation to lose weight, and the technical advice communication offers details of how to lose weight. The type of communication called for will vary with the type of obese person. This reasoning yields the joint classification of the obese and the communications required shown in Table 21.2.

Table 21.2
The relationship between type of communication
required and the categories of obese persons.

	Type of communication required by those whose own efforts are or would be:	
	Successful	Unsuccessful
Instigation to lose weight:		
Self generated	none	persuasive/motivational technical advice
Other generated and accepted	none	persuasive/motivational technical advice
Other generated and not accepted	persuasive/ motivational	persuasive/motivational technical advice
None	persuasive/ motivational	persuasive/motivational technical advice

The experiments to be described investigate the effects of various techniques in the persuasive/motivational category and the technical advice categories. However, as the subjects came in response to a newspaper appeal they are presumably drawn from the categories that are either self-generated, or generated by others and accepted. Further, as they had all tried to lose weight in the past, they can be categorized as those whose own efforts had been unsuccessful.

THE PERSUASIVE/MOTIVATIONAL TECHNIQUE

The persuasive/motivational techniques were chosen from those which social psychologists have demonstrated fairly conclusively to affect the success of persuasive communications. Brief non-technical accounts of these can be found in Ley & Spelman (1967), while comprehensive more technical reviews are provided by Berscheid & Walster (1969) and Insko (1966).

The first of these techniques is the use of group decision procedures. In these, instead of the information being presented in lecture fashion from an expert to an audience, the expert briefly presents information and advice to a group of subjects, who then discuss what has been said, and try to think of difficulties that people like them would have in following the advice.

After the discussion the subjects are asked to put up their hands if they are going to try the recommended technique. A series of studies reviewed by Lewin (1954) showed that group decision procedures were more effective in getting people to change their behaviour than were lecture methods. This was true even when the 'lecture' consisted of an expert and an audience of one. Thus, in one study a dietitian in a maternity hospital who had previously spent half an hour with each new mother advising on baby feeding, was able greatly to increase the effectiveness of her advice by using a group decision procedure in which she spent the half hour with a group of six mothers instead of just one. Although there are doubts as to which of the variables in group decision are critical, as a package the technique seems successful in inducing change in attitudes and behaviour.

Fear arousal

Another variable which has often been found to affect degree of compliance with advice is fear-arousal. Despite early findings in this field (Janis & Feshbach, 1953) it looks as though in most circumstances the more fear arousing a communication is the more compliance with advice there will be (Leventhal, 1970), although it is possible that the arousal of too much fear might be counter-productive (Janis, 1967).

One-sided and two-sided messages

A final variable is whether or not the persuasive communication is one-sided or two-sided. One-sided messages present only the case for following the advice and ignore possible counter-arguments. Two-sided communications also deal with the counter-arguments. The general finding is that two-sided presentations lead to more lasting change in attitude and greater resistance to later messages urging the opposite point of view.

TECHNICAL ADVICE

The commonest form of technical advice given to those trying to lose weight is a diet programme. However it is well-known that many people have great difficulty in keeping to their diets, and other techniques have been proposed to help people in this respect. Those used in the present series of investigations were self-control procedures based on operant conditioning principles, diet holidays and aversion classical conditioning.

Self-control procedures aim to teach the subject to control his own behaviour by applying well-established principles of learning. Specific programmes for the obese have been suggested by Ferster *et al* (1962) and Stuart (1967, 1971) who have claimed some success for these methods.

Their claims have been largely supported by other investigators (Hagen, 1970; Harris, 1969; Harris & Bruner, 1971; Wollersheim, 1970), but have required a great deal of the expert's time, sometimes even twice weekly contact. It would, therefore, be of interest to see if equally good results could be obtained by using leaflets as the main instructional device. The results obtained by Hagen (1970) suggest that this might be feasible.

AVERSION CONDITIONING

Classical aversion conditioning has also been included as a variable. There is ample evidence that aversion conditioning can sometimes affect behaviour (Yates, 1970), and there have been previous applications of such techniques to the problem of obesity. The aversive stimulus used can be a real one, e.g. an unpleasant odour (Kennedy & Foreyt, 1968), or an imagined one—a procedure known as covert sensitization or covert aversion technique (Cautela, 1966). Controlled studies using classical conditioning to affect weight reduction suggest that it might be a useful procedure (Foreyt & Kennedy, 1971; Janda & Rimm, 1972; Manno & Marston, 1972; Meynen, 1970).

REWARDS

Finally, the use of diet holidays was investigated. This was based on the view that eating carbohydrates is reinforcing to the obese. It should therefore be theoretically possible to increased adherence to a diet by rewarding such adherence by points which could be later traded for a diet holiday, on which extra carbohydrates could be consumed. No controlled study of this technique was found.

Table 21.3 provides a summary of studies using a no treatment control group. It is clear from the summary that further investigation is justified.

PERSONALITY

It seemed possible that certain personality variables might be related to compliance. Extraversion has been shown to be related to poor persistence and to desire for varied stimulation (Eysenck, 1967). It is often hypothesized that the obese eat in order to reduce anxiety. If this is so it might be expected that the more anxious individuals would have greater difficulty in losing weight. For this reason a measure of neuroticism was included.

There is now a substantial body of research suggesting that the internal-control dimension is an important factor in whether people

Table 21.3
Summary of behaviour modification studies
using no-treatment controls

Investigator	Average frequency of contact per week	Better than no treatment
A. Self control procedures		
Hagen (1970)		
(a) Personal contact	once	yes
(b) Correspondence	once	yes
Harris (1969)	twice	yes
Harris & Bruner (1971)		
(a) experiment 1	?	yes
(b) experiment 2	?	no
Stuart (1971)	twice	yes
Wollersheim (1970)	once	yes
B. Covert sensitization		
Janda & Rimm (1972)	once	no
Manno & Marston (1972)	twice	yes
Meynew (1970)	once	yes
C. Aversive conditioning		
Foreyt & Kennedy (1971)	?	yes

comply with advice (Lefcourt, 1972). This variable is derived from the work of Rotter (1954, 1955, 1960, 1966).

Some individuals see the locus of control of their actions as lying outside themselves, while others think that they control their own fate. The latter, the internally controlled, appear to be more successful in complying with advice.

METHODS

Recruitment and selection of subjects

The sample of subjects was obtained by a newspaper and television appeal for volunteers to help in slimming research. A local newspaper included a brief article on the proposed research and included an appeal for volunteers. This was followed by similar brief articles in national newspapers and one television item on a regional news programme. A total of 561 people wrote or telephoned asking for further details, and were sent various questionnaires to complete and a brief description of the general nature of the scheme. The questionnaire elicited information on age, sex, height, weight and eating behaviour in various circumstances. Subjects also provided written authorization for us to contact their general practitioner to ascertain whether there was any medical reason why the subject should not join the scheme. Of the 413 subjects who returned these questionnaires, 379 were female and 44 were male.

The general practitioners were then sent a letter explaining the nature of the project. A 'negative return' form was used. The doctor was asked to notify the team if he felt that his patient should be excluded on medical grounds. These were outlined as:

Suffering from a condition that might cause weight gain (e.g. congestive cardiac failure; renal oedema; endocrine diseases such as diabetes mellitus, thyroid dysfunction or Cushing's disease; pregnancy).
Receiving drugs such as appetite suppressants, corticosteroids, thyroid-active drugs, diuretics, etc.
Suffering from any mental or physical condition that might make dieting unsafe.

An additional check was provided by a brief screening interview conducted on the occasion of the subject's first visit. This interview revealed five subjects who were unsuitable. Altogether 64 subjects were rejected on medical grounds.

Another criterion for inclusion in the study was that the subjects should be at least 10 per cent above the average weight for their sex, age and height as assessed by the tables of Montegriffo (1968). Thirteen subjects were less than 10 per cent overweight.

As there were so few male volunteers it was decided to concentrate on the females.

Further complications in subject selection for experiments were introduced by subject holiday programmes, etc. If it was clear that subjects would not be able to attend sessions, for example because of holidays they were excluded from that experiment.

Experiment 1
Group decision, fear, sidedness of arguments, self control procedures and personality variables in the control of weight loss

This experiment was designed to investigate the effects of persuasive/motivational variables and a technical advice variable in the form of self-control procedures, on adherence to a dietary regime. The diet chosen was the Servier Unit Eating Guide, which is in an attractive presentation of the low carbohydrate diet. The Flesch

Reading Ease Formula was applied to the leaflet to ascertain its comprehensibility. This formula devised by Flesch (1948) gives an estimate of the percentage of the population likely to understand a given leaflet, and has been shown to have many practical correlates (Ley, 1973; Ley et al, 1972). The application of the formula suggested that the leaflet should be comprehensible to about 75 per cent of the population. It would have been desirable to have an easier leaflet, but as there was to be face to face instruction and opportunities to ask questions, this level of difficulty was regarded as acceptable.

The variables investigated in the experiment were degree of fear arousal, one-sided versus two-sided presentation, lecture versus group decision and self-control advice. Because of its nature the group decision method could not include the fear arousal and one-sided versus two-sided presentation variables.

A subsidiary purpose of the experiment was to provide correlational data on weight loss and various personality variables. These were extraversion, neuroticism, self-acceptance and internal-external control.

Subjects and Method

The subjects comprised 162 female volunteers selected from those in the pool of subjects who lived within evening travelling distance of the University, and who had indicated that they could attend over at least an eight-week period from their first visit. These subjects were invited to attend and 131 did so Table 21.4 shows the age and percent overweight distribution for these subjects.

Table 21.4
Ages and per cent overweight of
the subjects in Experiment 1

Per cent overweight	AGE (years)			
	20-29	30-39	40-49	50-59
10 - 19	3	8	3	—
20 - 29	5	22	16	—
30 - 39	4	13	10	1
40 - 49	6	9	5	1
50 - 59	3	7	2	1
60 - 69	1	3	1	—
70 - 79	1	2	3	—
80 - 89	—	—	2	—
90 - 99	—	—	—	—

Fear. The experimental conditions were made up of various combinations of the variables. There were three levels of fear arousal. The low fear lecture made brief factual mention of the risks to health of being overweight, listing examples of those diseases to which the obese are more susceptible. The moderate fear lecture referred specifically to the unpleasant nature of these diseases and to the reduced life expectancy of the obese. Finally the high fear version exphasized the crippling nature and extreme physical discomfort caused by these diseases, and the high death rate caused by them. Three levels of fear were used to increase the probability of detecting curvilinear relationships if they existed.

The effectiveness of these lectures in causing different levels of fear had been established in a preliminary experiment with three groups of subjects from the pool who had been randomly assigned to the three versions of the lecture. Nineteen heard the low fear, thirteen the moderate fear and nineteen the high fear version. None of these subjects was later included in Experiment 1. Immediately after listening to the lecture the subjects completed a check list measure of anxiety, the Multiple Affect Adjective Check-list (MAACL) (Zuckerman & Lubin, 1965) and rated the lecture for degree of fear arousal on a seven point bipolar scale: from comforting to frightening.

Analysis of the above measures showed that the three versions of the lecture from low to high fear produced significantly increasing anxiety amongst subjects, and that the three versions of the lecture were similarly rated by subjects as being increasingly more frightening. The conclusion is therefore that the attempt to manipulate fear arousal was successful.

One-sided and two-sided versions. Both the one-sided and two-sided versions of the lecture contained information on definitions of being overweight, the role of excessive input in causing obesity, the constituents of food and information about the recommended diet and its rationale, as well as the appropriate fear arousing section. In addition the two-sided version dealt with the ineffectiveness of alternative methods of losing weight such as slimming garments, massage, special drinks and the like; the suggestion that obesity was due to causes other than taking in more than one required; and arguments that there are benefits in being fat which outweigh the health risks. The lectures were always given by the same individual.

Self-control procedure. The self-control procedure consisted of a leaflet based on the work of Ferster *et al* (1962) and Stuart (1967, 1971) giving instructions in the application of self-control techniques. A placebo set of instructions was also invented called 'will-power' training. This contained advice which was not based on learning principles, and which indeed was sometimes contrary to the advice given to the self-control group. In the third condition subjects received only the diet sheet.

Group decision procedure. Three group leaders were available for the group decision procedure, and it had been intended that each would lead three groups of six people. In the event, due to the failure of some subjects to attend, some groups were of only three people. The groups were run on the lines indicated earlier. The leader briefly presented the same basic information as had been given in the lecture. The group then discussed problems associated with following the advice, asked questions and ended by each member making a public committment within the group to try to follow the advice.

Randomization. In the assignment of subjects to the experimental conditions some degree of matching was attempted. Four sub-groups were formed by dividing subjects into above or below median age, and above or below median percentage overweight. Subjects within the sub-groups were then assigned randomly to the experimental conditions. A summary of these conditions and the number of subjects who attended the lectures and group decision procedures is shown in Table 21.5.

Table 21.5
Number of subjects in the different experimental conditions attending the lectures and group decision procedures

	Fear level	*Self-control*	*Will-power*	*Diet only*
Lectures				
One-sided	low	6	4	6
	moderate	5	6	5
	high	5	6	4
Two sided	low	5	4	5
	moderate	4	4	5
	high	5	5	5
Group-decision				
Leader A		4	4	6
Leader B		5	6	4
Leader C		3	4	6

Subjects attended evening sessions, eighteen subjects being invited to attend each session. On arrival subjects were weighed and interviewed by the medical member of the team who used the brief screening procedure described earlier. They then filled in the various personality questionnaires. These were a short form of the Eysenck Personality Inventory (EPI) which provides measures of introversion and extraversion, and a modification of the Internal-External Control Questionnaire devised by Gurin et al (1969). When all had completed these preliminaries they attended one of the lectures or participated in a group decision procedure. After this they were given sealed envelopes to take home. These included either: the diet booklet for the diet only group, the diet booklet plus self-control instructions for the self-control group or the diet booklet plus will-power instructions for the will-power group. Subjects were asked not to compare their regimes with those of any friends or relatives in the scheme who might have received different instructions.

Follow-up visits were arranged two, four and eight weeks after the initial visit. These also took place in the evenings. Subjects were weighed, questions about the diet were answered and questionnaires were filled in. These included the MAACL to assess mood changes and a questionnaire designed to assess knowledge of the diet.

Results

The results can be summarized quite simply by saying that none of the main experimental variables exerted any significant effect. Analysis of variance was used to assess the significance of the results which are summarized in Table 21.6. The F-ratios presented are for subjects who attended all three follow-ups. This group was selected for analysis to avoid possible complications of interpretation arising from non-specific effects of attendance.

Table 21.6
Mean cumulative weight loss in the experimental groups

	Weight loss in lb at			F ratio and significance of 8 week loss
	2 weeks	4 weeks	8 weeks	
Group decision	5.88	6.94	9.06	0.85 (n.s.)
Lecture	5.21	6.03	7.69	
Low fear	4.13	5.19	6.75	
Moderate fear	5.90	7.70	8.10	0.23 (n.s.)
High fear	5.15	5.00	7.69	
One-sided	4.35	4.95	6.25	2.40 (n.s.)
Two-sided	5.53	6.63	8.63	
Diet only	4.89	5.58	6.79	
Will power	5.29	6.06	7.65	2.12 (n.s.)
Self control	5.95	7.40	9.90	
Numbers attending	92	77	68	

None of the interactions between variables was significant

Further analysis showed that attendance at follow-up was not related to the experimental variables. The conclusion is therefore that the persuasive and advisory communications used had affected neither weight loss nor attendance at sessions. The drop-out rate by the time of the eight week follow-up was 48.1 per cent. The data were examined to see whether drop-outs differed from those who stayed in. They did not differ in terms of initial weight and age, nor did they differ in any of the personality measurements. Further, those who attended the first follow-up but not others did not differ in initial weight loss.

The personality measures also yielded negative results except for the internal-external control scale. Correlations between the personality variables and weight loss are shown in Table 21.7.

Table 21.7
Personality variables and weight loss

Variable	Product-movement Correlation coefficient	Significance level
Extraversion (EP1)	0.06	n.s.
Neuroticism (EP1)	−0.08	n.s.
Internal-external control	0.31	$p < 0.05$

The relationship between internal-external control and weight loss was examined more closely. An analysis of variance showed that subjects obtaining high scores on this variable lost weight at a significantly faster rate than those with low scores. This is shown in Table 21.8.

Table 21.8
Differences in weight loss between internally and externally controlled subjects

| | Mean weight loss (lb) | | |
	2 weeks	4 weeks	8 weeks
Externally controlled	5.23	5.90	6.50
Internally controlled	5.32	6.68	9.96

F ratio for interaction = 9.89; df, 2, 107
$p < 0.001$

Lastly, mention should be made of some incidental findings. Knowledge of the diet was significantly related to total weight loss, ($r = + 0.29$, $p < 0.05$), but starting weight was not, ($r = - 0.06$) nor was weight loss at first follow-up related to subsequent weight loss. Of those who attended the third follow-up three had gained weight and one showed no change. Amongst those who lost weight a quarter lost between one and four pounds, a quarter between five and seven pounds, a quarter between eight and eleven pounds and a quarter more than twelve pounds. The range was from a gain of three pounds to a loss of twenty pounds.

Experiment 2
The effects of reinforcement by diet holidays

It is now well established that (a) the application of positive reinforcers increases the probability of the desired behaviour and (b) that partial reinforcement leads to habits having greater resistance to extinction and (c) that variable schedules lead to higher probabilities of response than fixed schedules (Honig, 1966). Premack (1971, 1972) has argued and demonstrated that reinforcing activities can be identified by their frequency of occurrence. On this basis it would be expected that eating foods containing carbohydrates would be reinforcing to our subjects. A variety of experiments have shown that points or tokens which can be exchanged for reinforcers become in themselves reinforcing (Ayllon & Azrim, 1968; Ullman & Krasner, 1969).

The aim of this experiment was therefore to see whether points given as rewards for complying with the diet, which were exchangeable for a diet holiday at some later stage, would be effective in increasing adherence to that diet.

Subjects and Method

All of the subjects who attended the eight week follow-up in Experiment 1 were invited to take part in the second experiment. All were told to continue to follow the advice that had been given up to that point, whilst also following any new advice to be given.

Subjects were also given a daily record sheet on which to record their intake of units, and if appropriate were informed about the diet holidays on which they could eat twice the daily allowance of units. Assignment was made at random to one of five conditions:

1. Control—carry on with diet and record daily number of units.
2. Fixed non-contingent holiday—carry on with diet, record daily number of units and take a diet holiday every thirteen days.
3. Non-contingent variable holiday—keep to diet, record daily

intake, and shake a pair of dice. If the dice showed one of three specified doubles of numbers a diet holiday should be taken the following day.
4. Contingent fixed ratio holiday—keep to diet, record daily intake. Every day daily units equal to or less than those prescribed a point is earned. When ten points have been earned a diet holiday can be taken the next day.
5. Contingent variable ratio holiday—keep to diet, record daily intake. Every day a point is earned shake a pair of dice. If one of four specified pairs of doubles was obtained a diet holiday could be taken the next day.

Previous data showed that subjects were compliant about 10 days in 13.

As well as verbal explanation of these procedures subjects were given instruction leaflets.

Subjects were seen on two follow-up visits, the first after three weeks and the second after seven weeks. At the first follow-up any problems in applying the procedure were discussed.

Results

Thirty-eight subjects were present at the seven week follow-up, and 22 of them produced records of daily intake. Analyses of variance were carried out on the number of days the subjects had complied with their diet in the previous week, and on total weight loss. Neither of these produced a significant result in the right direction. In fact subjects in the control group were nearly signifi-

Table 21.9
Mean weight loss at seven weeks by the various groups and mean number of days in the seventh week diet was kept

Group	Mean weight loss (lb)	Mean days compliant
1. Control non-contingent	3.33	4.80
2. fixed	4.44	3.50
3. variable	2.57	0.50
contingent		
4. fixed	0.83	2.80
5. variable	3.43	3.50
Significant differences:		
Weight loss:	2 v's 4, $p < 0.05$	
	1 v's 3, $p < 0.05$	
Compliance:	1 v's 2 + 3 + 4 + 5, $p < 0.1$	

cantly more likely to comply than those receiving diet holidays. Because of this the experiment was stopped. A summary of the results is shown in Table 21.9.

Experiment 3
OLFACTORY AVERSION, COVERT SENSITIZATION AND WEIGHT LOSS

The aim of this experiment was to see whether simple classical conditioning procedures could be used to avert subjects to high carbohydrate foods that they found difficult to give up. If successful this should result in further weight loss.

Subjects and Method

Thirty-four of the volunteer sample expressed an interest in a period of more intensive treatment. Twenty-eight of them turned up for this. The mean age of these subjects was 38.8 years with a standard deviation of 5.2 years. They had a mean percentage overweight of 35.4 (S.D. ± 14.1).

For each subject two foods were found which were still being eaten and which were high in carbohydrates.

Subjects were assigned at random to a smell aversion group, a covert sensitization or a control group. In both experimental groups subjects were told:

'You are unable to diet properly because you are still eating foods which are responsible for making you put on a lot of weight. Eating these foods has become a strong, learned habit. You have learned to eat them because they give you a great deal of pleasure. The way we are going to deal with this problem is by teaching you to associate these foods with an unpleasant experience. But don't worry about it. What we are going to do cannot possibly do you any harm'.

In the smell aversion group subjects were then given small sample tubes, each containing a different, unpleasant-smelling chemical (ammonium sulphide, acetamide and butyric acid). At a signal from the therapist all subject were asked to think of one of their individually selected foods and, as soon as it was clearly imagined, to open up one of the sample tubes, inhaling the fumes through their noses. Both foods and chemicals were paired in sequence so that each food was followed by each of the smells and to reduce olfactory adaptation effects no one chemical was sniffed in successive trials.

After the introduction subjects in the covert sensitization group were given a brief (15 minute) training in relaxation. After this the covert sensitization trials began. The instructions were as follows:

'I want you to imagine you are about to eat - - - - . The thought of eating - - - - is very attractive. You are looking forward to it. You are looking at it and thinking how good it will be. All of a sudden you begin to notice a slightly sick feeling in the pit of your stomach. As you reach for the food you are really beginning to feel sick. You have that unpleasant, queasy feeling in your stomach. You feel as if you are about to 'throw up'. As you lift up the - - - - to bring it to your mouth you can feel yourself sweating. You are now feeling really dreadful. There is vomit coming up your throat. You are just managing to choke it back by keeping your mouth tight shut. As you bring up the - - - - and prepare to open your mouth to put it in, the nausea gets even worse. Your stomach violently rebels. You retch and heave and can taste vomit in your mouth. As you open your jaw to put the - - - - in your mouth, you can't hold out any more. You vomit and puke all over the --- and down your clothes. The spew goes over the floor, furniture and even on a person standing next to you. You retch and vomit again and again. You feel terrible, but you can't stop. You can taste the vomit in your mouth. There are particles of food up your nose. There is a strong smell of sick. All this makes you heave and puke again. The person standing beside you is shocked. There is a dreadful mess and you smell. You decide to put the - - - - down and go to have a wash. Immediately you feel better. You have a good wash in clean water and put on fresh clothes. You stomach now feels calm, and you feel relieved and happy it's all over'.

Ten to 20 seconds was allowed between each trial and five minute rest pauses were inserted after each 10 minute period of aversion. Small electric fans were used constantly throughout a session, and a large booster fan was switched on during the five minute rest pauses.

Thirty six trials were completed in the first treatment session, 30 trials in the second session and 15 in the third and last session. Trials alternated between the two forbidden foods and the sessions lasted 40 minutes. The control group were told that they could not be

Table 21.10
Classical aversive conditioning and weight loss in pounds one and five weeks after treatment

Treatment	Time since end of treatment (lb)	
	One week	Five weeks
Olfactory aversion	2.4	1.4
Covert sensitization	1.7	2.1
Control diet only	−0.4	−0.4

treated immediately, and that they would have to wait for some weeks. At the end of that time they would be offered whichever of the two treatments turned out to be the more effective. In the meantime they should continue with their diet. In particular they should stop eating the two forbidden foods.

All groups attended weekly for four weeks, the first three sessions being treatment sessions, and the fourth a follow-up session. A further follow-up took place four weeks later.

Results

The results obtained for subjects who attended all sessions are shown in Table 21.10.

Dunnett's (1955) test for comparison of several treatments with a control was used to assess the significance of the results at each of the two follow-up times. At the first follow-up the differences between the control condition and each of the treatments was significant at the five per cent level. Both olfactory aversion and covert sensitization led to significantly greater weight loss than the control condition. By the time of the second follow-up however, these differences were no longer significant.

DISCUSSION

The findings of this series of experiments can be summarized as follows:
 1. group decision procedures produced no more weight loss than a lecture;
 2. degree of fear arousal did not affect weight loss;
 3. two-sided communications did not produce greater weight loss than one-sided communications;
 4. self-control instruction led to no greater weight loss than placebo instructions or diet alone;
 5. a points system leading to diet holidays had no affect on weight and, if anything, tended to decrease compliance with the diet;
 6. two classical aversion conditioning procedures produced significantly greater weight loss in the short term but not the long term;
 7. the subjects internal-external control characteristic was increasingly associated with success in losing weight as time went on;
 8. knowledge of the contents of the diet sheet was significantly associated with success.

The last of these is consistent with the hypothesis of Ley and

Spelman (1967) that failures in compliance are sometimes due to failures in comprehension and understanding.

The finding that the internal-external control dimension is related to success in losing weight is an interesting one. There is a growing body of evidence showing that this variable is associated with compliance and factors likely to affect compliance, e.g. reducing smoking (James, et al, 1965; Platt 1969), deferred gratification and reactions to failure (Lefcourt, 1972).

How this relationship could be utilized is more problematic. Perhaps a measure of internal-external control could be used to predict which subjects would have the greatest difficulty in losing weight. Those scoring at the external end of the scale should be more at risk than those at the other end. However, the correlation involved is not a high one and there are problems in using low relationships in selection for treatment (Ley, 1972b).

The classical aversive conditioning procedures produced a significant, albeit short term, effect. It should be possible by manipulation of frequency and number of trials to produce greater and more sustained effects. The techniques had the drawback of being expensive in terms of experimenter time. This problem might be overcome by the use of instruction leaflets, so that subjects could carry out the procedure themselves. This, indeed, was one of the aims of the use of self-control procedures in Experiment 1. Previous research establishing their effectiveness had with one exception involved frequent contact between slimmer and expert. It was therefore very disappointing to find that the use of a self-control instruction leaflet was no more effective than the placebo leaflet, or no leaflet at all. Nor did fear make any difference to weight loss. It might be thought that it was optimistic to hope for an effect. Most of the previous research had been on the effects of fear on attitude change or relatively immediate action such as having an X-ray or an anti-tetanus injection. However, studies have shown a long term effect of a fear arousing communication on smoking behaviour (Levanthal & Niles, 1964; Leventhal & Watts, 1966). In view of this it does not seem unreasonable to expect such effects in dieting.

The failures of self control, fear arousal, group decision and two-sided communications to have effects is suprising. Three hypotheses can be advanced to account for this. The first concerns the nature of the subjects, the second the nature of the diet and the third the analysis of the situation.

It could be argued that the subjects were a very highly motivated group and that therefore the persuasive-motivational manipulations were ineffective because of a ceiling effect. Indeed, it might be generally true that those who fall into the unsuccessful self instigated and other instigated and accepted groups summarized in Table 2 would not be expected to respond to motivational techniques because of already existing high motivation. This cannot, however, account for all of the findings. It does not explain the failure of the self control procedures, and the evidence in the form of the 48 per cent drop-out rate over the eight week period suggests that the level of motivation left something to be desired.

The second explanation concerns the nature of the advice to be followed. It would be expected that the easier it is to follow a piece of advice the more people would follow it. If the recommended diet was easy to keep to, then its very ease could obscure the effects of the motivational variables. It is possible, therefore, that the effects of increased motivation will be proportional to the difficulty experienced in following the advice. With advice which is hard to follow, increases in motivation within limits will be beneficial; with advice which is easy to follow, they will have no effect.

The qualification 'within limits' issued because in general, there is a curvilinear relationship between motivation and efficiency, efficiency rising with motivation up to a point, but decreasing thereafter (Eysenck, 1967). Similarly, the following of easy advice would not be expected to be facilitated by special techniques such as self-control procedures. As it stands this is a very *ad hoc* hypothesis. Without parametric data on the ease of adherence to various dietary schedules it is not possible to test it. For what it is worth, however, many of the subjects reported pleasurable surprise when they saw the diet, and nearly all who turned up at eight weeks had lost weight.

The hypothesis concerning the analysis of the situation is that there are a number of pieces of compliant behaviour that the subject must produce before the programme can be effective. These include activities such as reading instruction leaflets, and reading the diet sheet as well as following the advice therein. It is clearly possible that this programme was failing at this level, i.e. that self-control procedures were not working because they were not being tried. The effect of this would be to reduce the effective number of subjects and make a significant difference harder to detect. If subjects did not read the leaflets given to them, then even with effective procedures they would not lose weight, and it will be recalled that there was a positive correlation between knowledge of the contents of the diet leaflet and weight loss.

This explanation might or might not seem to be a plausible account of the failure of the technical advice communications, but it is hard to see how it can account for the failure of the persuasive motivational communications.

In designing future research these possibilities will all be borne in mind.

Acknowledgements

This research was part of a programme of research in doctor-patient communication financed by the Department of Health and Social Security.

The authors also wish to thank the Servier Research Institute for providing copies of the Servier Unit Eating Guide.

REFERENCES

AYLLON, T. & AZRIN, N. (1968) *The Token Economy*, New York: Appleton.
BERSCHEID, E. & WALSTER, E. (1969) Attitude change in *Experimental Social Psychology* Ed. Mills, J. London: Collier-Macmillan.
BOYLE, C.M. (1970) Differences between patients and doctors interpretations of some common medical terms. *Brit. Med. J.*, 2, 286.
CAUTELA, J.R. (1966) Treatment of compulsive behaviour by covert sensitization. *Psychol. Rec.*, 16, 33.
DUNNETT, C.W. (1955) A multiple comparison procedure for comparing several treatments with a control. *J. Amer. Stat. Ass.*, 50, 1096.
EYSENCK, H.J. (1967) The Biological Basis of Personality. Springfield: C.C. Thomas.
EYSENCK, S.G.B. & EYSENCK, H.J. (1964) An improved short questionnaire for the measurement of E and N. *Life Sci.*, 3, 1103.
FERSTER, C.B., NURNBERGER, J.I. & LEVITT, E.B. (1962) The control of eating. *J. Mathetics*, 1, 87.
FLESCH, R. (1948) A new readability yardstick. *J. Appl. Psychol.*, 32, 221.
FOREYT, J.P. & KENNEDY, W.A. (1971) Treatment of overweight by aversion therapy. *Behaviour Res. Therap.*, 9, 29.
GURIN, P., GURIN, G., LAO., R.C. & BEATTIE, M. (1969) A multidimensional I/E scale. *J. Soc: Issues*, 25, 29.
HAGEN, R.L. (1970) Group therapy versus bibliotherapy in weight reduction. *Dissertation Abstracts*, 31, 2985.
HARRIS, M.B. (1969) Self-directed programme for weight control: a pilot study. *J. Abn. Psychol.*, 74, 263.
HARRIS, M.B. & BRUNER, C.G. (1971) A comparison of a self control and a control procedure for weight control. *Behav. Res. Therap.*, 9, 347.
HONIG, W.K. (1966) *Operant Behaviour: Areas of Research and Application*, New York: Appleton.
INSKO, C. (1966) Theories of Attitude Change, New York: Appleton.
JAMES, W.H., WOODRUFF, A.B. & WERNER, W. (1965) Effect of internal and external control upon changes in smoking behaviour. *J. Consult. Psychol.*, 29, 127.
JANDA, L.H. & RIMM, D.C. (1972) Covert sensitization in the treatment of obesity. *J. Abn. Psychol.*, 80, 37.
JANIS, I.L. (1967) Effects of fear arousal on attitude change: recent developments in theory and experimental research. In *Advances in Experimental Social Psychology*. III. Ed. Berkowitz, L. New York: Academic Press.

JANIS, I.L. & FESHBACH, S. (1953) Effects of fear-arousing communications. *J. Abn. and Soc. Psychol.*, **48**, 78.

JOYCE, C.R.B., CAPLE, G., MASON, M., REYNOLDS, E. & MATHEWS, J.A. (1969) Quantitative study of doctor-patient communication. *Quart. J. Med.*, **38**, 183.

KENNEDY, W.A. & FOREYT, J.P. (1968) Control of eating behaviour in an obese patient by avoidance conditioning. *Psychol. Reports*, **22**, 571.

LEFCOURT, H.M. (1972) Recent developments in the study of locus of control. In *Progress in Experimental Personality Research VI*, Ed. Maher, B.A. New York: Academic Press.

LEVENTHAL, H. (1970) Findings and theory in the study of fear communications. In *Advances in Experimental Social Psychology V*. Ed. Berkowitz, L. New York: Academic Press.

LEVENTHAL, H. & NILES, P. (1964) A field experiment on fear arousal with data on the validity of questionnaire measures. *J. Personality*, **32**, 459.

LEVENTHAL, H. & WATTS, J. (1966) Sources of resistance to fear-arousing communications on smoking and lung cancer. *J. Personality*, **34**, 155.

LEWIN, K. (1954) Studies in group decision. In *Group Dynamica*, Ed. Cartwright, D. & Zander, A. London: Tavistock.

LEY, P. (1966) What the patient doesn't remember. *Med. Opinion and Rev.*, **1**, 69.

LEY, P. (1972a) Comprehension, memory and the success of communications with the patient. *J. Inst. Hlth, Ed.*, **10**, 23.

LEY, P. (1972b) The problem of assessing suitability for treatment. *Bull Brit. Psychol. Soc.*, **25**, 19.

LEY, P. (1973) The measurement of comprehensibility. *J. Inst. Hlth. Ed.*, **11**, 17.

LEY, P., BRADSHAW, P.W., EAVES, D. & WALKER, C.M. (1973) A method for increasing patients recall of information presented by doctors. *Psychol. Med.*, **3**, 217.

LEY, P., GOLDMAN, M., BRADSHAW, P.W., KINCEY, J.A. & WALKER, C.M. (1972) The comprehensibility of some X-ray leaflets. *J. Inst. Hlth, Ed.*, **10**, 47.

LEY, P. & SPELMAN, M.S. (1967) *Communicating with the Patient* London: Staples Press.

MANNO, B. & MARSTON, A.R. (1972) Weight reduction as a function of negative covert reinforcement (sensitization) versus positive covert reinforcement. *Behaviour Res. Therap.*, **10**, 201.

MEYNEW, G.E. (1970) A comparative study of three treatment approaches with the obese: relaxation, covert sensitization and modified systematic desensitization. *Dissertation Abstracts.*, **31**, 2998.

MONTEGRIFFO, V.M.E. (1968) Height and weight of a United Kingdom adult population with a review of anthropometric literature. *Ann. Human Genetics, London.* **31**, 389.

PLATT, E.S. (1969) Internal-external control and changes in expected utility as predictors of the change in cigarette smoking following role playing. Paper presented at the meeting of the Eastern Psychological Association, Philadelphia, April, 1969.

PREMACK, D. (1971) Catching up with common sense, or two sides of a generalization: reinforcement and punishment. In *On the nature of reinforcement*, Ed. Glaser, R. New York: Academic Press.

PREMACK, D. (1972) The effect on extinction of the preference relations between the instrumental and contingent events. In *Reinforcement: Behavioural Analyses.* Ed. Gilbert, R.M. & Millenson, J.R. New York: Academic Press.

RILEY, C.S. (1966) Patients' understanding of doctors' instructions. *Medical Care,* 4, 34.

ROTTER, J.B. (1954) *Social Learning and Clinical Psychology.* Englewood Cliffs: Prentice Hall.

ROTTER, J.B. (1955) The role of the psychological situation in determining the direction of human behaviour. In *Nebraska Symposium on Motivation,* Ed. Jones, M.R. Lincoln: University of Nebraska Press.

ROTTER, J.B. (1960) Some implications of a social learning theory for the preduction of goal directed behaviour from testing procedures. *Psychol. Rev.,* 67, 301.

ROTTER, J.B. (1966) Generalized expectancies for internal versus external control of reinforcement. *Psychol. Monographs.* 80, whole no. 609, 1.

STUART, R.B. (1967) Behavioural control of over-eating. *Behaviour Res. Therap.,* 5, 357.

STUART, R.B. (1971) A three dimensional program for the treatment of obesity. *Behaviour Res. Therap.,* 9, 177.

ULLMAN, L.P. & KRASNER, L. (1969) *A psychological approach to abnormal behaviour.,* Englewood Cliffs: Prentice Hall.

WOLLERSHEIM, J.P. (1970) Effectiveness of group psychotherapy based upon learning principles in the treatment of overweight women. *J. Abn. Psychol.,* 76, 462.

YATES, A.J. (1970) *Behaviour Therapy.* New York: Wiley.

ZUCKERMAN, M. & LUBIN, B. (1965) *Manual for the Multiple Affect Adjective Check List.* San Diego: Educational and Industrial Testing Service.

22. Untraditional Treatment of Obesity

F. QUAADE

The two permanent mainstays of traditional obesity treatment—diet and exercise—are based on a sound rationale; they are cheap, easy to explain and also certain of success, provided they are followed by the patient. All the same, the depressing experience is that in most cases, and in practically all those with pronounced obesity, they are doomed to failure. Why is it that these two therapeutic principles, so certain of success, if they are put into practice, so often fail? Why is it that new and drastic cures are constantly devised? There are two obvious answers. First the daily suppression of the urge to eat what one likes, an urge that feels as legitimate, and probably more so, to the obese as to the normal individual, imposes a strain so heavy that it cannot be withstood for more than a period of time too brief for the purpose and secondly a deep-rooted disinclination towards bodily exercise is often a primary cause of early-onset obesity, and once gross obesity has been established, for whatever reason, it will constitute a mechanical and psychological encumbrance of such dimensions that an effective programme cannot be put into practice.

It seems likely that any progress in the field of exercise will be confined to prophylaxis and to treatment of moderate obesity in younger, mobile persons.

It will follow from these cursory introductory remarks that what I propose to call 'untraditional' approaches to the treatment of obesity have, of necessity, not aimed at increasing physical performance. Instead, they have aimed at a decreased calorie intake through means other than diet, or at an increase in calorie output through channels other than that of exercise. Though widely different these untraditional treatments all have the same basic principle that is to put the regulation of calorie intake and output outside the patient's control; in other words to render the therapeutic results independent of the will-power and the collaboration of the obese individual.

It is possible to reduce the obese patient's food intake by means of anorectic drugs and I would like to give this brief consideration. These are all chemically closely related to amphetamine and other sympathomimetic amines, and to varying degrees most have central excitatory properties. Their mode of action must be classified as stimulation of the hypothalamic satiety centres, and although their reducing effect on appetite, food intake and body weight is well documented and superior to that of placebo, they tend to lose their effect after a few months.

My experience is that even fenfluramine is no exception to this rule, in spite of its alleged beneficial effects on the peripheral metabolism of carbohydrate and fat. We have been dissatisfied with all anorectic drugs and my collaborators and I have recently turned our attention to a frank emetic.

LEVODOPA

After the introduction of levodopa for the treatment of Parkinson's disease, nausea and vomiting were reported as conspicuous side-effects. This, in combination with our observation of considerable weight loss in some patients treated with levodopa for Parkinsonism, led us to conduct a trial of the effect of levodopa on body weight in obese patients without neurological disorders.

The study was double-blind and randomized, and as criterion of effect we chose the change in body weight after six months' treatment. Thirty-seven patients received levodopa and 21 served as controls. There were no differences in age, sex or initial body weight in the two groups. Weight varied between 74 and 212 kg. The initial dosage was 400 mg levodopa three times a day, gradually increasing until nausea and possibly vomiting occurred. When these side-effects occurred, the dosage was diminished. Maximal dosage was 4.8 g levodopa daily. No dietary or other treatment was given.

There were no statistically significant differences in weight alteration between the levodopa and placebo groups after six months' treatment or at any time during the trial (Fig 22.1).

In both groups there were individual cases with a weight loss of up to 13 kg, but average weights changed only a few hundred grams. In contrast to the placebo patients practically all members of the levodopa group periodically complained of nausea and vomiting. Nevertheless they stated that they were able to eat their usual meals.

The lesson we have learned from this otherwise purely negative trial is that in obesity daily nausea and even vomiting is compatible with an unaltered food intake and an unaffected body weight. We

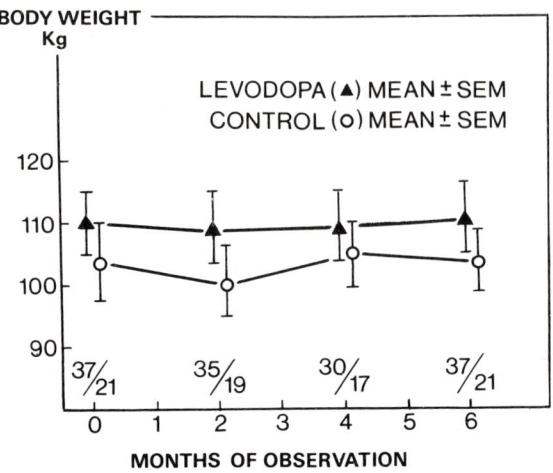

Figure 22.1
Average weight curves in 58 obese patients of whom 37 received levodopa, and 21 received placebo.

must conclude that a drug with effective hunger-reducing and not merely satiety-stimulating qualities is still lacking in the treatment of obesity.

STEREOTACTIC ELECTROCOAGULATION

Stereotactic electrocoagulation of the lateral hypothalamic area in humans with gross obesity is a new therapeutic experiment, which may be thought unethical and too drastic by some, but has been undertaken for a number of theoretical and practical reasons.

In animals abundant experimental evidence has been accumulating to demonstrate the presence of a dual mechanism in the hypothalamus for the regulation of food intake. Lesions of the ventromedial nuclei, either with electrocoagulation or goldthioglucose, lead to hyperphagia and obesity, whereas lesions in the lateral hypothalamic area are followed by hypophagia and weight loss. The latter phenomenon is transient after unilateral lesions, but bilateral electrocoagulation may result in total aphagia and cachexia. In human medicine, many clinical observations deal with the correlation between a hypothalamic lesion—mostly tumor or trauma—on the one hand, and an altered state of food intake on the other.

This evidence and the unsatisfactory therapeutic results produced in the very obese by conventional means combined to make me feel justified in effecting this therapeutic experiment in a small number of grossly obese human patients. Electrostimulatory exploration of the lateral hypothalamic area was undertaken, and when a positive stimulatory response, i.e. hunger sensation, occurred electrocoagulation of the presumed feeding centre was undertaken.

Five patients underwent this treatment, four women and one man, aged between 23 and 36 years. All were hyperphagic and had pronounced obesity which had resisted all previous conventional therapy. Body weights were between 118 and 180 kg. The patients were informed, and had accepted the experimental nature of the intervention and the uncertainty of its therapeutic benefit.

An extensive examination procedure, before and after the operation, revealed no endocrinological abnormalities in any of the patients. *Ad libitum* food intake was recorded by specially trained personnel before and after the operation. The second period of calorie counting began after the first postoperative week. The calorie calculations were made by an assistant who had no knowledge of the purpose and origin of the lists of ingested food and drink.

The operations, of which the first took place in December 1971, were performed by the Leksell technique. They were conducted on the non-dominant (right) hemisphere, except in the first patient (no. 1) who was operated on bilaterally. The target was the lateral hypothalamic nucleus. The coordinates were 2 mm behind the anterior commissure, 10 mm below the intercommissural line, where the optic tract was identified by stimulation 8-10 mm from the midline. From this point the electrode was withdrawn in steps of 3 mm. With a retractable protruding electrode each site was stimulated centrally and 3 mm laterally, medially, anteriorly and posteriorly from the electrode position. Stimulation parameters were: 1 mm, 5-8 volts, 50 cps in bursts of 10 and 20 seconds. The lesions were made by bipolar electrocoagulation, with the Leksell radio frequency generator. The size of the lesion was 4 x 4 mm, in one case 4 x 6 mm. Sound track and written recordings were made of the patients' verbal reactions during stimulation and coagulation.

The results of stimulation of the lateral hypothalamic region corresponded well to those reported from animal experiments and to previous experience in patients with behaviour disorders, such as aggressive psychotics and patients with temporal lobe epilepsy. This means that vegetative responses in the form of universal heat and cold sensations, and alterations in pulse rate and respiration, have been obtained. These responses, which were mainly elicited in the lower part of the stimulation track, were commonly coupled with feelings of fear. In the upper part of the region there were several responses of intense pleasure, bordering on euphoria.

In two cases (patients nos. 2 and 3) no convincing hunger

sensations were elicited; accordingly, no coagulation was made. These interventions, which may be termed negative explorations, serve as control operations with regard to the possibility of producing a non-specific decrease of food intake as a result of the craniotomy in itself. We received a convincing hunger response in the three other patients (nos. 1, 4 and 5). This was obtained 2-4 mm below the intercommissural line, 4-5 mm behind the anterior commissure and 6-9 mm from the midline. The electrocoagulation was centred at these coordinates, at the site of the maximal hunger response. In one patient (no. 1) a symmetrical, contralateral coagulation was performed three months later, although on that occasion the preceding stimulation elicited only epigastric discomfort and no convincing hunger feeling. The hunger reactions may be exemplified by the following utterances, 'I am so hungry that I could eat a whole fried chicken with chips', or 'I am so hungry that my entire belly feels like a vacuum'.

In the first postoperative week the three patients with lesions, but not the two others, stated that for the first time they were not very hungry and felt satiated at the beginning of their meals. Figure 22.2 shows that patients 2 and 3 whose lateral hypothalamus had been explored but not coagulated altered neither their spontaneous food intake nor their body weight after the operation. In the three remaining patients, two (nos. 4 and 5) with unilateral and one (no. 1) with bilateral lesions there was a significant decrease between preoperative and postoperative spontaneous calorie intakes ($0.01 < p < 0.05$). (Figs. 22.3 and 22.4). Body weight in these three patients was slightly and temporarily decreased, but not significantly.

In one patient (no. 4) there has been the rare complication of a subcortical abscess requiring a secondary operation. After her second coagulation patient no. 1 showed a slight reduction of spontaneity and initiative. This lasted for two to three months, after which she returned to her normal mental state.

CONCLUSION

The preliminary results may be summarized as follows:

In human subjects, as well as in experimental animals, the lateral hypothalamus is the site of nuclear or tract systems that are related to hunger. Electrocoagulatory lesions in this area may in man lead to a subjective feeling of an earlier satiety during meals and a significant but transient reduction of food intake. The lesions employed in this series did not produce weight loss in obese human subjects.

In view of the existing experience from animal experiments, the transient effect of a unilateral hypothalamic lesion on food intake

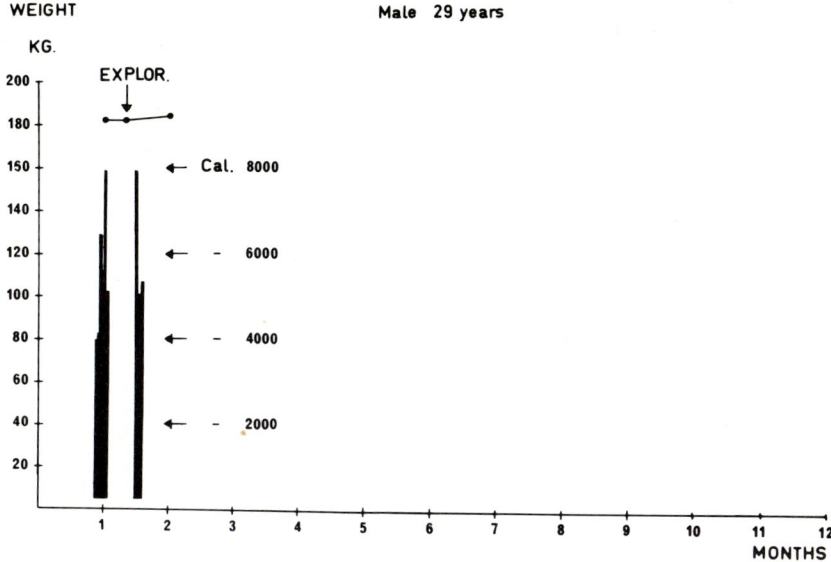
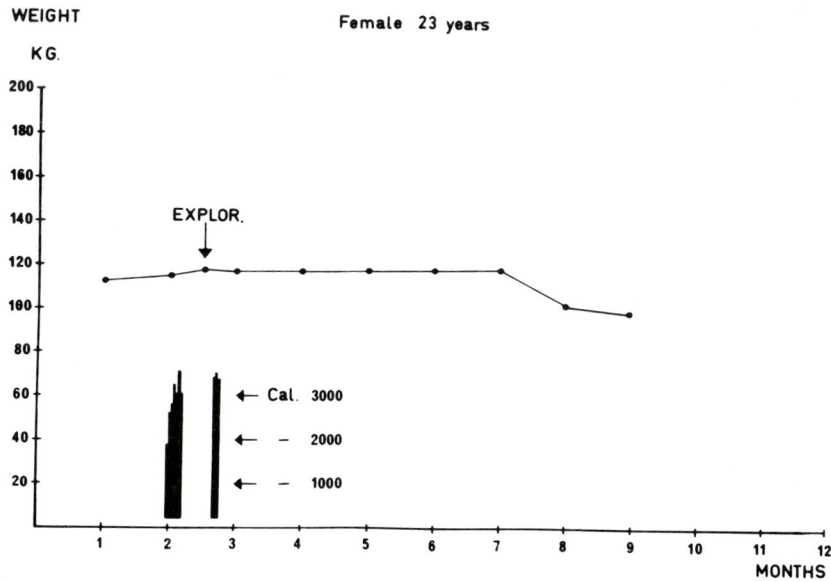

Figure 22.2
Body weight and spontaneous calorie intake in two obese patients before and after unilateral exploration of the lateral hypothalamus.

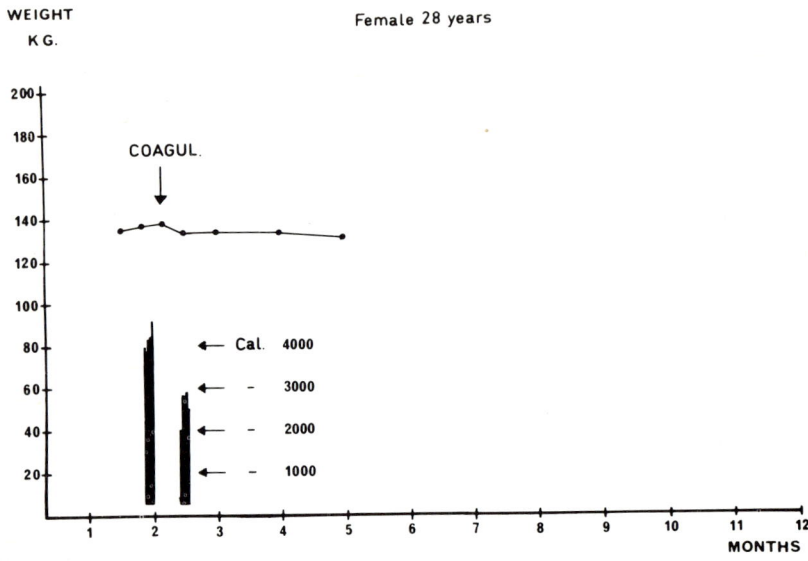
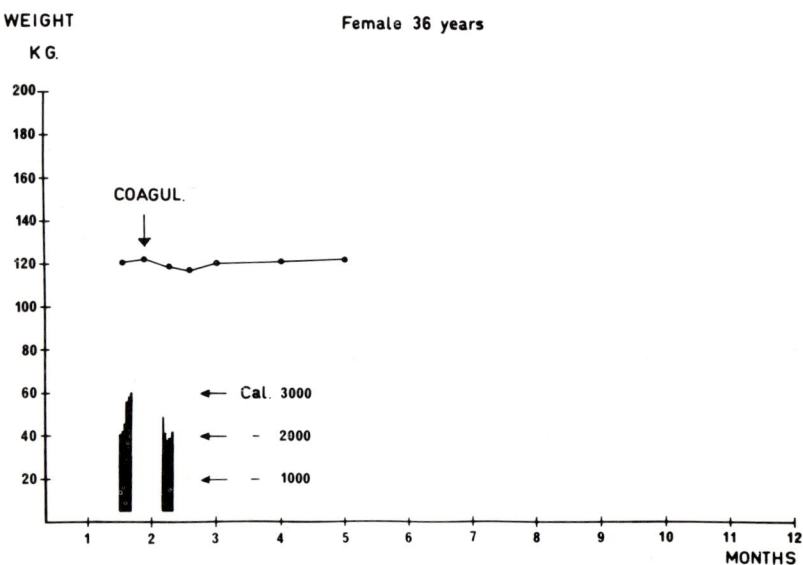

Figure 22.3
Body weight and spontaneous calorie intake in two obese patients before and after unilateral electrocoagulation of the lateral hypothalamus

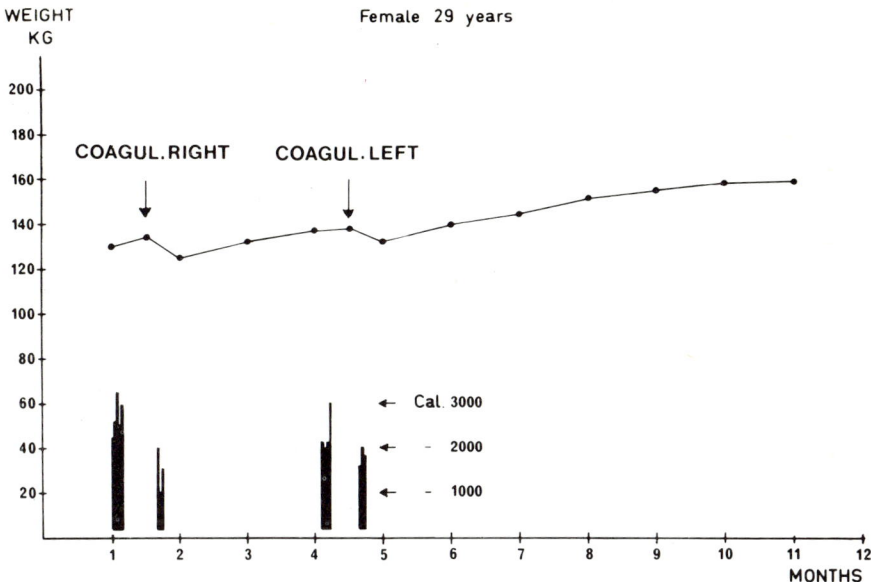

Figure 22.4
Body weight and spontaneous calorie intake in an obese patient before and after bilateral electrocoagulation of the lateral hypothalamus.

and body weight in humans was only to be expected. The lack of effect in one patient with bilateral lesions is more disappointing. It should, however, be noted that this patient did not respond satisfactorily to the second precoagulatory stimulation. I remain convinced that the lesion, if it is to have any lasting effect, should be bilateral. Future plans in this field will include attempts to make a more circumscribed and selective lesion, and the possibility of making the lesion through the stimulation electrode directly, at the site of maximal hunger response, is being considered.

CHOLESTYRAMINE

The possibility of increasing calorie output by means other than that of exercise must be considered. It would be valuable to induce steatorrhoea by means of a drug instead of by the drastic measure of an intestinal shunt operation.

Experiences with shunt operations indicate that the increased faecal loss of calories constitutes no feed-back signal to appetite regulation. Even small daily faecal losses are important because they are not compensated for by a correspondingly increased food intake.

Fat excretion in the faeces of six obese women (body weights ranged from 73 to 110 kg) has been measured during a three week period in which they received 2200 cal daily, 40 per cent from fat. During the second week the patients received 30 g of cholestyramine daily in three doses 30-45 min before meals. Cholestyramine is a resin which reduces fat absorption by binding the bile acids in the intestine. As shown in Figure 22.5, faecal fat excretion increased significantly during treatment, from an average of 27 g in the first week to 89 g in the second week.

Long-term treatment was then attempted using the same dosage of

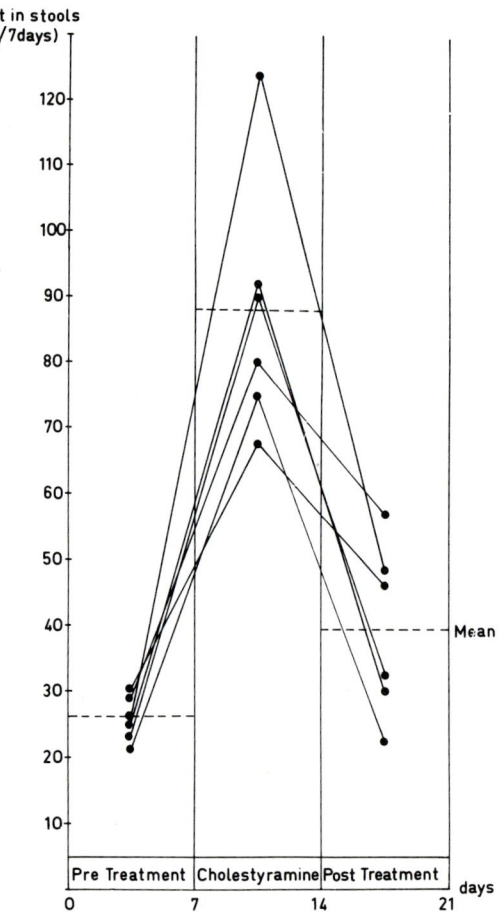

Figure 22.5
Faecal fat excretion in six obese patients before, during and after treatment with 30 g cholestyramine daily.

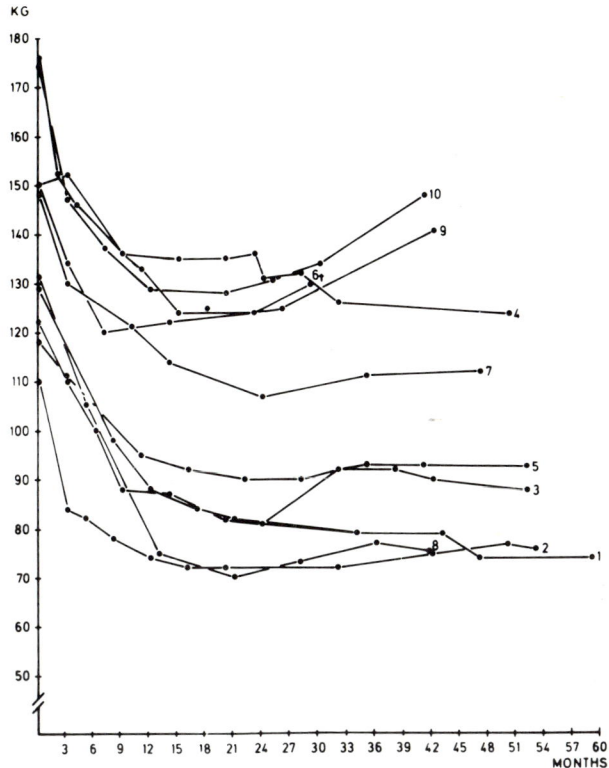

Figure 22.6
Weight loss in 10 obese patients after jejuno-ileostomy leaving 50 cm of small bowel in continuity. (Type I operation)

cholestyramine in association with a free diet. At 3-4 months faecal fat excretion remained high, between 90 and 95 g a week, indicating that no adaptation had taken place. During this time four of the six patients lost between 1 and 4 kg, one gained 3 kg and one patient did not alter her weight.

It had been realized beforehand that significant weight loss could only be hoped for after many months, or even years, of treatment. However, all patients discontinued the treatment before planned, because they could not accept the unpleasant smell and taste of the tablets, of which they had to take 60 a day. It was concluded that the answer to the old problem of a medicament which causes calorie loss without side effects had not been found.

INTESTINAL BYPASS

There remains only one really effective treatment of gross obesity,

348 OBESITY SYMPOSIUM

and that is the intestinal bypass operation. Unfortunately, it is also a treatment which is fraught with discomfort and even risk for the patient. It has therefore been my practice to keep the number of treated patients small and to follow them closely in the post-operative period.

During the last five years of my study jejuno-ileal anastomosis has been performed in 15 obese patients. In the first group of 10 patients, 37.5 cm of proximal jejunum was anastomosed to 13 cm of distal ileum leaving about 50 cm of small bowel in continuity (Type I operation). In the subsequent series of five patients (Type II

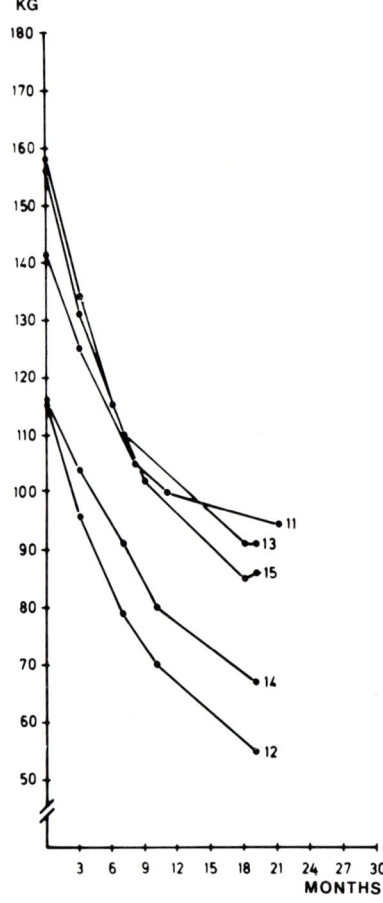

Figure 22.7
Weight loss in five obese patients after jejuno-ileostomy leaving 47 cm of small bowel in continuity. (Type II operation).

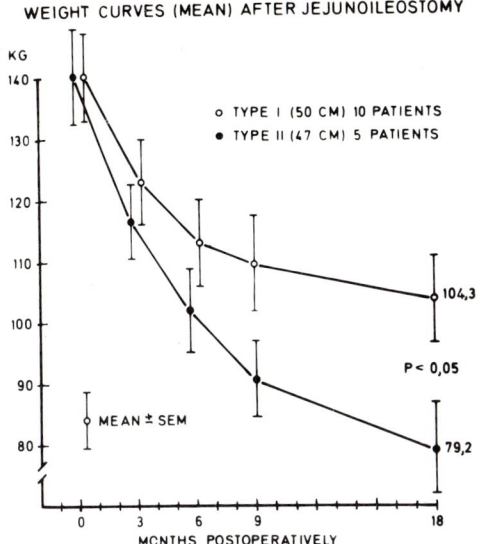

Figure 22.8
Average weight curves of obese patients operated on with Type I and Type II jejuno-ileostomy.

operation), the shunt was shortened by 3.5 cm to a total of 47 cm (34 cm of jejunum and 13 cm of ileum).

The results for the 10 patients with the Type I operation will be seen in Figure 22.6. The absolute weight loss was approximately the same irrespective of the patients' initial body weight. This means that the very obese patients stabilized their weights at too high a level, so that half of the Type I patients find themselves in the unfortunate situation of having a malabsorption syndrome while still remaining considerably obese.

Since weight loss was unrelated to the degree and duration of reflux to the excluded ileum (Quaade *et al*, 1971) the length of functioning small bowel was shortened in the next five patients to 47 cm (Type II). Figure 22.7 shows the individual weight curves of the five Type II patients, and Figure 22.8 the average curves of the two groups. The evident and statistically significant difference in weight loss has lead to the conclusion that the radicality of the surgical intervention should be adjusted individually according to the patients initial body weight. With this proviso I am confident that a satisfactory weight loss can always be ensured, even in gross obesity.

The adverse consequences of the treatment are the frequent bowel movements. This effect is an inevitable concomitant of the mal-

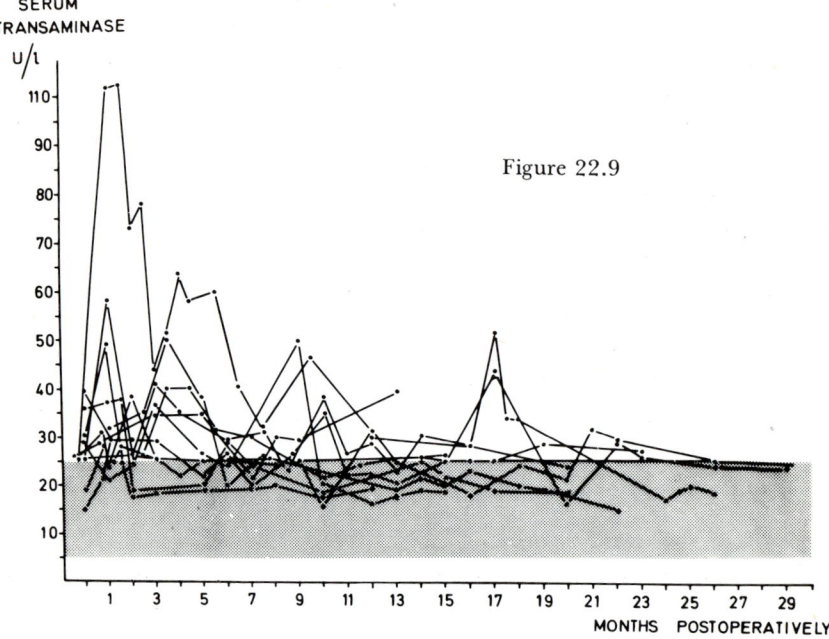

Figure 22.9

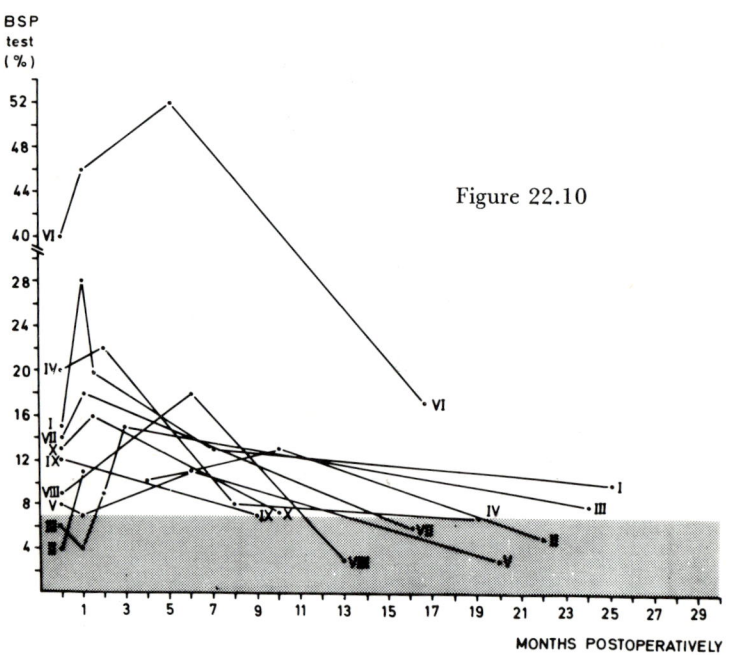

Figure 22.10

absorption syndrome and diminishes with time. It is also safe to say that electrolyte disturbances and vitamin B_{12} depletion should not constitute a problem (Juhl et al, 1973). A hitherto unexplained arthritis has been a problem in some patients, but it rarely necessitates reoperation with taking down of the bypass.

Serious postoperational liver injury has been described especially by Drenick et al (1970). However, when the possibility of liver damage caused by the shunt operation is considered, two facts should be borne in mind. The first is that varying degrees of disturbed liver function and of fatty degeneration are frequently connected with obesity *per se,* irrespective of treatment. Secondly, some impairment of liver function is often observed in obese patients on low calorie diets or during total fasting.

In our experience, patients with a postoperative elevation of serum transaminases and BSP retention show a return towards normal levels with increasing duration of postoperative observation (Figs. 22.9 and 22.10).

Histological appearances in the liver are summarized in Figure 22.11. Biopsies from seven patients during and after surgery showed an increase in fatty degeneration in three, a decrease in three and was no change in one. Extreme degrees of fatty changes were noted in

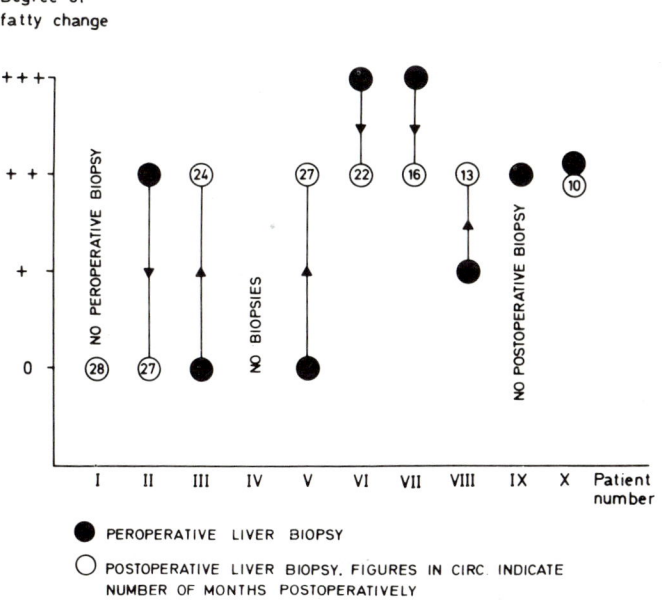

Figure 22.11

two patients at operation, but were not observed after surgery. Weight loss or duration of follow-up did not correlate with changes in the degree of fatty infiltration. Neither parenchymal fibrosis nor proliferation of the bile ducts were demonstrated in any specimens.

In the 15 patients described, one has died two years after operation from acute pulmonary thrombosis.

With the available experience from jejuno-ileal bypass procedures I would advocate it for selected cases of gross obesity. There remains the problem: is the life expectancy better for the operated than for the non-operated patient with gross obesity? No retrospective data are available to solve this problem. In order to produce a reliable answer, I have become a participant in a prospective, multicentre study, in which it is planned to randomize well-defined cases of severe obesity into two groups, one treated conventionally and the other operated upon with jejuno-ileal bypass. There is no doubt what the result will be with regard to weight loss, and it is also likely that after operation most patients have a happier existence. But it is ethically imperative to find out whether their lives are shortened by the operation.

REFERENCES

DRENICK, E.J., SIMMONS, F. & MURPHY, J.F. (1970) Effect on hepatic morphology of treatment of obesity by fasting, reducing diets and small-bowel bypass. *New Eng. J. Med.*, 282, 829.

JUHL, E., BRUUSGAARD, A., HIPPE, E., KORNER, B., QUAADE, F. & BADEN, H. (1974) Vitamin B_{12} depletion in obese patients treated with jejunoileal shunt. Scand. J. Gastroent. In press.

QUAADE, F., JUHL, E., FELDT-RASMUSSEN, K. & BADEN, H. (1971) Blind-loop reflux in relation to weight loss in obese patients treated with jejunoileal anstomosis. *Scand. J. Gastroent.*, 6, 537.

23. Treatment of Obesity: Round Table Discussion

G. A. BRAY (Chairman), P. LEY, JOHN YUDKIN, JOHANNA T. DWYER, J.F. MUNRO, W.J.H. BUTTERFIELD, J.T. SILVERSTONE, J.S. GARROW and F. QUAADE.

Dr. Bray. We will start with a brief comment by each of the panellists to the following question: when do you treat obesity?

Dr. Ley. When the overweight is a danger to the patient's health or when the patient is overweight and wishes to lose weight for reasons best-known to themselves.

Dr. Quaade. Obesity is, by definition, an accumulation of fat which poses problems to the individual's psychological, or physical well-being. As soon as problems arise in these two spheres, the individual should be treated. That means that moderate degrees of obesity in people with no problems are better left alone in many instances.

Dr. Silverstone. I agree with everything that has been said, but I would include another group—the very overweight adolescent, because they have considerable psychological problems, as a result of their social isolation.

Dr. Garrow. I think that obesity should be treated when we believe that the benefits of treatment will outweigh the difficulties. I agree that the exception is the obese adolescent, who is often unwilling to undertake the rigours of dieting. These are the people I try hard to persuade. However, in adults in general, I would be guided by whether the patients agreed that they stood to gain more than they might lose.

Dr. Munro. I should like to re-emphasise that it is not only when we believe treatment is advisable but when we have persuaded the patient to believe this.

There are situations in which more harm than good can be done by trying to achieve weight loss in a patient who is not motivated appropriately in that direction, in particular, the patient referred by his general practitioner, or because a close relative has made him come. If the patient himself does not want to lose weight, we are wasting time.

Professor Yudkin. The first treatment for obesity is prophylaxis. It is a public health problem. If we could find ways by which more people could be persuaded not to become overweight, our task as physicians would be less difficult.

Secondly, having agreed in broad terms with what has been said previously, we should remember that we do not really treat obesity— it is the patients who treat themselves. This is a condition par excellence in which we try to persuade people to undergo self-treatment.

Dr. Dwyer. I agree with Professor Yudkin; the time to treat obesity is when the patients are ready to be treated. Some of the follow-up work we did indicated that the eight or nine year old girls and boys did much better. Again about the age of fifteen it is possible to capitalize on their self interest in dieting, especially among the girls.

Dr. Bray. Dr. Silverstone and others have mentioned adolescence. Are there some ways in which these adolescents can be motivated to succeed? Are there some variables which can be identified when treatment is begun to give some idea of who will be successful, and who will not? Dr. Ley pointed out internalization versus externalization. Are there any other criteria which would be helpful in aiding us to motivate people, or are there any criteria and characteristics by which we can identify those likely to succeed?

Dr. Ley. Before we did our research I would have said that in order to motivate patients you should frighten them, use group decision and two-sided communications. Having obtained negative results, I am not sure this is correct!

Dr. Silverstone. The under-twenties are the most difficult to treat—I think Dr. Ley found it to be so, but I still think this is the group with which to try the hardest.

Dr. Bray. What do you do for them?

Dr. Silverstone. We might try some of the techniques mentioned by Dr. Ley. I know he said that, in practice, none of these techniques was better than any other, but looking at his data, he achieved nearly 50 per cent greater weight loss with the Stuart and Nurnberger approach. We have not tried this with adolescents nor, as far as I know, have other workers. We have done it with adults in a slightly different way—not using a questionnaire or an instruction sheet, but exactly as Stuart did it by giving programmed instructions week by week. We did this for twelve weeks, comparing it with a control group who were given equal interviews, talking traditionally about their weight problems, psychological problems, etc. I have data showing that the Stuart form of treatment was more effective in the short-term. We have no follow-up data.

I studied a small group of housewives who are among the most resistant in our community to this form of treatment. I wanted to see whether the method was successful with working class women, not unintelligent but certainly not sophisticated people. It seemed to succeed when they were treated individually but when we tried it again in groups it did not work at all well.

The mean weight loss was not startling, but the difference was obvious. We switched round therapists so that each patient was treated by 'psychotherapy' by one therapist, and then changed to 'Stuart treatment', and *vice versa*.

Dr. Bray. Can I ask you to extend this a little? We have been seeing a number of the grossly obese adolescents, aged between thirteen and seventeen, weighing 300 lb or more, who do not generally profit by this kind of therapy or by dietary advice. How vigorous are you willing to be? Are these individuals subjects for coagulation of the lateral hypothalamus, or by-pass surgery, or intensive psychoanalysis? What can be done with this group?

Dr. Silverstone. Dr. Quaade has convinced me that hypothalectomy is not very good. By-pass surgery in a young adolescent can lead to extraordinary problems. We have heard elsewhere that the problems of flatus are so great that wives refuse to sleep in the same room as their husband and workmates refused to work in the same place. As far as I can gather, there are considerable social problems arising from this procedure.

In-patient treatment, such as practised by Dr. Munro and his colleagues, would seem to be a much safer procedure. I wondered whether Dr. Garrow would apply a dental splint; we have not heard him discuss this interesting, untraditional form of treatment.

Dr. Garrow. I have persuaded one of my dental colleagues to fit a dental splint to the teeth of a small number of patients who agreed that they found themselves unable to control their eating. With this in place, it is possible to drink but not eat. This is a desperate attempt to find an alternative to by-pass surgery; it is more readily reversible and, in principle, less dangerous.

In our present state of knowledge, I would not embark on such procedures in adolescents because I think that the psychological harm might outweigh any physical benefits.

Dr. Munro. One thing we can do for patients is to give them a realistic concept of the expected rate of weight loss. Adolescents, in particular, have a very unrealistic approach, and expect to lose weight very rapidly. They become disheartened when they do not achieve this.

They must be convinced that theirs is a life-long problem, and that slow but steady weight loss is much more satisfactory than drastic weight reduction, with subsequent weight regain.

Professor Yudkin. I am surprised that no-one has used the word 'motivation'. The patient clearly needs to want to lose weight sufficiently. I have never seen a fat ballet dancer, or a fat jockey or boxer.

Dr. Dwyer. First, motivation. We have found, in working with children and adolescents, that it is often the patient's mother who requests the treatment, not the patient who is usually a girl. The mother does all the talking: we circumvent this by interviewing both separately. Frightening them into losing weight does not work very well with young children or adolescents because they are not frightened of dying of a heart attack, for example, although adolescent girls may be frightened of not having a date the following Saturday night.

Another extremely important aspect is that during the course of therapy the child, or young adolescent must learn more about himself and what to expect. There is confusion between fatness and other aspects of the body form. We hope to leave the patients understanding their own growth, and perhaps themselves, better at the end of their treatment.

Dr. Quaade. I should like to comment on by-pass operations in adolescents. Our view is that the patient should be of age before this operation can be contemplated, even in cases of gross obesity. There are a number of reasons for this, including medico-legal aspects and, most important, our ignorance of the really long-term consequences of the operation. However, the operation is not as irreversible as has been stated. It is always possible to remove the shunt.

I have some experience with drug-induced anorexia as treatment of obesity in childhood. I have done this in controlled studies with amphetamine. It is effective, as in adults, for a short time. Amphetamine did not produce dependence in the children; it seems that the young child is not prone to addiction, but the treatment does not help the obesity for more than a short period of time.

Dr. Bray. May we extend that a little further to another question: does the Panel know any scientific reasons why tolerance develops to the anorexic drugs in adults?

Dr. Silverstone. I wonder whether tolerance does develop. Miss Samuel quoted one study, and Dr. Munro's work with fenfluramine also showed that it takes a long time for tolerance to develop.

McKay's work on diethylpropion seemed to show that it was still having some effect almost one year after treatment had commenced.

I think tolerance is not just a matter of pharmacological effect, but also a matter of adhering to the diet, with or without the drug.

Dr. Bray. To extend this a little, the Food and Drug Administration (FDA) in the United States has examined all the data from clinical trials which have been submitted by pharmaceutical companies in order to confirm the effectiveness of their agents. The FDA indicated two months ago that provided sufficient patients have been retained in the trials in them for analysis, the effectiveness of the anorexic drug has remained clearly evident for as long as twenty weeks. There is no evidence of any decrease of effect of any one drug, or of superiority of any one drug. The main problem is the high drop-out rate of patients from the studies; few of them maintain sufficient subjects for analysis at twenty weeks. Those which did showed significantly greater effect with anorexic agents than with non-anorexic agents.

Dr. Munro. This is not in keeping with the Edinburgh experience. Figure 23.1 shows the experience covering a number of years in Edinburgh, on patients defined as suffering from refractory obesity. Each is a double-blind study. The control group either gained a little weight, or there was no change in weight.

In patients with refractory obesity, irrespective of the drugs used, the mean anorexic effect is lost after six to eight weeks.

When we compared the weight losses on continuous and intermittent phentermine (one month on and one month off) there was no significant difference between the two dosage regimes over a thirty-six week period. The placebo group lost a little weight to start with but then their weight loss flattened out at about 12 weeks.

If phentermine or any of the other similar amphetamine analogue is being used, it should be given intermittently only, on the grounds that this is cheaper, as effective and, presumably, is less likely to lead to drug addiction. The interesting difference is between this and fenfluramine. With intermittent fenfluramine employing acute withdrawal, the results were bad. There was a high incidence of withdrawal depression. The results are comparable to the placebo effect in a similar group of patients; whereas fenfluramine given continuously appears to have a different effect. If fenfluramine is being prescribed, it should be given to the patient until the value of the drug has been lost, at which stage it should be discontinued.

Dr. Silverstone. I do not question your findings, but what you may be showing is not drug tolerance but diet tolerance. Continuous phentermine could work continuously. It is not better or worse than the other. We should take people on continuous drug treatment and determine the anorexic effect, using for example the linear analogue scale at monthly intervals. We could then see whether it still has the same potential anorexic effect. It may not have the same weight reducing effect because patients may not be adhering to their diet, or for other reasons.

Dr. Garrow. Dr. Munro and his colleagues carried out measurements at four-week intervals. (Fig. 23.1) In the last eight weeks of continuous fenfluramine treatment there was perhaps a little more than 1 kg weight loss. To say that the effect continued for thirty-six weeks is only marginally true but I accept that trials up to twenty weeks have shown that the anorexic effect continues. The drop-out rate tends to produce reports of continuous activity—for example, in a recent long-term study on diethylpropion the mean weight loss of the group continued for a very long time simply because the less successful patients dropped out.

Dr. Bray. Could I give another interpretation? A paper published in 1948 showed the results of a forty-week study with dextroamphetamine. The discussion was that if tolerance or loss of effectiveness develops, there would not be a plateau of body weight but a re-accumulation of weight to the level seen with the placebo. It was argued that the plateau, as seen with all these drugs, occurring after six weeks, or longer, was a reflection of

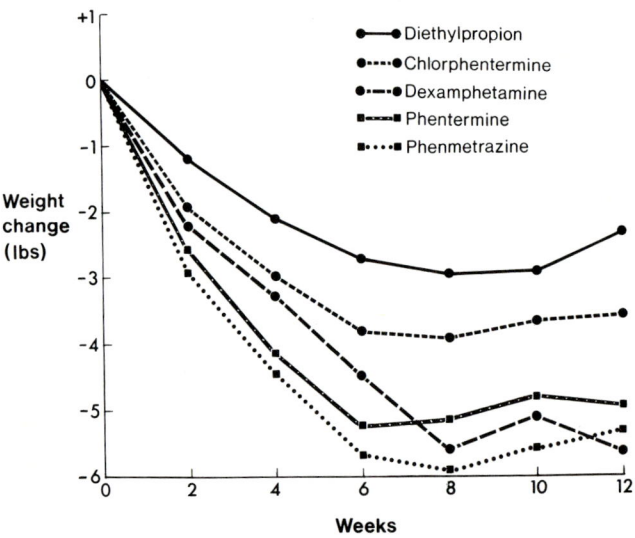

Figure 23.1

continued activity and a readjustment between the calorie intake and body requirements. This is in contrast to a re-accumulation of weight if the drug has lost effect. I believe this was a reasonable interpretation of the studies, and would fit with those present studies.

Dr. Craddock. I do not believe we should stop drug treatment after twenty weeks. For example, I have a patient who has lost 115lb during eleven months continuing drug treatment and he is still losing weight. Of my last ninety-six patients treated with anorexic drugs, twenty-seven have continued to lose weight after three months and nine have continued to lose weight after six months. Intermittent treatment presents practical problems.

Dr. Bray. There has been a question on both sides of the Atlantic about the effectiveness of commercial slimming groups, relative to what is offered by physicians. Does anyone have any evidence or thoughts about whether these groups are more or less effective than physicians as a group?

Dr. Ashwell. When we were compiling the 'Which?' slimming guide, commercial slimming groups were covered. We sent out a questionnaire to about two thousand people who said they had experience of slimming. They were asked whether they had been to a slimming club and how much weight they had lost there, which club it was, what they thought about it, which were its best factors and which its worst. There was a summary question at the end and it was clear that dieting, with the help of a slimming group, was the best method—better than diet alone, better than diet and exercise and better than dieting with the advice of a physician.

It was the people who had been to commercial slimming groups who were the most enthusiastic slimmers. This was in 1971 and Weight Watchers was a very active group, whereas the other slimming groups were only just starting. We found that 80 per cent of the people who told us about groups had attended Weight Watchers, and only 20 per cent belonged to other groups.

We asked them which were the most important factors in the group that made it successful for them. The two most frequently quoted were constant encouragement given by the lecturer, and the feeling of being part of a group of people with similar problems.

Another response to this question was that money was paid each week. I was very impressed by the success of these groups though the most they are usually granted is grudging approval!

Dr. Silverstone. We must, first, compare like with like. I mentioned yesterday that the hospital attender is in a different category from the general practitioner attender and, in turn, is probably in a different category from the Weight Watcher attender. Many of the last will have already been to their physician. A thorough epidemiological study needs to be done, with patients allocated randomly to all sorts of treatment before any conclusions can be drawn.

If Weight Watchers could show that 40 per cent of their population got down to goal weight, they will have done much better than anybody could ever claim for any other method. The answer may come out of the Oxford analysis of their data.

Dr. Dwyer. I have some experience of various slimming clubs in the Boston area.

The disadvantages of the slimming groups are that they are related specifically to adult obesity rather than to childhood and adolescent obesity. The diets are geared to adult needs and preferences rather than to the way children eat and the life they lead. The emphasis is on weight loss rather than loss of fat; this comes across very strongly week after week. Inactivity is given almost no emphasis in the groups which I have attended. Psychological support is inadequate and not directed towards children and adolescents, who need far more psychological support than do middle-class, stable ladies.

The nutrition information is sometimes incorrect. The goals are usually set by the patient herself. With adolescents, we find that they invariably set their ideal weights lower than we would set them. Finally, false impressions are created of the many brands of low calorie foods which these groups promote and sell.

The advantages of these groups are many and should not be neglected. Certainly, the reducing diets, at least among the most popular commercial clubs in the United States, are adequate in nutrients other than calories—at least for adults. Usually the permission of a physician is required before advice may be given although this varies from state to state. They foster group support and friendly competition and furnish a social outlet against the boredom at home—especially for adult women. They also provide some way of constantly monitoring the food intake and weight, with rewards for success. Of course, the patient is involved socially in her own therapy. Cooking hints are also provided. They have been much more ready to explore some of the behaviour techniques which traditionalists have neglected. Their costs are probably lower in terms of effectiveness, but this remains to be seen. All other aspects connected with group therapy, which have been explored today, are also important.

Professor Yudkin. The fact remains that, having said all this, we do not have hard information about the success rate of any of the slimming clubs do we? We do not know that number of people who went, what their problem was, how overweight they were, how long they stayed and what was their success.

Dr. Bray. Indeed, we do not have very satisfactory comparative data. Doctors Stunkard and McLaren provided one of the few sets of criteria for comparisons between various groups and methods. Most others are not satisfactory. Methods are needed for standardizing comparisons so that clinical judgements may be made.

Dr. Garrow. That is extremely important. If we say that slimming clubs ought to publish their results and make them comparable, this is equally true of obesity clinics and private physicians.

Professor Keen. Most of the discussion has been on the subject of treatment of obesity. We are talking about a group of people who have exceeded some threshold of normality which either they appreciate themselves or which is appreciated by their parents or others for them.

Could the Panel concern itself a little with the question of the establishment of norms in the population as a whole? Are we all too fat? Should we be setting new patterns of body weight and body size, if we are going to make a serious attempt to reduce the frequency, for example, of atherosclerosis, of diabetes mellitus and of a number of other conditions? The techniques adopted by us must be very different; with the chronically failed case of obesity we are dealing with the wreckage of the situation. How can this be tackled in the general population?

A word of reassurance and optimism. We have taken a group of ostensibly normal men in whom obesity is represented no more frequently than in the population at large. We have given them instruction to restrict their carbohydrate intake to 120g daily and put some effort into their education. We also have a randomly selected control group who have been given no such instruction. As a result, compared with the placebo group there has been a mean fall of 14lb in weight in the carbohydrate restricted group, which has been maintained for four-and-a-half years now.

Dr. Durnin. It is high time that we started to look at the distribution of fat in the community and here I have to return to my basic premise that we should start measuring fat rather than measuring body weight. If the amount of fat is known, then, by means of community studies, we can determine the prevalence of different degrees of fatness in the population. We can then assess this in relation to disease processes, or psychiatric disorders, or whatever particularly interests us.

The obvious standards we have are those which appertain to people who universally would be considered able to do hard physical work; athletes are a good example. We could therefore say that this is a desirable norm, and there is no reason why as we become older, we should become fatter; perhaps we might reduce our body fat with increasing age. This is exactly what was found in an active population in New Guinea. There was a uniform fat content at all ages, equivalent both in men and women to the amount present in athletic Caucasian males and females. This was a community doing moderately hard physical work.

Professor Yudkin. One must ask, standards for whom? If it is recognised that obesity is a public health problem, we need people to recognise for themselves that they need to reduce their adiposity, or prevent their adiposity. There needs to be some sort of criterion which is not so much a precise standard but good enough for the general population.

Dr. Dwyer. I would like to agree but beauty is in the eye of the beholder. We have found too that fitness is in the eye of the beholder. We have interviewed many subjects who feel they are extremely active since they walk to their cars in the morning! In the programme I have discussed obese girls who were being treated and were driven to school in cars. I am not sure that it is possible to count on an individual's perceptions, or on the perceptions of the general public. Our data suggest that adolescent girls tend to aim at a figure less than their physician would accept and middle-aged gentlemen the reverse.

Dr. Ashwell. I can confirm Dr. Dwyer's comments. In a study of attitudes to weight we found that 15 per cent of young women, aged 15 to 29, were actually classed as underweight on the Metropolitan Life Insurance figures, yet thought they were overweight.

In the survey 2000 people who, it must be admitted, were interested in their weight in that they claimed slimming experience, were asked what would be their ideal weight. This was classified according to the Metropolitan Life Insurance figures. Eighty per cent gave a figure which would be classified as suitable i.e. ± 10 per cent of the Metropolitan Life Insurance figures for middle frames.

It seems that the general public are aiming at near ideal figures and I think we will have to have something very good to replace them.

Dr. Bray. The Gallup organisation which does polls in the United States completed one about two months ago on the number of people who either thought they were overweight, or who were doing something about it. I think 46 per cent of the population either considered themselves overweight or were actively doing something about it. This meant that they had some standard against which they compared themselves. I think you are right, and that the general public use standards, usually the Metropolitan Life figures and it would be difficult to displace them.

Dr. Howard. Does Dr. Munro think that starvation is feasible on an out-patient basis? It is a common experience among these in-patients receiving low calorie diets that they do not feel hungry. Why do they not feel hungry? Would they feel hungry at home, in free-living conditions and completely starved?

Dr. McLean Baird and I have recently succeeded in using very low calorie diets, 200 to 300 cal/day for out-patient treatment of obesity.

Dr. Munro. We have tried but only two of our patients managed to adhere to the regime for any length of time. In retrospect, I regretted having starved them. They were peculiarly obsessional people who had become extremely disturbed and obsessed by their weight at the end of the treatment.

Altogether we have starved 11 out-patients, all of whom had had experience of in-patient starvation. However, I never starve them for more than three weeks.

Dr. Galton. I have seen two patients on therapeutic starvation who after a few days became severely ketoacidotic. This was accompanied by nausea and vomiting. If they had not been under supervision in hospital, this might have had serious consequences.

Dr. Munro. I agree entirely. We see all patients who are being starved at home twice weekly.

Dr. Howard. It has often been claimed that in complete starvation the lack of hunger is due to ketonaemia. Dr. Silverstone disagreed with this point of view because patients without ketosis receiving an 800 Kcalorie diet in hospital did not feel hungry either. Our experience is that when patients are put on to complete starvation they are not hungry, and when they are given carbohydrate to prevent ketosis they are still not hungry.

Dr. Silverstone. Patients were given a questionnaire twice a day just before normal meal times for a period of three days. When they were having control measurements taken during a period when they were receiving eight hundred calories per day, they felt normally hungry. They were then starved for two weeks. They were very hungry on the first day, and showed a reversal on the second day with the appearance of quite severe ketosis, and then their hunger fluctuated around the original level. The hunger did not disappear. When they were re-fed their hunger reduced, i.e. they became satiated rather easily at the end of the starvation period.

Dr. Garrow. There is one possible hazard to out-patient starvation.

I have seen one patient who developed an acute magnesium deficiency. This may also apply to other nutrients.

Mr. Miller. Let me return to the argument of the effectiveness of anorexic agents. It seems to me that to determine effectiveness one needs to measure food intake.

Since, within a given population, people are able to maintain weight at different levels of food intake, it seems reasonable that those who show no further weight loss may have settled for a new balance at a new calorie intake level.

Professor Adadevoh. The discussion is very heavily biased towards hospital-based treatment. Obesity is a public problem and the approach should be similar to that adopted for any infectious disease, or immunization scheme. We should place the emphasis on a public health approach and measures should be directed towards prevention. The climate now is such that the problem should be recognised.

Dr. Garrow. People need to be motivated but it is easy to be glib about motivation. How can we motivate people? People with painful osteoarthritic knees can be overweight and understand that relief from pain could be obtained by losing weight. They are as motivated as anyone can be, in a reasonably free society, yet they still cannot lose weight.

By all means let us try to motivate people but it is not always easy to do this.

Dr. Kannel. We have to conceive of obesity, like any other major problem, as consisting of a number of categories. One is the general problem in which we have about one-third of the general population estimated to be 20 per cent above some ideal weight. Physicians cannot deal with that.

Secondly, there are those who are massively obese. They have a special problem connected with their body bulk, they have special metabolic problems and they may require drastic treatment measures.

Thirdly, there are those in whom overweight is one feature of a general medical problem. In other words, they need to reduce their weight because they have diabetes or hypertension or heart failure, etc.

For the general problem in the general population, we do not need to lose hope. Epidemiological data tell us that theirs is not a medical problem, but a social one. We have lost sight of the fact that women are much lighter nowadays than they used to be. I cannot help but feel that this must be response to social pressure. It is more fashionable to be lean.

Mr. Harvey. What does Professor Yudkin consider are the low cost, low carbohydrate, high protein and nutritious foods in 1973 which we can advise our patients to buy and eat?

Professor Yudkin. First, it is often forgotten that reduction in carbohydrate frequently means a reduction in expensive foods which people buy—such as soft drinks, confectionery, cakes and biscuits.

Secondly, there are some high protein foods which are less expensive than others; for example, cheddar cheese and eggs.

Thirdly, patients on carbohydrate reduced diets have been shown to be eating less than previously. In practice, I find that the cost of low carbohydrate diets are marginally less, on average, even today, than the average diet of an uncontrolled food pattern of an average obese patient. One study showed that whilst it was substantially less than the average cost of the normal diet consumed by such people, it was a little more than a very carefully calculated calorie counted diet. Thus, it does not have to be an expensive diet.

The most important thing is to remind people that they will save, in most cases, on the carbohydrate-rich foods. When people are told to reduce their carbohydrate intake, they think of cutting out bread and do not calculate the saving in terms of manufactured foods, mostly sugar-rich foods.

Dr. Munro. Many patients drift insidiously into obesity. One of the positive steps which we should try is to ensure that all manufactured food has its calorie content on the label. Some people do not appreciate the calorie content of their food or drinks.

Dr. Richards. I agree. If we consider the high pressure advertising to which we are exposed, we should be directing our attention to the public health aspect. Advice to parents, and particularly in terms of food values, might perhaps do far more than anything that we can offer as physicians.

I want to return to discuss the severe naturesis which occurs during periods of starvation. It is clear now that a large proportion of this is probably due to increased glucagon secretion and may result in severe postural hypotension. There is a marked sodium retention and oedema when the patient is re-fed. This is another reason why it is perhaps inadvisable to treat out-patients on starvation regimes.

Dr. Burland. We have concentrated on treating the obese adult. Whether one believes in critical periods in infancy and childhood, and whether one believes in the importance of the numbers of adipocytes acquired in childhood, the problem must surely go back to childhood. If we can prevent or treat obesity early in infancy or childhood, this must drastically reduce the numbers of obese patients presenting in adult life. In order to achieve that we would have to spend some considerable time rearing a population of lean children who would become discerning parents and eventually discerning grandparents, because mothers and grandmothers have a marked influence on food intake and obesity in childhood.

Surely we should direct our attention not only to the prevention and treatment of adult obesity, but much more seriously to education and understanding of the development of obesity in infancy and childhood.

Perhaps we should practice dietary education in 'Well' Baby Clinics.

Dr. Bray. Dr. Dwyer dealt most with the potential for educating the group. Is there anything more that we can do? Dr. Burland is right, I am sure; many obese adults started their obesity during childhood.

SUMMARY

W.J.H. BUTTERFIELD

The round Table Discussion has been of great interest: it has touched on a large number of topics related to the treatment of obesity.

Anthropologically, obesity is a relatively new problem. Man has been evolving for 30 million years, but only in the last 10 thousand has he had agriculture to provide a steady source of food, and it is only in the last, perhaps, two thousand years that it has been possible for many people to become obese.

With regard to Dr. Burland's comments on children, one of my paediatric friends has scales in his department, which weigh from 5 to 20 lbs. When he started to use them almost all the one year old babies could be weighed on those scales, now not all of the six month old babies can be weighed on them. I am sure that mothers encourage overeating in pregnant daughters, who themselves by using new baby foods add to the tendency in their offspring; perhaps we should motivate mothers differently and encourage them by means of prizes to keep their babies weights within the proper range. Prophylaxis is certainly better than treatment as far as obesity is concerned.

It is now well known that overfeeding in early infancy increases not only the total amount of adipose tissue, but also the total number of adipocytes. We need, first of all, a simple diagnostic procedure which will give us an indication as to whether there are excessive numbers of adipocytes as well as enlarged cells. Confirmation may come from the history, particularly if the patient or a senior relative knows that they have been fat since infancy. In such cases we shall need to devise diets which take not only fat from the adipocytes, but also treatments which affect the whole cell, including the nuclear DNA content so that, in fact, we are attacking the number of cells as well as their size. Otherwise because smaller fat cells are now recognised to be more insulin sensitive than larger ones, as soon as the dieting ends the fat mass will promptly increase again as, alas, we all know too well!

Is starvation the answer to this problem of looting the storage cells in the adipose mass not only of their energy, but also of their nucleic acids? We obviously need much more information on this and follow-up of strict starvation versus other dietary regimes as regards the number of fat cells.

Dr. Howard mentioned the idea of starvation as a dietary treatment for out-patients. There are risks, of course, depending on the basal nutrition and the presence of mineral deficiencies, including those which follow from naturesis and magnesium loss, which could lead to complex circulatory, hormonal, and metabolic problems.

For a long time actuaries in insurance companies have realised that overweight is a serious problem and it is recognised that weight loss in obese people is associated with a decrease in mortality. The doctor in practice is faced with problems of morbidity and he needs to know how much morbidity can be prevented by treating obesity. Not all fat people become diabetic, or hypertensive, or osteoarthritic, and doctors need to know how to be able to identify those at such risk. Will this come from the family history? Do all forms of morbidity follow a similar pattern to mortality and improve with weight loss, or do they return later, as ageing proceeds?

Besides these deceptively simply clinical questions we have much more to learn about the interaction between the gastro-intestinal tract and the hunger and satiety centres, about the psychology of eating and how it is related to depression in some patients, or aggressive instincts in others. We remain ignorant of the motivation of people who lose weight, which is particularly important since we will probably need to adopt the appropriate approach to each individual obese person coming for treatment. Some will need group psychotherapy, others need a pill, others psychotherapy on an individual basis, and for others there may be more effective treatments still to be worked out. One hopes that eventually therapy will be related to the cause—too many fat cells in infancy, wrong setting of the appetite centre, before or after childbearing, and so on.

In closing, therefore, may I thank the speakers for a very stimulating occasion, and the organisers of the symposium for reminding us that obesity is a large field with many aspects still remaining for investigation.

24. Summary of Meeting

C. C. BOOTH

I am a gastro-enterologist, mostly interested in people who are underweight as a result of gut disease, and my task is usually to make them put on weight.

I have been impressed by the degree of socio-economic and political overtones which go with obesity and which have emerged from this meeting. Only an American could say that the most common nutritional problem in the world today is obesity, whereas most of us would take a different view, in relation to other parts of the world. Only a contributor from an English hospital would have been so emphatic about the differences among social classes.

Usually when I hear cells being discussed at a meeting, I am involved in detailed discussions about the functions of lyzozomes and, if energy is involved at all, mitochondria and the role of inner and outer membranes. To have spent two days without hearing either of those organelles mentioned is a remarkable thing in this modern cellular era. The absence of any mention of the word 'immunology' is also remarkable.

This leads me on to talk about the adipose organ. Dr. Widdowson made the point that it is a fundamental and fascinating organ, in a comparative sense, particularly if one considers the function of the adipose organ in the migrating bird, or the Pacific or Atlantic salmon when it is travelling up river. Its physiology has been touched on remarkably little in discussion. Themes have tended to be developed relating either to experimental models or to the different types of obesity which occur in man.

I have heard the term 'adipocyte' from time to time, but find the adipocyte extremely difficult to define. I was confused by the inability of any of the speakers to present a definition of what is an adipocyte. Many people think it is a fibroblast which takes up lipid, but what does that mean, and is it specific? What of this question of numbers, and whether it is possible to measure the numbers of adipocytes or their size? I have the impression that there is considerable difference of view between what happens in experimental animals and what happens in man. A number of people showed that adipocytes in different sites can be of different sizes—in biological terms that would not surprise me at all. It is also clear that different sites will yield different sorts of adipocytes.

I like Dr. Galton's idea that the adipocyte is following in the wake of the erythrocyte, but the erythrocyte has three major areas of clinical interest: one is its main protein, haemoglobin, and all the diseases associated with that; secondly, there are enzyme defects associated with the erthyrocyte; thirdly, there is the immunology of the red cell membrane, the first area in which autoimmune disease was postulated. I do not think that Dr. Galton has made the case yet that the adipocyte has reached that degree of sophistication—whether it will in future remains to be seen.

Immunologically speaking, there are a number of disorders of lipid tissue which occur. One is the curious lipodystrophy which occurs in people with hypocomplementaemic nephritis, which appears to involve the upper part of the trunk rather than the lower. Whether this involves an immunological reaction which affects adipocytes is not known, but I suspect that it is the adipocytes rather than the nucleic acids which are affected since if they are involved, it could almost certainly occur in all the other cells in the body which have the same nucleic acid content.

The discussion of the control of appetite has been fascinating. Dr. Anand has done outstanding work in this field, and the work from other sources which has been presented at this meeting intrigues me greatly. It seems sad that the specific therapeutic manoeuvres which Dr. Quaade and his colleagues have made have not led to an effective form of therapy. That makes me wonder whether, physiologically, we are not missing something. I am sure that we are missing out the influence of the gastro-intestinal tract.

As a gastro-enterologist, I was fascinated that although there is interest in what is laid down in tissue, how it arrives there by way of the membrane of the gut has received remarkably little attention. I do not know what mechanism controls this in the gut, or the small intestine, but I am convinced that such mechanisms as exist are extremely subtle, that we know nothing about them at present, and that we will within the next ten or fifteen years. It may be that there are receptors in the gut which induce reactions of various sorts hormonally, and are vital to appetite control and to what the gut is called upon to do. Clearly, this is theory at present but, as far as hyperphagia is concerned, there is some evidence available. For example, it is known that in hyperphagic animals who become obese, the villi show hyperplasia. They do not show hypertrophy; the cells do not enlarge, but there are more cells, and longer villi. I do not know what it is that causes this to occur but clearly something which is present in food and which goes through a group of cells which have a transport function. They then respond by hyperplasia. This is interesting because it is comparable to what is being postulated in relation to lipids being deposited in the adipose organ.

Gut cells are extremely interesting to study in this sense. It is possible to work out the effect of removal of an area on hyperplasia in another area. The answer for surface membranes, in general, is that if a piece of tissue is removed, there is no general increase in terms of hyperplasia. Thus, if a piece of gut or skin is removed, hyperplasia in the residual tissue does not usually result. Hyperplasia in gut occurs only in proportion to the hyperalimentation which may develop as a result of that procedure. This is different from what happens with organs which are internal. Dr. Galton made the point that if half of the liver is resected, then the other half develops hyperplasia. With the adipose organ, if half is resected what happens to the other half? Is it an organ, like the liver, which then develops hyperplasia? I do not believe we have the answer.

This Symposium has been very interesting in terms of making me think about other aspects of biology in relation to adipocytes, and their action. Intestinal function is interesting in the sense that our intestine is oriented to a nutritional scheme of things, which goes back into the mists of time. Man being not only an omnivore, but an obligatory carnivore, and being—certainly in Caucasian races—predominantly carnivorous in his background, he has been involved in a form of nutrition which is totally different from that to which he is now exposed. There is no doubt that a lion who kills, then sleeps for three days and kills again, needs a long and effective intestinal tract to deal with a large amount of food which he takes in at any one time. On the other hand, the human intestine is adapted now to taking regular meals, in a civilized sense, and receives more food than it would under any other circumstances. In these terms, it is possible to look upon the distal intestine, the ileum—the part that Dr. Quaade's group is trying to short-circuit—as the reserve area, not normally needed except for the transport of vitamin B_{12} and the bile acids.

I am not sure that I am so uninterested in the question of short-circuiting operations for severe obesity as some others. I look at it as one who sees many patients who have had massive resections of intestine for clinical reasons. Post operatively, it is astonishing how well they are, in a nutritional sense, with remarkably little intestine. The problem of flatus can be dealt with usually by dietary management.

Postgraduate education, in contrast to undergraduate education, teaches what is not known, rather than what is. I have had a very enjoyable two days. I should like, finally, to say something about Lord Rothschild. He is a member of a very famous European banking family, and a biologist of notable distinction who has spent most of his life as a basic scientist. He was called in by the government of this country two years ago to report on research funding. Nowadays, whenever I am asked to look at somebody's research fund application, I have to bear in my administrative mind constantly the thought of what Lord Rothschild would say about their proposals. In other words, could your research be undertaken on a contractual basis, with value for investment being the hallmark of success. Listening to the discussions today, I do not know what Lord Rothschild would have said. If it could be said that all the money which has been used over the last ten years had really done something for obese people, particularly in Western society, that would be worthwhile. I think it has been suggested that it would be difficult to prove that anything physicians and nutritionists have done has had any real effect yet. But it may well be that you have done all the basic work and so there is no reason for us to lose hope.

Index

Absorption, intestinal, compounds altering, 294, 295
Adenyl cyclase, 204
Adipocyte (Adipose cell), enlarging, triglyceride in, 211
  deranged metabolism of, 18
  failure to define, 369
  function, 192
  hormones, effects on, 204–216
  human and its disorders, 192–202
    changes in diabetes, 194–196
    excessive release, 199–202
    storage, 196–199
    failure of storage, 193–196
    glucose entry to, 194, 195
  hyperplasia and insulin insensitivity in, 33
  in obesity, 91–95
  lipid content, 87
  lipogenesis in, 17, 18
  lipoma, 198, 199
  number and age, 88, 89
    and age at obesity onset, 92, 98
    infancy overnutrition and, 93
    weight loss and, 92
  number and marasmus, 81
    in obesity, 15
    and size with high fat diet, 103
    and size in rats, 16
  size and
    adipose tissue mass changes, 231
    exercise, 176, 178–185
    glycerol release, 16, 17
    metabolism, 178–185, 206–208, 210
      glucose, 181

  nutritional state, 209
  plasma insulin, 177
  subcutaneous $v.$ deep sites, 215
  surface area and fat stores, 167
Adipose organ (see also Adipose tissue)
  cellular growth, 87–90
  critical development periods, 92, 93
  growth, 85–87
  hypercellularity, 98, 99
  nature of, 99
Adipose tissue (see also Adipose organ)
  distribution in African, 83
  function and regulation, 211
  glycerol and fatty acid release from, 201
  hyperinsulinaemia in obesity in, 177, 178
  mass and cell size changes, 231
    changes and metabolism, 205, 210
    energy balance in, 205
  metabolism and exercise, 178–185
Adiposity and coronary heart disease, 27
  and weight, 26
  measurement of, 264–265
Adrenaline, and glycerol release from adipocytes, 17
  metabolic effects, factors influencing, 204–216
Adrenergic sensitive mechanisms in hypothalamic control, 136
Adrenocorticotrophic hormone (ACTH) in lipolysis, 204
Aerobic power of muscle and exercise, 173

in rats, 179
Afferent nerves, gastrointestinal, and feeding control, 124
African, obesity in, 60—71
  adipose tissue distribution, 83
  dietary habits, 62—64
  physique, 64—68
    biochemical correlates, 66—68
  variations in, 69
  treatment, 70
Age and obesity, 26, 27, 32
  of West Indians, 77
  at onset of obesity and adipocyte number, 92
Alcohol and thermogenesis, 168
  carbohydrate content, 271
  in energy intake, 4, 162
Alimentary tract signals to hypothalamus, 124
Alloxan-induced diabetes, 150, 152
Amino acids, insulin-sensitive and weight gain, 244
  serum and appetite, 135
Aminorex, 298
Amphetamine and related compounds in obesity treatment, 297—303
  addiction, 300, 303
  effect on feeding centres, 137
  side effects *see* various drugs
  stimulant properties, 297, 302
  tolerance, 297
Amphetamine psychosis, 300
Amygdala lesions and feeding behaviour, 123
Analytical procedures in Framingham Study, 25
Angina pectoris and obesity, 41, 42, 47, 49, 55
  weight loss effect, 56
Anorectic drugs, 168, 295—305
  intermittent usage, 357—359
  mode of action, 339
  non-phenylethylamine agents, 306, 307
  tolerance to, 356, 357
Anorexia nervosa, food intake in, 114
  weight gain in, 251
Ante-natal obesity, 100, 101
Antibiotics and malabsorption, 294, 295

Antidiabetic agents and peripheral glucose metabolism, 226
Anti-insulin serum, 150
Anthropometric measurements of adolescent girls, 257, 259
  West Indians, 75
Appetite and hunger, 4
  and smoking, 168
  control and gut receptors, 370
  drugs affecting, 137—141, 295—305
  effect of bile on, 295
  neurological regulation of, 116—143
  regulation and exercise, 185
Aphagia and lesions of amygdala, 123
  lateral hypothalamus, 118, 120
  and stereotactic electrocoagulation, 340
Arteriosclerotic process and age, 55
Arterio-venous glucose levels and hunger, 107, 219
Arthritis and overweight, 48
Atherogenic traits, cardiovascular disease and weight, 28, 35—37, 47, 48
  weight loss effect, 44
Atherosclerotic cardiovascular disease and obesity, 28, 40, 49
Aversion conditioning and weight loss, 320, 330—332

Basal metabolic rate, 165
  depression of, 3, 166
Benzphetamine, 299
β-cells, abnormal insulin output by, 23
  chronic stimulation, 249
  stimulation and diet, 233
  sulphonylurea effect on, 227
Biguanides in obesity treatment, 226, 296
Bile acids and appetite, 295
Biological accompaniments of obesity, 35—38
Birthweight and childhood obesity, 102
Blood gluocose and weight, 36
  pressure and weight, 35, 36
  sugar levels in diabetes, 217
  uric acid, weight and height, 68
Body composition and exercise of non-obese, 174, 177

INDEX 375

obese, 173
   fat, and exercise of non-obese, 176
      obese, 173, 174
   and skinfold measurements, 85
   as an organ, 85
   estimation, 163
   failure to lose, 182–185
   growth in childhood, 85
   temperature and food, 136
   weight and fat, 361
Brain infarction and obesity, 40, 47
Bulk fillers in obesity treatment, 296

Cachexia, 143
   and stereotactic electrocoagulation, 340
Caffeine and energy balance, 162
   thermogenesis, 168
Caloric inefficiency and overfeeding, 231
Calorie content of foods, labelling of, 365
Calorific constituents of low-carbohydrate diet, 273
Calorimetry in food estimation, 162, 163
Carbohydrate and nutrient content of foods, 273
   —constant study, 240
   dietary and hyperinsulinaemia, 235–239
   —free diet, 274
   —high diet and β cell stimulation, 233
      and insulin sensitivity, 182
      and obesity, 60, 62
      in West Indies, 79
   intake and weight changes, 239–246
   low-diet, 271–280, 322
      advantages of, 278
      calorific constituents of, 273
      cost, 365
      criticisms, 273–275
      exercise and adipocyte metabolism in, 180
      food intake regulation, 279
      low K values in, 189
      nutrient content, 275–277
      terminology, 250
   metabolism and exercise, 176
   peripheral metabolism in obesity

   and diabetes, 217–227
   refined, in diabetes, 81
   —rich snacks, 277
   —variable: fat study, 239
      insulin resistance in, 240, 241
Cardiovascular disease and artherogenic traits, 36, 37
   and obesity, 24–51
      in West Indians, 79
      mechanisms of, 47, 48
   and weight, 25, 37
   discriminant function analysis, 45
   risk factors, 28, 47
Cardiovascular morbidity, 40–42
   profile to reduce risk, 43
   weight in, 44
Central nervous regulation of feeding, 116, 117, 123–128
Cerebrovascular disease and hypoglycaemia, 59
Chemosensitive receptors in intestine, 128
   regulation of feeding centre, 129–136
Childhood malnutrition, 74, 79
   obesity, adipocyte size and number in, 15, 91–95
      adipose organ growth, 85–87
      and birthweight, 102
      cellular growth in, 87–90
      critical periods in, 85–95
      in Africans, 70
      preventive measures, 85, 95
      types of, 266
Cholecystokinin in obesity treatment, 295
Chlorphentermine, 304
Chlortermine, 304
Cholesterol, plasma and diet, 249, 274
Cholestyramine, 345
   mode of action, 346
Chylomicron-triglycerides, hydrolysis, 193
Claudication, intermittent, and weight, 41
Cold-induced thermogenesis, 166
Congestive heart failure and hypertension, 43
   and obesity, 40
Control of obesity, psychological variables in, 316–335 (see also

Psychological variables in obesity control)
Cornell Medical Index, 112
Coronary heart disease and obesity, 24–51, 41, 42
  hormonal changes in, 55
  risk and obesity status, 43, 52–59
Coronary occlusive disease and diabetes, 59
Cortisol and diabetes, 194
  in obesity, 233
Covert sensitization and weight loss, 320, 330–332
Craniopharyngioma, 13
Crash diet, 271
Critical flicker frequency and fenfluaramine, 305
Cyclic-AMP, insulin effect on, 200
Cyproheptadine and feeding centres, 140

Dental splint in obesity treatment, 355
2-Deoxy-D-glucose and feeding centres, 140
  hyperphagia, 147
Depression and dieting, 115
Developing countries, obesity in, 74–84
Diabetes (mellitus), adult, 193, 199–202
    adipocyte metabolism in, 194–196
    lipoatrophic, 196
    plasma fatty acids in, 201
    phosphofructokinase impairment in, 195
  and coronary occlusion, 58
  experimental, 150
    glucose tolerance test, 217
    glucose uptake, 222, 223
  hyperphagia and hyperglycaemia in, 146
  insulin,
    hypoglycaemia and exercise, 226
  in pregnancy, 102
  juvenile, exercise in, 174
  and obesity, 28, 48
    genetic association, 81
    in African, 60, 61, 66
    in Jamaican, 74, 78, 79
    refined sugar in, 81
    peripheral carbohydrate metabolism in, 217–227
  insulin resistance in, 223
Diet, β-cell stimulation and, 233
  change in obesity treatment, 1, 2
  development for man, 275, 276
  high-carbohydrate and obesity, 60, 62
    and insulin sensitivity, 182
  high-fat and adipocytes, 103
  holidays, 319, 328–329, 332
  imbalance due to prejudice, 62
  insulin levels and, 233–235
  low calorie, 70
    glucose disposal in, 217
  low-carbohydrate, 271–280
    exercise and adipocyte metabolism, 180
    nutritional adequacy of, 272
  low K values in, 189
  palatability of, 279
  plasma cholesterol, triglyceride and, 249
    glucose and, 235
  reducing, attitudes to, 262, 278
  success rate and social class, 110
Dietary education, 253–268
  habits of Africans, 62–64
  —induced thermogenesis, 166, 167
  obesity, 7
Diethylpropion, 301
Dieting and depression, 115
  attitudes of adolescents, 262
  self-control in, 319
Digestion products and feeding centre regulation, 129
Dinitrophenol in obesity treatment, 294
Diuretics in obesity treatment, 2, 295
Drug-induced obesity, 7
  thermogenesis, 166
Drugs affecting feeding behaviour, 137-141, 165

Easy gainer, 250, 251
Economic status and obesity, 78
Electrical stimulation of hypothalamus, 121
  of limbic lobe structures, 123
Electrocoagulation, stereotactic, 340–345
Emotional changes, energetics of, 162
  factors in aetiology of obesity, 106

Endocrine alterations and obesity, 6, 229-247
   experimental and spontaneous, 229
   insulin changes, 232-246
Energetics of fat gain and loss, 160, 161
Energy balance, and obesity, 160-169, 163
   content of weight changes, 160
   cost of tissue synthesis, 160
   effects of stress and drugs on, 162
   feeding and, 116
   homoeostasis, 161, 167, 168
   intake and expenditure, 3, 4, 162
      restriction and weight loss, 271
   —low, nutrient-high diet, 272-275
   over-eating and, 113
   tissue production, estimation, 215
Exercise and adipose tissue metabolism, 178-185
   summary, 185
   and peripheral glucose uptake, 224
      hypoglycaemia in diabetes, 226
      role of liver, 225
   in human obesity, 171-186
      juvenile diabetes, 174
Eysenck personality inventory, 112, 325

Faecal fat excretion, drug-induced, 345, 346
Familial hypertriglyceridaemia, 193
Fasting state, glucose uptake in, 218
   therapeutic, 281
Fat and body weight, 361
   and myocardial infarction, 55
   estimation of, 163
   cells (*see also* Adipocyte)
      hypertrophy, 9
      size and number in obese, 52
   dietary, and plasma cholesterol, 274
      and plasma glucose, insulin and growth hormone, 241-244
   gain and loss, energetics, 160, 161
   store control and adipocyte size, 167
   synthesis, efficiency in obese, 166
Fatty acid, cell associated, nonesterified (CAFA) adipocyte size, 207, 208
   physiological significance, 213

free in acquired obesity, 231
   release from adipose tissue, 201
Fear arousal in obesity control, 319, 322, 324, 332
Feeding and water exchanges in body, 143
   behaviour, and limbic status, 123
      drugs affecting, 137, 141, 295-305
   central nervous regulation of, 123-128, 142
      long-term, 137
      short-term, 124
      signals during meals, 124-128
   centre, 118-121
      damage to, 157
      EEG activity with hunger, 122
      location in rat, 121
   genetic determination of, 116
   homoeostatic nature of, 116
   reflexes, 141
   regulation of, 116
Fenfluramine in obesity treatment, 304-306
   abuse, 305
   and feeding centres, 137-139
   mode of action, 306
Fetus fat, 85
Flesch Reading Ease Formula, 322
Food, attitudes of obese girls, 261-263
   cues, sensitivity to, 112
   habits, questionnaire on, 255
   intake and hunger, 117
      control of, 3
      determinants of, 164
      drugs in control of, 165, 295-305
      hypothalamic control, 164, 165
      lesions of amygdala and, 123
      regulation of, 124-128
      reticular formation and, 123
   preferences, hypothalamic control, 141
   tables and energy intake, 162
Foods, carbohydrate and nutrient content of, 273
Force-feeding, 158
Forearm technique for peripheral glucose uptake estimation, 217
Framingham Study, 24-51

Gallbladder disease and overweight, 48
Gastric afferents and food intake, 125—128
   distension, satiety centre response, 125—127
   motility and hunger, 107, 114
      hunger-satiety complex, 117
Genetic association of diabetes, 81
   determination of feeding, 116
   obesity, 6, 13—19
      high-fat diet and, 103
Glucagon and feeding centres, 139, 140
   in lipolysis, 204
   in obesity, 233
Gluco-receptor cells in satiety centre, 150
   mechanism, 135
   —sensitive regulation of feeding centre, 130—135
Glucose blood levels and hunger, 107, 130, 114
   diet and, 235—245
   hypothalamic centre activity and, 134
   disappearance rate (K), 243
   disposal in low calorie diet, 217
   entry to adipocyte, 194, 195
   homoeostasis, 221, 222
   metabolism in adipose tissue, 181
      defects in diabetes, 194
   sensitivity in satiety centre, 156
   tolerance, carbohydrate-high diet and, 240
      carbohydrate kind and, 190
      exercise and, 179, 180
      impaired, hormones implicated, 232, 233
      test for diabetes, 217
      weight and, 35
   transport inhibition, 147, 148
   uptake, exercise during, 224
      in diabetes, 222, 223
      in fasting state, 218
         lean and obese, 218, 221
         skinfold thickness and, 219, 222
      insulin resistance in, 221, 223
      liver function in, 220, 223
   utilization in hyperinsulinaemia, 11
Glucostat hypothesis, 146
Glucostatic feeding centre regulation, 129, 130—135

Glycerol release from adipose tissue, 201
   effect of adipocyte size, 16, 17
Glycogen storage disease, 197
Gold thioglucose, 147, 152, 155
Gout and obesity, 61
   overweight, 48
Group decisions in obesity control, 318, 322, 325, 332
Growth hormone and diabetes, 194
   in lipolysis, 204
   in obesity, 232
   of an organ, model, 93
Guar gum, 296

Haemodynamic threat of obesity, 37
Hard gainer, 250, 251
Heart, effect of overweight on, 37
   rate and energy expenditure, 163
Hexokinase, feedback inhibition of, 196
Homoeostasis, energy, maintenance of, 161
   glucose, 221, 222
   in feeding, 116
Hormonal changes and coronary heart disease, 55
Hormones and the adipocyte, 204—216
   in obesity treatment, 2, 293
Human adipocyte and its disorders, 192—202 (*see also* Adipocyte, human and its disorders)
   obesity (*see also* Obesity)
      exercise, effect of, 171—186
      genetic, 13, 15
      hypothalamic, 11—13
      varieties of, 6—19
         classification, 7
Hunger and appetite, 4
   contractions and feeding centre, 127, 128
   inhibition of, 127
   factors influencing, 107, 114
   maximum feeling of, 114
   —satiety complex and gastric motility, 117
   sensation and food intake, 117
      central theory, 117, 118
      EEG activity of feeding centre, 122

peripheral theory, 117
Hypercellular obesity, 98, 99
   in rats, 16, 18
Hypercholesterolaemia and obesity, 32, 274
Hyperglycaemia and satiety centre activity, 131
   cause of, 193—196
   cerebrovascular disease and, 59
   hyperphagia and diabetes, 146
Hyperinsulinaemia in obesity, 9—11, 23, 171
   adipose tissue and, 177, 178
   dietary carbohydrate and, 235
   in rats, 19
   insulin resistance and, 232—246
   sequence of, 248
   physical training and, 171—177
Hyperlipidaemia and hyperinsulinaemia, 171
   and obesity, 28
   type I, 193, 196
Hyperphagia, gold thioglucose-induced, 147
   in obesity, 6—8
      insulin changes in, 22
      effect on, 10, 11
      in rats, 19, 23, 118
   lesions of amygdala and, 123
   hypothalamus and, 118, 120
Hyperplasia of fat cells, 9, 16
   insulin insensitivity, 33
Hyperplastic obesity and exercise, 185
   in infancy, 185
   villi in hyperphagic animals, 371
Hypertension and obesity, 28, 61
   in West Indians, 78
Hypertriglyceridaemia and adipocyte size, 177
   familial, 193
Hypertrophy of fat cells, 9, 13, 16
   exercise in diabetes and, 226
   feeding centre activity and, 131
   hyperinsulinaemia and, 11, 23
Hypothalamic feeding centres, 121
      between-meal information to, 129—137
         chemosensitive regulation, 129—136
         thermosensitive regulation, 136
   drugs affecting, 137

hunger and satiation, activity with, 132
   intestinal afferent nerves and, 128
   signals from alimentary tract, 124
      hunger contractions, 127
Hypothalamic injury in obesity, 6
   abnormalities following, 8, 9
   experimental, 6—11
   human, 11—13
   hyperphagia in, 6—8
   model of, 11
   mechanisms and feeding, 118—123
   regulating signals, 123, 124
   during meals, 124—128
Hypothalamus activity and blood glucose and insulin, 147
   and food uptake in rats, 118

Inactivity, physical, in obesity, 6
Infancy, obesity in, 4, 52, 101
   adipocyte number in, 52, 93
   nutrition, effect of, 80, 81, 96
   weight gain and bone age, 96
Insulin alteration and obesity in animals, 19, 22
   and hyperphagia, 10, 11, 23
   antilipolysis, 200
      lipogenesis and adipocyte size, 209
   insensitive muscle, 171, 182
   insensitivity and adipocyte hyperplasia, 33
   levels, plasma in obese, 171
      adipocyte size in, 177
      diet, effect of, 233—239
      dietary fat, effect of, 240—243
      exercise, effect of, 173, 180, 189, 225
      juvenile diabetics, 174
      myocardial infarction patients, 176
   metabolism in hypothalamic obesity, 9
   factors influencing, 204—216
   peripheral fixation, 221, 223
Insulin requirements for satiety centre activity, 146—154
   resistance and hyperinsulinaemia, 232, 246
   sequence of, 248
   peripheral glucose uptake and, 221, 223

weight gain and, 244
—sensitive amino acids, 244
Insulinogenic index, 174
Intermittent claudication and weight, 41, 48
Internal control, 320, 323
   and weight control, 327, 332
   —External Control Questionnaire, 326
Intestinal absorption, compounds altering, 294, 295
   afferent nerves and food intake, 128
   chemosensitive receptors, 128
   bypass, 347–352
     adverse consequences, 349, 351, 355, 372
     reversibility, 356
Intracranial hypothalamic disease, 13

Jejuno-ileostomy, 348–352
   adverse consequences, 349, 351, 355, 372
   and life expectancy, 352
   degree of weight loss, 349
Juvenile-onset diabetes, 193

Ketonaemia, 363
Ketosis, 274, 275
Kwashiorkor, 81

Lateral hypothalamus, feeding centre, 118, 119
   electrical stimulation, 122
Levodopa, effect on body weight, 339
Limbic status and feeding behaviour, 123
   system and modulation, 114
Lipid content *per* adipocyte, 87
   metabolism and exercise, 176
Lipoatrophic diabetes, 196
Lipodystrophic tissue, 214, 370
Lipogenesis, 17, 18, 204
   carbohydrate-high diet and, 80
Lipolysis, 204
   activation by fasting and isoprenaline, 216
   in obese kindred, 197
   rate and adipocyte size, 207, 208
Lipoma adipocyte, 192, **198, 199**
Lipoprotein lipase defect, 193
Lipostatic regulation of hypothalamus centres, 135
Liver function and shunt operation, 351
   in glucose tolerance test, 220–223
   role in exercise, 225
Low calorie food, commercial, 360
   —carbohydrate diet, 271–280
     advantages, 278
     criticisms, 274
     food intake regulation, 279
     nutrient content, 275–277
     nutritional adequacy, 272
   —fat diet and coronary heart disease, 56
Luxuskonsumption, 166

Malabsorption, antibiotics causing, 294, 295
Malnutrition in infancy, 74, 79
Marasmus, 81
Maturity attainment and obesity, 55, 267
Mazindol, 306
Medial hypothalamus lesions and obesity, 118
Medical advice, factors in non-compliance, 316
Medicinal treatment of obesity, a review, 293–308
   biguanides, 296
   bile, 295
   bulk fillers, 296
   dinitrophenol, 294
   diuretics, 295
   intermittent treatment, 300, 302
   intestinal absorption, compounds affecting, 294, 295
   non-phenylethylamine anorexiants, 306, 307
   phenylethylamines, 297–306
   thyroid hormone, 293, 294
Menarche in obese girls, 259
Metabolic alterations and obesity, 35, 229–247
   adipocyte changes, 18
   hypothalamic injury and, 8
   experimental and spontaneous, 229
   with age and exercise, 174, 175
   differences of obese and lean, 168
   effects of insulin and adrenaline, 204–216

pathways, defects in, 192
parameters and exercise, 173—177
regulation errors, 14, 192
acquired, 199
Metabolism of adipose tissue and exercise, 178—185
Metformin, 296
Methyl cellulose, 296
Microelectrodes, stereotactically guided, 131
Montegriffo, tables of, 322
Morbidity of obesity in West Indians, 78—80
Mortality and weight, 39
Myocardial infarction and obesity, 41, 42, 55
   body fat changes and, 184
   exercise and metabolic changes and, 176
   weight loss, 56

Neurological mechanisms regulating appetite, 116—143
   diagram, 142
   historical, 117, 118
   regulation of central nervous control, 123—128
   tests on anatomical substrates, 118—123
Neurones single, blood glucose changes and, 132
   electrical stimuli and, 131
Neuroticism and obesity, 106
   assessment of, 112
Nialamide and feeding centres, 139
Nicotine and energy balance, 162
Non-phenylethylamine anorectic agents, 306
Nutritional adequacy in a diet, 272
   knowledge questionnaire, 254, 263
   obesity, 6

Obese families, 32—34
   girls, attitudes to food, 261—263
   menarche in, 259
   year of maximum growth, 261
   reduced and weight regain, 168
Obesity, acquired, calorific maintenance, 231
   free fatty acids in, 231
   adipose tissue and hyperinsulinaemia in, 177, 178

ante-natal, 100, 101
categories, 364
childhood, critical periods in, 85-95
   maturity attainment in, 267
   types, 266
control, preventive programme, 253—268
   psychological variables, 316—335
   (see also Psychological variables in obesity control)
definition, 353
diabetes and, 60, 194
diet change in treatment, 1
endocrine and metabolic changes in, 229—247
Obesity, energy balance in, 160-169
   exercise and, 171—186 (see also Exercise in human obesity)
hypercellular, 98, 99
hyperphagia and, 23
hyperplastic in infancy, 185
in Africans, 60—71
in developing countries, 74—84
in girls, 255
Obesity index and age, 54
infant, 4, 52
   need to prevent, 365
medicinal treatment of, 293—308
   (see also Medicinal treatment of obesity)
pathogenesis, factors in, 105—115
pattern in Africans, 68—70
peripheral carbohydrate metabolism in, 217—227
post-partum, 62, 64
prevalence, 1, 52—59
response to hyperphagia, 159
socio-economic status and, 54, 82, 109, 110
symbol of beauty, 65
thermodynamics of, 160
treatment, general discussion, 353—368
   untraditional, 338—352
varieties of, 6—19
   classification, 7
   genetic, 13—19
   hypothalamic, 11—13
Obesity and cardiovascular disease, 24—51
   biological accompaniments, 35—38

data, sources of, 26, 27
determinants of, 32—35, 52—59
familial, 32—35
inactivity, overeating in, 49
prevalence, 26—31
preventive implications, 48—50
survival, 26
weight, effect of, 26
Oestrus abnormalities and hypothalamic injury, 9
Olfactory aversion and weight loss, 330—332
Organ growth, model for, 93
Oropharyngeal afferents and food intake, 124
Osteoarthritis and obesity, 61
Out-patient starvation, therapeutic, 282
Over-feeding, caloric inefficiency during, 231
endocrine and metabolic changes in, 229—247
energy balance and, 113

Pathogenesis of obesity, psychological and social factors in, 105—115
emotional factors, 106
perceptual disturbances, 107, 108
Peripheral metabolism of carbohydrate in obesity and diabetes, 217—227
exercise and, 224—226
fixation and plasma levels of insulin, 221, 223
exercise and, 225
forearm technique in, 217, 218
glucose uptake and insulin resistance, 221
in diabetes, 222
in fasting state, 218
in lean and obese, 218—221
oral antidiabetic agents on, 226
weight reduction, effect, 223, 224
Peripheral theory of hunger sensation, 117
Personality and dieting success, 320, 322, 327
Persuasive/motivational technique in obesity control, 318, 319
group decisions in, 318, 322

Phendimetrazine, 301
Phenformin, 296
Phenmetrazine, 300
and feeding centres, 137
Phentermine, 300
Phenylethylamines in obesity treatment, 297—306
addiction, 300, 303
side effects (*see* various drugs)
stimulant properties, 297, 302
tolerance, 297
Phlorizin binding in satiety centre, 148—150, 158
Phosphofructokinase impairment, 195
citrate effect on, 198
Physical activity, and obesity, 6
attitudes of adolescents, 262
education of girls on, 253—268
insulin levels and, 233
in obese men, 171—174
metabolic parameters and body composition, 173
Physique of African, 64—68
biochemical correlates, 66—68
Post-partum obesity, 62, 64
Pregnancy and diabetes, 102, 194
and postpartum obesity, treatment, 303, 304
Preventive programme for obesity control, 253—268
conclusion, 267, 268
Prolonged therapeutic starvation, 281—292 (*see also* Starvation)
Prophylaxis of obesity, 354
Psychological factors in pathogenesis of obesity, 105—115
disturbance and dieting, 115
emotional factors, 106
variables in obesity control, 316—335
aversion conditioning, 320, 330
discussion of findings, 332—335
personality, 320, 327
Psychological factors
persuasive/motivational technique, 316—335
rewards, 320
technical advice, 319
Pubertul growth spurt, 259
Puberty and body fat increase, 86

Reserpine and feeding centres, 139
Respiratory quotient, 163
Reticular formation and food intake, 123

Satiety centre, activity, and gastric distension, 125
  insulin requirement for, 146—154
  inhibition of hunger contractions, 127
  location in rats, 121
  necrosis, experimental, 147, 152
780 SE and feeding centres, 139
Self-control in dieting, 319, 322, 324, 332
Seltzer-Mayer criteria, 257, 265
Serum lipid levels and weight, 35, 36
Servier Unit Eating Guide, 322
Sex and obesity of West Indians, 77
Shunt operation, 345—352
  reversibility, 356
Skin temperature and hypothalamic centres, 107
Skinfold thickness, body fat and, 85, 99, 163
  in Africans, 65, 66
  coronary heart disease and, 49
  glucose uptake and, 219, 222
Slimming groups, 359, 360
Smoking and appetite, 168
Social factors in pathogenesis of obesity, 32, 105—115, 108
  status, diet success rate and, 110
    eating habits and, 55
    obesity and, 54, 109, 110
Socio-economic status and obesity, 82, 109
Specific dynamic action of food, 136
Spouse aggregation of obesity, 32
Starvation, therapeutic, failure of, 283, 290
  follow-up, effect of, 291
  magnesium deficiency in, 364
  naturesis in, 365
  out-patient, 282, 363
  permanent value, 281
  prolonged, 281—292
Starvation, therapeutic, refeeding, 282
  weight loss during, 283
  other benefits, 291

Steatopygia, 65
Stereotactic electrocoagulation, 340—345
  bilateral stimulation, 340, 342
  exploration, effect of, 342
  unilateral stimulation, 342
Stomach distension and satiety centre activity, 126, 127
Sucrose, dietary, adaptation to, 276
Sulphonylureas, 226
Summary of meeting, 369—372
Sympathomimetric drugs, 139

Tachycardia due to mazindol, 307
  phendimetrazine, 301
Therapeutic starvation, prolonged, 281—292 (*see also* Starvation)
Thermodynamics and obesity, 160
Thermogenesis, 3, 161, **166—168**
Thermogenic drugs, 168
Thermosensitive control of hypothalamus centres, 136
Thyroid hormone in obesity treatment, 293, 294
Thyrotoxicosis, 294
Tissue synthesis, energy cost of, 160
Tolbutamide and feeding centres, 139
Treatment of obesity, chance of success, 354
  diet change, 1, 2 (*see also* Diet)
  diuretics, 2
  hormones, 2
  motivation, 356
  prophylaxis, 354
  requirement for, 353
  round table discussion, 353—368
    summary, 366—368
  untraditional, 338—352
    cholestyramine, 345—347
    intestinal bypass, 347—352
    levodopa, 339
    stereotactic electrocoagulation, 340—345
Triglyceride levels, plasma and diet, 249
  exercise and, 176
  metabolism, 192, 204
    adipocyte size and, 179, 206—209
  mobilization pathway defects, 197
  storage disease, 196, 197

in enlarging adipocytes, 211
Tumours in hypothalamic obesity, 12, 13

Untraditional treatment of obesity, 338–352 (*see also* Treatment of obesity, untraditional)

Vagal afferent nerves and satiation, 126
Ventromedial hypothalamus, electrical stimulation, 121
   injury and obesity, 6–9
   insulin requirements, 146–154
   satiety centre, 119, 121

Water balance and body weight, 189
   retention in overweight, 2
Weight and cardiovascular disease, 25, 28, 35
   age, 32
   biological and weight changes, effect of, 35, 36
   heart weight and, 37
   mortality, 39
   obesity, 26
   trends in, 28–31
Weight, changes, adipocyte metabolism in, 206, 207, 210
   energy content of, 160
   control, guidance on, 262
   excess and ability to reduce, 283
   gain, diet and plasma cholesterol, 249
   in anorexia nervosa, 251
   insulin changes and, 240–244
   varied carbohydrate intake and, 239
   loss, adipocyte number and, 92
   aversion conditioning in, 320, 330–332
   benefits of, 44–47
   coronary heart disease and, 55
   dietary carbohydrate and glucose and insulin levels, 235–239
   in therapeutic starvation, 282
   motivation, 356
   peripheral carbohydrate metabolism and, 223, 224
   physical training and, 174
   maintenance and hypothalamic function, 146
Watchers, 359
   water balance and, 189
West Indies, obesity, in 74
   age distribution, 77
   morbidity, 78–80
   prevalence, 74–78
   sex distribution, 77, 78
Wetzel grid, 254, 264

Xanthomata eruptive, 193

8129937
3 1378 00812 9937